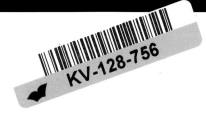

Sports Nutrition for Paralympic Athletes

TP 13008355
SOS

Sports Nutrition for Paralympic Athletes

Edited by
Elizabeth Broad

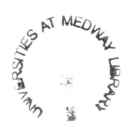

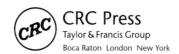

CRC Press
Taylor & Francis Group
Boca Raton   London   New York

CRC Press is an imprint of the
Taylor & Francis Group, an **informa** business

CRC Press
Taylor & Francis Group
6000 Broken Sound Parkway NW, Suite 300
Boca Raton, FL 33487-2742

© 2014 by Taylor & Francis Group, LLC
CRC Press is an imprint of Taylor & Francis Group, an Informa business

No claim to original U.S. Government works

Printed on acid-free paper
Version Date: 20131202

International Standard Book Number-13: 978-1-4665-0756-2 (Hardback)

Library of Congress Cataloging-in-Publication Data

Sports nutrition for paralympic athletes / editor, Elizabeth Broad.
   p. ; cm.
   Includes bibliographical references and index.
   ISBN 978-1-4665-0756-2 (hardback : alk. paper)
   I. Broad, Elizabeth, editor of compilation.
   [DNLM: 1. Sports for Persons with Disabilities. 2. Nutritional Requirements. 3. Sports Nutritional Physiological Phenomena. QT 260]

   GV445
   796.04'56--dc23
                                                2013046968

Visit the Taylor & Francis Web site at
http://www.taylorandfrancis.com

and the CRC Press Web site at
http://www.crcpress.com

Contents

List of Figures

List of Tables

Foreword

Lord Sebastian Coe declared that the recent 2012 London Paralympic Games resulted in a "seismic effect in shifting public attitudes" to sport for athletes with an impairment. The Paralympic Movement can no longer be ignored as a legitimate competitive sporting event. Sports science and performance management supporting these athletes is a rapidly growing body of knowledge. Only in very recent times has a comprehensive handbook been published on sports medicine for Paralympic athletes.

What fuels our Paralympians nutritionally is vitally important and this book addresses this essential area. Currently the most well-credentialed and acknowledged person in sports nutrition for the impaired is Dr Elizabeth (Liz) Broad. I have worked with Liz for over 15 years and she has demonstrated an unrelenting dedication to improving the science base in this area. I have been privileged to work and collaborate with Liz both during and since my retirement from my 25 years of involvement as an Australian Paralympic team physiotherapist and international Paralympic classifier.

Liz has provided a much-needed volume on an essential part of any athlete's competitive edge. As one of the most prolific authors in this area, she has assembled an international team of collaborators, all experts in this field. *Sports Nutrition for Paralympic Athletes* provides information on the broad subcategories of all physical impairments (grouped as spinal cord injuries, amputees, cerebral palsy and les autres), along with visual impairments, hearing impairments and intellectual impairments. Specific areas such as body composition, supplements and practical issues are discussed comprehensively. Case studies enhance and illustrate a direct and first-hand application to managing Paralympic athletes. While it might be argued that for the most part sports nutrition for the impaired may be no different from that for regular athletes, the required expertise to ensure the best science is utilised in some areas needs to be explored and highlighted. Hopefully this book will challenge and stimulate current and future research in this area to improve the delivery of this intrinsic component of athlete preparation.

Sports Nutrition for Paralympic Athletes is an essential addition to the resources for anyone interested in the sports nutritional requirements for our Paralympic athletes. Sports nutrition can be the difference in being competitive and making the podium. As a resource this book is vital in the armory of sports medicine teams and with the Paralympic profile rapidly increasing it will be required reading for professionals endeavouring to give their athletes a competitive edge.

Jane Buckley
Australian Paralympic Team Physiotherapist 1984–2000
IPC International Classifier 1992–2009
Medical Director of the Australian Paralympic Team for Sydney 2000

Preface

When I was first approached by Ira Wolinsky as to whether I was interested in editing a book on sports nutrition for athletes with an impairment, I was grateful that finally the unique needs and challenges of these athletes were being recognised and were believed to be worth devoting more than a chapter to. Throughout the ensuing (and daunting) process of collating all the information presented in this book, I have been reminded of how little we know in some areas, while being buoyed by the enthusiastic researchers and practitioners who have a lot to contribute.

Individuals with an impairment constantly have to adapt to progress in the world we live in—our challenge is to come up with ideas about how they can do this in sport. The scope of this book was not to rewrite a range of excellent comprehensive resources already devoted to various aspects of sports nutrition, but rather to provide a more expansive set of knowledge, considerations and tips that a practitioner might need to consider when applying this knowledge to an athlete with an impairment. In doing so, I believed it was important to provide as much background information about impairments and para-sport as necessary and practical. In my professional experience, I have become very comfortable with the fact that many athletes with an impairment are "an N of 1" who have their own unique needs and challenges, and have embraced the problem-solving process that is often required to help them optimise and adapt to training, compete at their desired level (whatever that may be), remain healthy and above all, enjoy their sport. If there's one thing I've learnt, it's to *never* think that something may *not* be possible.

This book is aimed at students interested in working within para-sport and sports nutrition, sports practitioners and coaches who are searching for information to help them adapt their practice if necessary, and researchers who may want some ideas as to some cool research projects to involve their students in!

Acknowledgements

Ira Wolinsky initiated the concept of this book, and I am honoured that Ira and the reviewers of the initial proposal believed that I could pull this together! I thank Kari Budyk (project coordinator), Randy Brehm (senior editor), and the staff at Taylor & Francis and CRC Press for their support throughout the production process.

This book would not have been possible without the support of all the contributors, athletes, coaches and scientists. Thank you all for your passion, time and willingness to share knowledge, especially in a Paralympic year! A special note of gratitude and admiration goes to Jeanette Crosland, who despite experiencing a tumultuous year herself remained determined to fulfil her commitment to this project. The Australian Paralympic Committee is recognised for having enabled me to be more fully involved with the Australian Paralympic sports programs and London 2012 Paralympic team over a 2-year period—a rare opportunity for any sports dietitian and a highlight of my career. I also owe enormous thanks to the sports nutrition team at the Australian Institute of Sport. You are a daily source of inspiration and enthusiasm and have been gracious in allowing me some 'time out' to complete this project.

To my husband Darren for your constant challenging and red penning, and my family and friends for everything that you do to support me in my crazy endeavours!

Finally, I devote this book to all the athletes and coaches I have worked with over the past 20 years. It's been an absolute pleasure!

Editor

Dr Elizabeth Broad, B.Sc., Dip.Nut.Diet, MAppSc, PhD, Level 3 Anthropometrist, APD, FSDA. Liz has been a sports dietitian for over 20 years, working with elite and developing athletes from a wide range of sports in Australia and in the UK. Liz's interest in athletes with an impairment was sparked early, through working with the Australian Institute of Sport Athletics program (paralympic athletes) and undertaking her masters dissertation on 'The Effects of Heat on Shooting Performance in Wheelchair Shooters'. While having always worked in some capacity with athletes with an impairment, during 2011–2012 the Australian Paralympic teams were the primary focus of her work. Liz has been fortunate enough to work at two Olympic Games with canoe/kayak, and was the lead sports dietitian for the Australian Paralympic Team at London 2012.

In addition to sports nutrition, Liz has experience in exercise science, team management, and has lectured in sports nutrition and in biochemistry of exercise at several universities. She has also authored several book chapters, lay and scientific publications.

Liz has recently commenced working at the US Olympic Committee with their Paralympic Program.

Contributors

Craig Boyd, BSc (Hons), MSc, PGCE
Sheffield Hallam University
Sheffield, United Kingdom

Elizabeth Broad, PhD, APD, FSDA
Australian Institute of Sport
Canberra, Australia

Louise Burke, PhD, APD, FSDA
Australian Institute of Sport
Canberra, Australia

Siobhan Crawshay, BNutrDiet, APD
Australian Institute of Sport
Melbourne, Australia

Jeanette Crosland, MSc, RD, SENr
Registered Dietitian and Sports
    Nutritionist
Lancashire, United Kingdom

Stephanie Edwards, MS, RD
University of Colorado
Colorado Springs, Colorado

Victoria Goosey-Tolfrey, PhD
Peter Harrison Centre for Disability
    Sport
Loughborough, United Kingdom

Jennifer Krempien, MSc, RD
University of British Columbia
Vancouver, Canada

Nanna L. Meyer, PhD, RD, CSSD
University of Colorado/U.S. Olympic
    Committee
Colorado Springs, Colorado

Claudio Perret, PhD
Swiss Paraplegic Centre
Notwil, Switzerland

Mike Price, PhD
Coventry University
Coventry, United Kingdom

**Greg Shaw, BHSc (Nutr & Diet), Dip
Sports Nutrition IOC, APD**
Australian Institute of Sport
Canberra, Australia

Gary Slater, PhD, APD
University of the Sunshine Coast
Maroochydore, Australia

Matthias Strupler, MD
Swiss Paraplegic Centre
Notwil, Switzerland

Peter Van de Vliet, P.T., PhD
International Paralympic Committee
Bonn, Germany

CONTRIBUTIONS BY WAY OF COMMENTARY

Scientists

Keith Baar, University of California Davis
Ron Maughan, Loughborough University
Romain Meussen, Vrije University
Kevin Tipton, Stirling University
Luc Van Loon, Maastricht University

Coaches

Peter Day, Cycling
Iryna Dvoskina, Athletics
Ben Ettridge, Basketball
Emily Nolan, Strength and Conditioning

Athletes

Carol Cooke, Cycling
Hamish McDonald, Athletics
Michael Milton, Triathlon
Richard Nicholson, Athletics

Abbreviations

AB	Able-bodied
AD	Autonomic dysreflexia
ADL	Activities of daily living
BIA	Bioelectrical impedence analysis
BM	Body mass
BMD	Bone mineral density
BMI	Body mass index
BMR	Basal metabolic rate
CHO	Carbohydrate
CP	Cerebral palsy
DXA	Dual-energy x-ray absorptiometry
EA	Energy availability
EE	Energy expenditure
EEE	energy expenditure of exercise
FFM	Fat-free mass
FM	Fat mass
GI	Glycaemic index
MS	Multiple sclerosis
RMR	Resting metabolic rate
SCI	Spinal cord injury (injured)
TBW	Total body water
TEF	Thermic effect of feeding

1 Introduction

Elizabeth Broad

CONTENTS

"There is little point in training hard without taking advantage of the opportunities that nutrition support can offer" (Maughan and Burke 2011) is a strong statement but in today's world of elite sport it is well founded. The principles of sports nutrition have evolved substantially over the past two decades, whereby present day recommendations are individualised to the athlete's specific goals and periodised according to the time of the week, macrocycle and stage of an athlete's development and sporting career. The core goals are to maximise the adaptations to training to therefore optimise performance on the day of competition. These outcomes are underpinned by the need to achieve an appropriate body composition, to promote health and wellbeing, minimise the time lost to illness and injury and maintain the enjoyment of food. The goals of sports nutrition can be applied across the spectrum of athletic endeavour; from the developmental athlete through to the 'elite' performer, as well as the individual who exercises for general fitness and weight control. In this way, our definition of *athlete* is an expansive one that describes any individual who is undertaking regular exercise or involved in sport, regardless of the intended outcomes.

Sport for individuals with an impairment has grown progressively over the last century from its early beginnings as a component of rehabilitation following injury. Interestingly, at one stage the risk of injury to an athlete with an impairment was thought to be too great that they should refrain from physical activity. Research has disproven this claim. Ferrara and Peterson (2003) found that injuries endured by an athlete with an impairment (9.3 injuries per 1,000 athlete-exposures (AE)) are less common than those endured by able-bodied athletes in specific sports like American football (10.1 to 15/1000 AE) and soccer (9.8/1000 AE); basketball exhibited a lower injury rate (7.0/1000 AE). Not only do athletes with an impairment have a lower injury rate when competing in sport, they also exhibit a higher quality of life associated with physical activity. The opportunities for individuals with any form of impairment to participate in sport and exercise have increased substantially over recent decades, with specialist coaches/trainers, sporting events, national and international competitions, and opportunities to become an elite level athlete competing at the Paralympic Games. As a consequence, many athletes with an impairment are now undertaking committed training programs which are similar to those undertaken by their able-bodied counterparts, and seeking a high standard of competition performances. However, the opportunities for athletes with an impairment to receive funding to support them competing at an elite level has not necessarily kept pace with that of able-bodied athletes. Therefore it is not uncommon to have athletes at the elite level who still work full-time, who have limited opportunities to train regularly with their team-mates and who have to travel long distances (including overseas) to take advantage of opportunities to compete. In addition, many coaches are still learning how best to balance training type, frequency and load required to optimise training for an athlete whose physiological capabilities may be altered. Creating a support team that includes the coach and athlete can be useful for generating ideas around how best to manage all components of training, including their sports nutrition requirements.

Whereas dietary advice based on general health principles may have been sufficient for the past preparation of athletes with an impairment, we now recognise the benefits of specialised nutrition support for achieving training and competition goals. The role of the sports dietitian/nutritionist is to assess an individual athlete's current dietary practices and provide advice regarding how this can be improved to support training capability, training adaptations, body composition goals and competition performance. Adapting general sports nutrition guidelines to develop individual, periodised approaches for athletes with an impairment is no different to an able-bodied athlete. Practitioners should aim to develop a sound knowledge of both the athlete's impairment and the events in which they compete so that the specific physiological requirements, practical challenges and culture of the sport can be appreciated and integrated into the sports nutrition plan. The plan must be fine-tuned to the individual through practice and feedback. Applying sports nutrition principles to some forms of impairment (such as visual impairment, high-functioning cerebral palsy, intellectual impairment) and sporting activities is fairly straightforward, since their physiological functioning is not substantially different to that of an able-bodied individual. In contrast, some impairment types have substantially altered physiological and physical capabilities, and many para-sports

---

COMMENTARY BOX 1.1

ATHLETE INSIGHT: To upcoming sports nutritionists.

Don't treat us any differently! Yes, in the long run some athletes with an impairment may have to do something different than our able-bodied counterparts, but don't start out thinking we are any different. It is important to listen, be supportive, and sometimes you may have to "think outside the square"!

—**Carol Cooke, cyclist, Paralympic medallist;**
ex-rower and able-bodied swimmer

have unique physiological demands (such as goalball, boccia, wheelchair rugby), all of which have very little research available to help understand how best to apply sports nutrition principles. This book aims to assist practitioners working with athletes with an impairment by presenting the research that is available, and by providing practical tips and guidelines for problem solving when research is not available.

1.1 OUTLINE OF THIS BOOK

The book commences with a description and short history of sport for athletes with an impairment (or para-sports, both of which are the accepted terms; International Paralympic Committee 2010), including the concept of classification. It is acknowledged that not all athletes with an impairment will be participating at a level that requires them to be classified, however the principles are useful to understand for individuals who may be involved in organising, running or officiating in local sporting events where individuals with an impairment may participate.

Chapter 3 reviews current principles of sports nutrition for both training and competition. Since there are very few scientific studies specifically undertaken on athletes with an impairment, this chapter will outline the guidelines developed for able-bodied athletes and highlight areas that can be challenging for athletes with an impairment. Subsequent chapters (4–9) will further investigate these challenges within specific classes of impairment and outline solutions.

Chapters 10–13 then explore areas associated with sport and exercise which a sports nutrition practitioner may require a more in-depth understanding of, or utilise tools associated with, in their assessment of athletes' needs and may influence the advice which is given.

Since many athletes with an impairment are so unique, case studies and comments from athletes and coaches are utilised throughout the book to provide practical examples of the process which may be required when advising an athlete. In addition, commentaries from experts in the field of sports nutrition research are

---

COMMENTARY BOX 1.2

COACH'S INSIGHT: What are the differences between coaching athletes with an impairment compared to able-bodied athletes?

> The athlete's education of the elite sport process. Elite sport mentality is not developed at a young age or while the athlete is beginning when they have an impairment. Also, athletes can enter the elite sport pathway at an older age [due to acquiring their impairment] and have no prior background in sport or knowledge of elite sport requirements. Habits, good and poor, have already been formed and this is very hard to break.

**—Ben Ettridge, wheelchair basketball coach of 8 years,
coach of Paralympic medal-winning teams**

presented to answer specific questions on how their field of research could be adapted to this population. Throughout this book, it is assumed readers have a pre-existing understanding of basic exercise physiology, exercise biochemistry and nutrition—where this is not the case, several key readings have been recommended. While we have attempted to outline the majority of impairments that practitioners are likely to come across, it is acknowledged that not every single impairment can be explored. However, it is our hope that we have provided sufficient detail and breadth of information that the practitioner understands where to look when presented with a more unusual case.

1.2   THE SPORTS NUTRITION PATHWAY—FROM REHABILITATION TO HIGH PERFORMANCE

The spectrum of impairments can be subdivided into two main categories: those that are inborn or present at a very early age and those that have been acquired. Individuals who have acquired their impairment, especially via trauma or from health-related issues such as cancer, will usually have undergone a period of rehabilitation which may have involved substantial periods of time in hospital. Indeed, an increasing number of athletes with an impairment come from a military background, having acquired their impairment while on 'active duty'. Depending on the time frame between the onset of their impairment and entry into sport, the individual may also be having to deal with a wider range of practical and psychological issues, such as adjusting back to home, managing their impairment itself and its clinical manifestations, changing occupation, having to get carers to look after essential needs, etc. Information such as this should be asked early on as it assists in understanding the framework that the athlete is currently operating within.

From a clinical perspective, individuals who have acquired their impairment have likely been exposed at some point to nutrition education and support, since nutrition needs are elevated immediately post trauma for healing of wounds and at other times may have decreased substantially due to periods of inactivity. Indeed, there is a substantial range of scientific literature regarding many clinical aspects of impairments. There is a lot to be learnt from this literature which remains relevant to athletes with an impairment, such as the nutritional management of pressure wounds, prevention of urinary tract infections, and the understanding of bladder and bowel management for spinal cord injuries. However, it is also important to acknowledge the context of this work, which is generally embedded in acute post-injury/illness or long term institutionalised practice. For example, studies of energy expenditure of, or body composition changes in, sedentary spinal cord injured (SCI) individuals may present results that are substantially different to the SCI athlete population; pressure wound management research is generally undertaken in bed-ridden, potentially undernourished, individuals; and energy expenditure assessments in cerebral palsy have generally been undertaken in children whose activity levels are not reported.

Part of the challenge to a sports nutritionist working with these athletes can be changing their mindset from that of rehabilitation to that required for high

---

COMMENTARY BOX 1.3

COACH'S INSIGHT: What sports nutrition practices have had the biggest impact on the training capability or performance of your athletes?

> Practical intervention by a sports nutritionist. Also, the athlete's personal understanding and acceptance that their commitment and adherence to the advice is essential in order for the benefits to be achieved.

—Peter Day, Paralympic cycling head coach

---

performance. This can be a substantial shift in nutrition focus in terms of volume, type, and timing of food and fluid intake and, in fact, the whole reason for consuming food. For example, it is not uncommon, particularly early in their involvement with sport, for energy requirements to be underestimated by the athlete, especially when weight control has been a focus and the individual was not an athlete prior to their injury/illness. Another example is the deliberate restriction of fluid intake by a spinal cord injured individual when travelling longer distances due to restrictions in accessing a bathroom. When changing an athlete's diet or hydration practices, it will therefore be important to explain why these changes may be beneficial, with the focus on optimising performance and health. Any changes should be undertaken progressively, and the practitioner may require some patience to allow the process to evolve, especially where the athlete is having to manage a whole range of new scenarios. The outcomes will inevitably be worth it!

KEY READINGS

Ferrara, M.S., and Peterson, C.L. 2003. Injuries to athletes with disabilities: identifying injury patterns. *Sports Medicine* 30:137–143.

International Paralympic Committee. 2010. *IPC style guide*. http://www.paralympic.org/sites/default/files/document/120201082521458_IPC_Style_Guide+July+2010.pdf (accessed March 14, 2013).

Maughan, R.J., and Burke, L.M. 2011. *Sports nutrition: more than just calories—triggers for adaptation. Nestle Nutrition Institute Workshop Series*, vol. 69. Vevey: Nestec and Basel: S. Karger AG.

McArdle, W.D., Katch, F.I., and Katch, V.L. 2000. *Exercise physiology; energy, nutrition and human performance*. Philadelphia: Lea and Febiger.

Vanlandewijck, Y.C., and Thompson, W.R. 2011. *The Paralympic athlete*. West Sussex: Wiley-Blackwell.

2 Sport for Individuals with an Impairment

Peter Van de Vliet

CONTENTS

This chapter provides an overview of the history and growth of the Paralympic Movement with particular emphasis on the Paralympic-specific elements of the sports that are on the Paralympic (Winter) Games program and the development of Paralympic classification.

2.1 HISTORY OF SPORT FOR INDIVIDUALS WITH AN IMPAIRMENT

Sport for athletes with an impairment has existed for more than 100 years. In the 18th and 19th centuries new contributions proved that sport activities were very important for the rehabilitation of injured persons. The first Sport Club for the Deaf was founded in Berlin in 1888 and the Comité International des Sports des Sourds (CISS; International Sports Federation for the Deaf) was founded in 1922 (Gold and Gold 2007). In 1924 the first International Silent Games were held. Amongst the earliest sports organizations for people with physical impairments were the Disabled Drivers Motor Club (1922) and the British Society of One-Armed Golfers (1932) (Brittain 2010).

    Following World War II, traditional methods of rehabilitation could not meet the medical and psychological needs of large numbers of injured soldiers and civilians. At the request of the British government, Dr. Ludwig Guttmann, a Jewish medical doctor with specialty in neurology and neurosurgery who was forced to leave his post in a German hospital in war time, founded the National Spinal Cord Injuries Centre at the Stoke Mandeville Hospital in Great Britain in 1944. Guttmann introduced sport as a form of recreation and as an aid for remedial treatment and rehabilitation. Inspiration for incorporating sport in the rehabilitation program came from the patients themselves who had developed their own 'active' programs.

On July 28, 1948—the day of the opening ceremony of the Olympic Games in London—the Stoke Mandeville Games were founded, and the first competition for athletes with spinal cord injury took place on the hospital grounds in Stoke Mandeville, just 35 miles away from London. Two British teams with 14 former servicemen and 2 former servicewomen competed in archery. In the next year's edition, Dr. Guttmann, inspirer and organizer of the event, gave an opening remark in which he declared his hope that the Games would become international and achieve 'world fame as the disabled men and women's equivalent of the Olympic Games' (Bailey 2007). In 1952, the event became 'international' with the participation of ex-servicemen from the Netherlands. In 1960, the International Stoke Mandeville Games were staged for the first time in the same country and city as the Olympic Games, i.e. in Rome. They went down in history as the first Paralympic Games. The first Paralympic Winter Games took place in Örnsköldsvik, Sweden in 1976 (Bailey 2007; International Paralympic Committee 2006). From that early beginning, the movement grew into a professional organization, now known as the International Paralympic Committee (IPC), which is the global governing body of the Paralympic Movement as well as the organizer of the Paralympic Summer and Winter Games. This event today involves 4200 athletes competing in 20 summer sports and 600 athletes in 5 winter sports. The historical growth is presented in Figure 2.1.

The word *Paralympic* was originally a combination of the words *paraplegic* and *Olympic*; however, with the inclusion of other impairment groups at later stages and the closer association of the Paralympic Movement with the Olympic Movement, it now refers to *parallel* (from the Greek preposition *para*) to the Olympic Games to illustrate how the two movements exist side by side. Paralympics has been the official term of the Games since 1988 (Tweedy and Howe 2011). In the lead-up to the 1988 Games the International Olympic Committee (IOC) agreed to the term *Paralympic* being used for the Seoul Games and all Games from then onward, and in 2001 the relationship between the IPC and the IOC was formalized in a detailed cooperative agreement (Bailey 2007).

Over the course of the first decades, rehabilitation remained an important driver for the development of Paralympic sport (Tweedy and Howe 2011), but little by little sports participation started to grow beyond that stage, mainly by patients who had completed their hospital program and been discharged into the community. Their drive was no different from others in the community: to have enjoyment, social interaction, recreation, competition and enhanced health and well-being (Vallerand and Rousseau 2001).

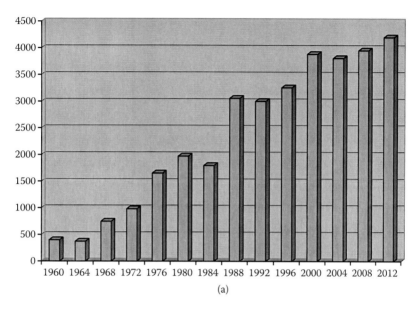

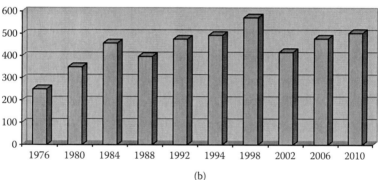

FIGURE 2.1 Growth of the Paralympic Movement. (a) Number of competitors at the Paralympic Summer Games. (b) Number of competitors at the Paralympic Winter Games. (Continued)

2.2 THE PARALYMPIC MOVEMENT

Until 1952, the Stoke Mandeville Games were organized by Guttmann and his hospital staff, with a group of doctors, nurses, physiotherapists, trainers, and administrators deciding on rules, classifications, and all other factors. In 1961 the International Stoke Mandeville Games Committee was founded and took over responsibility for organizing the Games until 1972 when the constitution was amended to form the International Stoke Mandeville Games Federation (ISMGF). In the 1990s, the ISMGF would become the International Stoke Mandeville Wheelchair Sports Federation (ISMWSF).

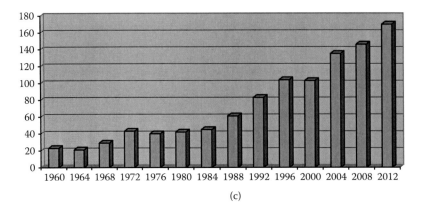

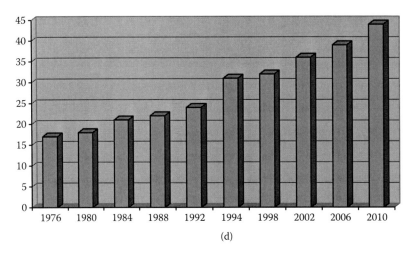

FIGURE 2.1 (CONTINUED) Growth of the Paralympic Movement. (c) Number of nations at the Paralympic Summer Games. (d) Number of nations at the Paralympic Winter Games.

In the beginning only athletes with a spinal cord injury participated in Paralympic sport, but through the 1970s and 1980s the scope of the movement had expanded to include athletes with other types of impairment, ultimately leading to the creation of an international umbrella organization for Paralympic sport. This process was initiated in 1960 when an international Working Group on Sport for the Disabled was set up to study the challenges facing persons with an impairment who wanted to become involved in sports. Its aim was to establish an organization that included all impairment groups. It resulted in the creation in 1964 of an international sport organization called the International Sport Organization for the Disabled (ISOD). ISOD offered opportunities for those athletes who could not belong to the ISMGF, including athletes with visual impairment, amputation and cerebral palsy. ISOD achieved its inclusion in the Toronto 1976 Paralympic Games (athletes with visual impairment and amputation) and in the Arnhem 1980 Paralympic Games (athletes with cerebral palsy).

From these initial structures, different impairment groups established their own international sports organizations that arranged various competitions, ultimately leading to today's International Organizations of Sport for the Disabled:

- CPISRA: Cerebral Palsy International Sport and Recreation Association
- IBSA: International Blind Sports Federation
- INAS: International Sports Federation for Persons with an Intellectual Disability (previously named INAS-FID)
- IWAS: International Wheelchair and Amputee Sports Federation (amalgamation of ISOD and ISMWSF in 2004)
- CISS: Comité International des Sports des Sourds (member of the Paralympic Movement from 1986 to 1995)

These international organizations recognized the need to coordinate both the Paralympic Games and other international and regional sports competitions. Therefore ISOD, ISMGF, CPISRA and IBSA created the International Coordination Committee of World Sports Organizations for the Disabled (ICC) in 1982 to govern the Paralympic Games and to represent the participating organizations in dialogues with the IOC and other global organizations (Bailey 2007). This need for a united voice in negotiations with organizing committees was reflecting Dr. Guttmann's philosophy that an attempt should be made to organize the Paralympic Games back-to-back with the Olympic Games.

The member nations demanded more national and regional representation in the ICC and this finally led to the foundation in 1989 of a new, democratically organized institution: the International Paralympic Committee (IPC). Initially headquartered in Bruges, Belgium, the organization moved to Bonn, Germany, in 1999 and with that move professional management team structures were introduced. Currently the Olympic and Paralympic Movements have become so closely aligned that it is reasonable to posit that Dr. Guttmann's 1948 vision—that the Paralympic Games would become the "disabled men and women's equivalent of the Olympic Games"—has been realized (Tweedy and Howe 2011).

2.3 PARALYMPIC SPORTS

The Paralympic Games represent an international, multisport competition for athletes with an impairment that reflects the highest standards of athletic excellence and diversity. The goal of the Paralympic Sports Program is to provide exciting and inspiring events in the Paralympic Games that allow athletes to achieve competitive excellence while engaging and entertaining spectators.

The IPC conducts a quadrennial review of which sports, disciplines and medal events are included in the Paralympic Games. Each sport and discipline applying for inclusion must meet specific minimum eligibility conditions and must have a level of organizational infrastructure and professionalism that is sufficient to manage and sustain its sport.

The following criteria are considered:

- The sport is governed by an International Federation which is a member of the Paralympic Movement. Criteria for membership are explicit in the *IPC Handbook* (www.paralympic.org). This governing body can be the IPC itself, an international federation governing an Olympic sport, an International Sport Organization for the Disabled, or an international sport federation specifically for athletes with an impairment. An overview of sports governance (for 2013) is presented in Table 2.1.
- The sport is organized for athletes with an impairment, with wide and regular practice across nations and regions (for individual sports, a minimum of 24 nations in 3 regions (Summer Games) and a minimum of 8 nations in 2 regions (Winter Games); for team sports, a minimum of 18 nations in 3 regions (Summer Games) and a minimum of 8 nations in 2 regions (Winter Games)).
- Statutes, practices and activities are in conformity with the *IPC Handbook* and contribute to the IPC vision and mission, including the adoption and implementation of codes and guidelines of fair play (including Anti-Doping Code, Classification Code, Medical Code, Code of Ethics).
- The sport has a structure of national organizations each recognized by its own country.
- The sport can demonstrate a regular quadrennial competition program including two world championships over the last eight years.
- The sport has a sustainable governance and organization structure that effectively manages the sport.

The final decision on the Paralympic Games sports program lies with the IPC Governing Board and is based on the assessment of three core characteristics which broadly outline the philosophical priorities of the Paralympic program within the boundaries of the overarching IPC-IOC agreement (defining maximum number of sports and athletes). These characteristics are presented in Table 2.2.

The sport-technical rules of Paralympic sports are tailored—where needed and appropriate—to the needs and demands of the athletes competing in the sport. A systematic overview of all modifications falls outside the scope of this chapter, but examples include:

- Two bounces of the ball in wheelchair tennis before returning
- Guide runners connected to athletes with visual impairment via tethers
- Skiing guides using acoustic systems to assist skiers with visual impairment
- Use of technical aids to steer horses
- Ball-bouncing rules in wheelchair basketball
- Use of soft springs in pistol shooting, use of supportive devices to hold rifles

When sports do not have an Olympic or able-bodied equivalent, as is the case with goalball and boccia for example, the sport's governing body has developed its own set of sport-technical rules. For a full and comprehensive overview, the reader

TABLE 2.1

Governing Bodies of Sports on the Paralympic Games Program (as of March 2013)

Sport	International Federation	Impairment Types
Alpine skiing[a,b]	International Paralympic Committee (IPC)	P/V
Archery	World Archery (WA)	P
Athletics	International Paralympic Committee (IPC)	P/V/I
Boccia	Boccia International Sports Federation (BISFed)[c]	P
Canoe[d]	International Canoe Federation (ICF)	P
Cycling	Union Cycliste Internationale (UCI)	P/V
Equestrian	Fédération Internationale d'Equitage (FEI)	P/V
Football 5-a-side	International Blind Sport Federation (IBSA)	V
Football 7-a-side	Cerebral Palsy International Sport and Recreation Association (CPISRA)	P
Goalball	International Blind Sport Federation (IBSA)	V
Ice sledge hockey[a]	International Paralympic Committee (IPC)	P
Judo	International Blind Sport Federation (IBSA)	V
Nordic skiing[a] (cross-country + biathlon)	International Paralympic Committee (IPC)	P/V
Powerlifting	International Paralympic Committee (IPC)	P
Rowing	International Rowing Federation (FISA)	P/V
Sailing	International Foundation for Disabled Sailing (IFDS)	P/V
Shooting	International Paralympic Committee (IPC)	P
Swimming	International Paralympic Committee (IPC)	P/V/I
Table tennis	International Table Tennis Federation (ITTF)	P/I
Triathlon[d]	International Triathlon Federation (ITF)	P/V
Volleyball (sitting)	World Organization for Volleyball for Disabled (WOVD)	P
Wheelchair basketball	International Wheelchair Basketball Federation (IWBF)	P
Wheelchair curling[a]	World Curling Federation (WCF)	P
Wheelchair fencing	International Wheelchair and Amputee Sports (IWAS)	P
Wheelchair rugby	International Wheelchair Rugby Federation (IWRF)	P
Wheelchair tennis	International Tennis Federation (ITF)	P

Note: P, including athletes with physical impairment; V, including athletes with visual impairment; I, including athletes with intellectual impairment. Note: All athletes must meet classification criteria as defined by the sport.

[a] Winter Games program.

[b] Including para-snowboard (discipline of alpine skiing for the purpose of Paralympic Winter Games).

[c] Sport previously governed by CPISRA but independent since January 2013 (formal approval by the IPC due in November 2013).

[d] New sport in the Rio 2016 Paralympic Games program.

TABLE 2.2

Paralympic Sports Program Core Characteristics

Quality: The essential principles with respect to degree of excellence, accomplishment, or attainment.	Fair play	Driving the collective values of the IPC; ensuring that the spirit of fair play prevails, the health risks of athletes are managed, fundamental ethical principles are upheld, prejudice and discrimination are not tolerated, and all forms of cheating are discouraged and dealt with sternly
	Inspirational	Creating a distinct opportunity for personal experience/reflection that acts as a catalyst for change through showcasing the extraordinary perseverance of the human spirit through athleticism
	Exciting	Providing a vibrant and energizing atmosphere that is entertaining in the context of each sport, yet creates a collective motivational atmosphere that is attractive to spectators and media
	Elite	Representing the highest athlete performance in the context of the specific sport
Quantity: The principles that establish parameters and/or conditions necessary for success.	Viable	Ensuring operational and programmatic capability in the context of the IPC's obligations to its relationship with the IOC and considering the impact on the organizing committee (cost-effectiveness, infrastructure, operational safety. and risk management)
	Sustainable/ Dynamic	Ensuring a healthy and stable program that allows forecasting and ongoing evaluation; stable enough to be sustainable and dynamic enough to meet the needs of the present and the future
Universality: The collective principles or conditions that ensure and reflect a diverse movement.	Equitable	Ensuring that gender representation and the type and extent of impairments represented at the Games are taken as a fundamental factor in establishing the Games framework
	Global	Establishing a framework that strives to ensure regional representation and the global nature of the Games
	Balance	Weighing and positioning the types of sport and competitions included based on the nature of the sport/disciplines (e.g. individual versus team, power versus precision, speed versus endurance, combat versus artistic)

Source: International Paralympic Committee, internal communication, 2008.

is referred to the sport-technical rules of each sport on the IPC website (http://www.paralympic.org/Sports).

The introduction and continued development of Paralympic-specific equipment has been part of the evolution of the Paralympic Movement. Since standard devices could inhibit sporting performance or create a safety issue, sport-specific wheelchairs and prostheses, modifications to sailing and rowing equipment, and the design of sport-specific equipment such as sledges (ice-sledge hockey) or sit-skis (alpine/Nordic skiing) have been developed. Whilst having significantly enhanced the ability and safety of the user, technological developments in sport have created some controversy (Burkett 2010). An example of such controversy is the frequently publicized debate relating to Oscar Pistorius before the 2008 Beijing Olympic and Paralympic Games and the 2011 IAAF World Championships (Jones and Wilson 2009; Lu 2008). The sporting bodies do need to consider equipment matters in a holistic approach (Burkett 2010); striving to ensure progress in technological developments goes hand in hand with an even playing field that ensures safe sport participation and equity of access to technology-driven equipment. Consequently, the Paralympic Movement has developed an IPC equipment policy which all sports are required to implement (International Paralympic Committee 2011). In the best interest of the athletes and to avoid potential legal problems and unwarranted issues for any party involved, the role of so-called assistive equipment will be the subject of continued open debate.

2.4   CLASSIFICATION

Efforts to promote Paralympic sports as elite must be clear about what elite performance is in the Paralympic context, and classification is a critical component of Paralympic sports. Hence understanding Paralympic sports requires a minimal introduction to classification.

Different forms of classification exist in sport, including events by gender, weight category or age (youth series, master classes). Grading systems to organize competition (e.g. soccer leagues) are also classification systems. The Paralympic Movement provides competitive sporting opportunities for athletes with a range of impairments, and as such, interrelates a concept of 'health and conditioning' with 'sport' (Tweedy and Vanlandewijck 2011). This relationship constitutes the basis of Paralympic classification.

2.4.1   HISTORICAL PERSPECTIVE

A first reference to classification can be found in Joan Scruton's biography on the origins of the Paralympic Movement when conclusions were drawn from the 1955 International Stoke Mandeville Games: "consideration must be given to whether it would not be fairer to divide the netball competition into at least two classes—higher and lower lesions" (Scruton 1998, p. 77). The outcome of the discussion was a change from netball to wheelchair basketball with a division of the competition into two classes: (1) for complete spinal cord lesions and (2) for incomplete spinal cord lesions (Scruton 1998). When Dr. Guttmann started to incorporate sports in rehabilitation programs, impairment-based systems of classification were developed. Athletes started to receive a single 'class' based on their medical diagnosis and competed in that class for all sports. This basis of classification meant that impairments resulting from different medical conditions (e.g. spinal cord injury resulting in lower limb paralysis versus double-above-knee amputation) yet resulting in roughly the same activity limitation in wheelchair propulsion were not considered in the classification process (Tweedy and Vanlandewijck 2011). As the Paralympic Movement matured and turned into a sport-driven organization over a medical system extending from rehabilitation, 'functional' classification systems began to be implemented. Initial efforts hereto date from the late 1970s and the 1980s. In functional systems, the main factors that determine class are not diagnosis and medical evaluation, but how much the impairment of a person impacts upon sports performance. Consequently, functional classification systems are sport-specific (Tweedy and Howe 2011) because any given impairment may have a significant impact in one sport yet a relatively minor impact in another.

2.4.2 Current Paralympic Classification

As an outcome of this historical development and with the growth of the movement, there are currently >25 Paralympic systems of classification. Given the absence of relevant scientific evidence or specific guidance/frameworks, the initial systems developed were based on expert opinion provided by 'classifiers' with a diverse range of backgrounds—medical doctors, therapists, athletes and coaches. While the majority share the above key features there is considerable variability on a range of fundamental issues, including the definition of key terms and the basis for determining minimum impairment criteria.

Step 1 in the classification process is to identify if an athlete holds an eligible impairment for a certain sport. The Paralympic Movement offers sport opportunities for athletes with physical, visual and intellectual impairments and these can be divided into 10 eligible impairment types (impaired muscle power, impaired passive range of movement, limb deficiency, leg length difference, short stature, hypertonia, ataxis, athetosis, vision impairment, and intellectual impairment) (International Paralympic Committee 2013). Each sport decides which impairment type(s) their sport will cater to. Some sports are only designed for athletes with one impairment type. Goalball, for example, is only open for athletes with visual impairment. Other sports, such as athletics and swimming, are open to athletes in any of the 10 impairment types. Athletes will need to submit medical diagnostic information to prove the existence of an eligible impairment type.

Step 2 is to decide how severe an impairment has to be in order for an athlete to be eligible to compete in their sport. This severity is identified by the impact on the sport performance as explained above. The process of classification involves a physical (medical) assessment and a technical (sport-specific) assessment, mostly complemented by observation in training and/or competition, and done by classifiers. These are specialists trained and certified by the international federation that governs the sport. Their profile is different depending on the impairment types they assess (e.g. (para-)medical background and/or technical expertise in a sport for athletes with physical impairment, opthalmologist or optometrist for athletes with visual impairment, and psychologists and/or technical expertise in a sport for athletes with intellectual impairment). It is crucial to understand that the presence of an eligible impairment is a prerequisite but not an inclusive criterion. Inclusion only is a fact when the severity of the impairment impacts on the sport performance (a so-called minimal impairment) and when the impairment is considered permanent.

Step 3 is the allocation of a sport class to group athletes together depending on how much their impairment impacts performance in a particular sport. Although there is no common standard to identify sport classes, classification systems can more or less be categorized in four groups:

- Open classes: All athletes competing only need to meet the minimal impairment criterion.
- Letter-number combinations: Most sports have a letter code (referring to sport or discipline, e.g. S in swimming stands for freestyle, backstroke and butterfly, and SB stands for breast stroke; T in athletics stands for running/wheelchair racing and jumping, and F stands for throwing events).
- Point scores: Typically in use in team sports, athletes are given a point score with lower points indicating more severe activity limitations. A maximum number of points is allowed on the field of play at any given time, ensuring a spread of athletes competing with diverse activity limitation.
- Some sports use sport-specific language, such as rowing which groups athletes in A (arm use only), TA (trunk and arm use) and LTA (leg, trunk and arm use).

Details can be found in the sport-specific classification rules of each sport (see http://www.paralympic.org/Classification/Introduction).

A distinct exception to the above is the classification system for athletes with visual impairment which has remained medical over time. As a consequence, the same criteria (current assessment only for visual acuity and visual field, leading to sport class B1, B2 or B3) apply across sports. This system will need to change over time (see next section).

2.4.3 SCIENTIFIC PRINCIPLES OF CLASSIFICATION IN PARALYMPIC SPORT

The actual classification situation is mainly due to the absence of a theoretical or conceptual model to guide Paralympic classification (Sherrill 1999; Tweedy 2002). The IPC has recognized the need to coordinate classification under these provisions and in 2003 the IPC conducted a classification audit, which recommended the development of a universal classification code "to support and co-ordinate the development and implementation of accurate, reliable and consistent sport focused classification systems" (International Paralympic Committee 2007). The outcome of this process is the IPC Classification Code which was approved by the IPC General Assembly in 2007. The purpose of this document is to harmonize classification over all Paralympic sports on the basis that it will contribute to sporting excellence for all athletes and sports in the Paralympic Movement, providing equitable competition through classification processes that are robust, transparent and fair. Crucial to this is Article 2.1.1 that "classification is undertaken to ensure that an Athlete's impairment is relevant to sport performance" (International Paralympic Committee 2007). It is well recognized that the sport class an athlete is assigned has a significant impact on the degree of success they are likely to achieve.

All Paralympic systems of classification in future need to be based on the code provision (Article 2.1.1) to promote participation in sport by people with impairments by "minimizing the impact of eligible impairment types on the outcome of competition." This requires all classification systems to describe eligibility criteria (who is in?) in terms of type and severity of impairment, and to describe methods for classifying eligible impairment according to the extent of activity limitation they cause in a particular sport or sports discipline, based on scientific evidence. These criteria are further elaborated upon in a scientific publication by Tweedy and Vanlandewijck (2011). The IPC Governing Board adopted its publication as the official IPC Position Stand on classification in Paralympic sport.

A crucial and critical aspect of Paralympic classification is that enhancement in performance through training may *not* lead to class changes. Similarly, the number of classes defined in a sport may not be driven by the number of athletes in a sport at a single point in time (Tweedy and Vanlandewijck 2011).

Classification in Paralympic sport is a complex and dynamic process, and a full analysis of the underlying principles would lead us too far for the purpose of this publication. As a general principle, however, one can state that all sports currently look into how they can improve and scientifically validate:

- To measure impairment by means of simple, readily available, objective tests that account for the greatest variance in sports performance.
- To measure activity limitation by defining the key components of the sport.
- To gain insight in training history and personal and environmental factors affecting how well an athlete will do the activity.
- To identify intentional misrepresentation of abilities. It is inherent to the human being and thus athletes to try to obtain favourable outcomes of testing and anecdotal evidence suggests that athletes may not cooperate fully during testing or attempt to exaggerate the severity of their impairment—hence the development of detective tools.

The direction to develop evidence-based classification systems implies the engagement of individuals that know the sport (administrators, officials—including classifiers—as well as athletes) and sports scientists, whether or not they are currently working with Paralympic athletes. More recently, this has driven the instigation of expert meetings in which academics experienced in assessing impairment and sports scientists involved in the development of able-bodied equivalents of Paralympic sports have been brought together with experts in Paralympic sports. The complementary expertise, knowledge, and resources of these key players ensures that further development of Paralympic classification systems will focus on the development of objective, reliable methods for measuring both of the core constructs in the model: impairment and activity limitation.

Already several initiatives based on the above theoretical or conceptual model have been launched in different sports. The work in IPC athletics, reported as *IPC*

Athletics Classification Project for Physical Impairments: Final Report—Stage 1, by Tweedy and Bourke (2009) is considered instrumental in this regard, and generated follow-up investigations reported by Vanlandewijck and colleagues (2011a, 2011b) on the role of abdominal muscles and the importance of seat positions in wheelchair propulsion, and by Beckman and Tweedy (2009) on muscle coordination in athletes with coordination impairment (CP). Further initiatives include Nordic skiing (Pernot et al. 2011) with the development of a test table for abdominal balance in cross-country sitskiing, swimming (Evershed et al. 2012) with an analysis of standardized measures of muscle testing, and wheelchair rugby (Altmann et al. 2011) which focuses on the role of trunk function in wheelchair maneuverability. Over the past years, the Paralympic Movement has successfully reintroduced athletes with intellectual impairment (in the sports of athletics, swimming and table tennis) and this was under the condition that a new sport-specific and evidence-based classification system, following the conceptual model of Tweedy and Vanlandewijck (2011), was developed. In 2010 the IPC approved the inclusion of para-triathlon and para-canoe on the condition that the current classification system be revised and aligned with the scientific principles of Paralympic classification and both international federations have initiated the work hereto. Most recently, sport-specific classification for athletes with visual impairment has been looked into as mentioned before.

The above is all indicative of the dynamic, though complex, matter of Paralympic classification so that ultimately the success of an athlete is determined by skill, fitness, power, endurance, tactical ability and mental focus, no different to any able-bodied counterpart.

2.5 CONCLUSION

From its origin in the 1940s, the Paralympic Movement has undergone multiple changes with a shift from disability-centered structures to sport-specific ethos. This advancement was greatly enhanced by sustained affirmative assistance from the IOC, and the development of criteria for sustainable Paralympic sports which set standards to ensure both further growth and sporting excellence. With the growth of the Paralympic Movement the concept of classification has undergone a shift. From an initial medical model, the Paralympic Movement has now mandated its membership to develop sport-specific evidence-based systems of classification. The IPC Classification Code and IPC Position Stand on scientific principles of classification in Paralympic sport now guide the sports to develop a system that promotes participation in sport by individuals with an impairment by minimizing the impact of eligible impairment types on the outcome of competition. This requires research that develops objective, reliable measures of both impairment and activity limitation and investigates the relative strength between these constructs. All sports have initiated this process, in an initial phase by a critical self-audit of their current classification system and through the engagement of sport scientists from different disciplines in the review and further development of classification. The outcome is a continued critical reflection on how classification—the cornerstone of the Paralympic Movement—can be improved to ensure that the athlete with the best sportive skills, independent from his or her impairment, ultimately is the one that wins.

COMMENTARY BOX 2.1

COACH'S INSIGHT: Differences between coaching athletes with an impairment and able-bodied athletes.

The coach of an athlete with an impairment must be fully aware of the real limitations and the daily difficulties that the athletes may need to overcome. Obviously this is dependent on the classification of the athlete and their desired level of achievement in competition, and whether this is commensurate with their ability and/or coaching style. The coach must have greater empathy and demonstrate understanding and acceptance of the issues. However this does not mean allowing shortcuts or lack of training commitment, but rather developing an excellent process to ensure the best is being achieved considering the potential obstacles. Does this differ between different disabilities? Yes—obviously a C5 man (least impairment) will be less resource demanding than a handcyclist or a high disability single bike rider who really requires assistance getting on and off the bike, and therefore requires coverage at all training sessions.

—Peter Day, Paralympic cycling head coach

I have found with more individualised and hands-on coaching of the athlete you can get some very significant results and performances; small group or one-on-one sessions are best, and allow you as the coach to observe and learn how their impairment impacts on their movement and performance.

—Emily Nolan, strength and conditioning coach

REFERENCES

Altmann, V.C., Groen, B.E., Keijsers, N.L.W., Hart, A.L., Van Limbeek, J., and Vanlandewijck, Y.C. 2011. Reliability of the revised trunk classification system for wheelchair rugby. Abstractbook VISTA2011, Bonn, Germany. http://www.paralympic.org – Events – VISTA2011 (accessed March 11, 2013).

Bailey, S. 2007. *Athlete first. A history of the Paralympic Movement.* Hoboken, NJ: John Wiley & Sons.

Beckman, E., and Tweedy, S.M. 2009. Towards evidence-based classification in Paralympic athletics: evaluation of the validity of activity limitation tests for use in classification of Paralympic running events. *British Journal of Sports Medicine* 43:1067–1072.

Brittain I. 2010. *The Paralympic Games explained.* Abingdon: Routledge.

Burkett, B. 2010. Technology in Paralympic sport: performance enhancement or essential for performance? *British Journal of Sports Medicine* 44:215–220.

Evershed, J., Frazer, S., Mellifont, R., and Burkett, B. 2012. Sports technology provides an objective assessment of the Paralympic swimming classification system. *Sports Technology* 5:1–2, 49–55.

Gold, J.R., and Gold, M.M. 2007. Access for all: the rise of the Paralympic Games. *Journal of the Royal Society for the Promotion of Health* 127:133–141.

International Paralympic Committee. 2006. *Paralympic Winter Games 1976–2006.* Bonn: International Paralympic Committee.

International Paralympic Committee. 2007. IPC classification code and standards. http://www. paralympic.org – The IPC – IPC Handbook (accessed May 31, 2012).

International Paralympic Committee. 2011. IPC equipment policy. http://www.paralympic.org – The IPC – IPC Handbook (accessed March 11, 2013).

International Paralympic Committee. 2013. IPC policy on eligible impairments in the Paralympic Movement. http://www.paralympic.org – The IPC – IPC Handbook (accessed March 11, 2013).

Jones, C., and Wilson, C. 2009. Defining advantage and athletic performance: the case of Oscar Pistorius. *European Journal of Sport Science* 9:125–131.

Lu, A. 2008. Science at the Olympics: do new materials make the athlete? *Science* 321:626–627.

Pernot, D.H.F.M., Lannem, A.M., Geers, R.P.J., Ruijters, E.F.G., Bloemendal, M., and Seelen, H.A.M. 2011. Validity of the test-table-test for Nordic skiing for classification of Paralympics sit-ski sports participants. *Spinal Cord* 49:935–941.

Scruton, J. 1998. *Stoke Mandeville: road to the Paralympics*. Aylesbury, UK: Peterhouse Press.

Sherrill, C. 1999. Disability sport and classification theory: a new era. *Adapted Physical Activity Quarterly* 16:206–215.

Tweedy, S.M. 2002. Taxonomy theory and the ICF: foundations for a unified disability athletics classification. *Adapted Physical Activity Quarterly* 19:220–237.

Tweedy, S.M., and Bourke, J. 2009. *IPC athletics classification project for physical impairments: final report—stage 1*. http://www.ipc-athletics.paralympic.org – classification (accessed May 31, 2012).

Tweedy, S.M., and Howe, P.D. 2011. Introduction to the Paralympic Movement. In *The Paralympic athlete*, ed. Y.C. Vanlandewijck and W.R. Thompson, 3–30. Hoboken, NJ: Wiley-Blackwell.

Tweedy, S.M., and Vanlandewijck, Y.C. 2011. International Paralympic Committee position stand—background and scientific rationale for classification in Paralympic sport. *British Journal of Sports Medicine* 45:259–269.

Vallerand, R.J., and Rousseau, F.L. 2001. Intrinsic and extrinsic motivation in sport and exercise. In *Handbook of sport psychology*, ed. R.N. Singer, H.A. Hausenblaus, and C.M. Janelle, 389–416. 2nd ed. New York: John Wiley & Sons.

Vanlandewijck, Y.C., Verellen, J., Beckman, E., Connick, M., and Tweedy, S.M. 2011a. Trunk strength effects on track wheelchair start: implications for classification. *Medicine and Science in Sports and Exercise* 12:2344–2351.

Vanlandewijck, Y.C., Verellen, J., and Tweedy, S.M. 2011b. Towards evidence-based classification in wheelchair sports: implications of seat position in wheelchair acceleration. *Journal of Sports Sciences* 29:1089–1096.

3 Principles of Sports Nutrition

Elizabeth Broad and Louise Burke

CONTENTS

3.1 INTRODUCTION

The principles of sports nutrition have evolved substantially over the past two decades, whereby present-day recommendations are individualised to athletes' specific goals and periodised according to the time of the week, macrocycle and stage of athlete's development and sporting career. The core goals are to maximise the adaptations to training and to optimise performance on the day of competition. These outcomes are underpinned by the need to achieve appropriate body composition, promote health and wellbeing, minimise the time lost to illness and injury, and maintain the enjoyment of food. The goals of sports nutrition can be applied across the spectrum of athletic endeavour; from the developmental athlete through to the elite performer, as well as the individual who exercises for general fitness and weight control.

The aim of this chapter, therefore, is to set the scene for sports nutrition guidelines from which other chapters in this book can draw. Since there are very few scientific studies specifically undertaken on athletes with an impairment, this chapter outlines the guidelines developed for able-bodied athletes and highlights areas that can be challenging for athletes with an impairment. Subsequent chapters further explore these challenges and outline solutions. Adapting general guidelines to develop individualised periodised approaches for athletes with an impairment is no different to doing so for the able-bodied population. Practitioners should aim to develop a sound knowledge of the events in which their athletes compete so that the specific physiological requirements, practical challenges and culture of the sport can be appreciated and integrated into the sports nutrition plan. Finally, the plan must be fine-tuned to the individual through practice and feedback.

In undertaking this review, we will assume readers have a pre-existing understanding of basic exercise physiology, exercise biochemistry and nutrition. We cover a range of contemporary issues of sports nutrition, including a focus on principles that have been recently updated or have become a source of debate. Readers are advised to seek more detailed information from the recommended reading material provided at the end of the chapter.

3.2 GOALS OF TRAINING NUTRITION

3.2.1 ACHIEVING OPTIMAL ENERGY REQUIREMENTS FOR TRAINING SUPPORT AND HEALTH

Assessing an athlete's diet for nutritional adequacy will require, at some point, an assessment or estimation of daily energy requirements. Assessing energy balance is also important when there is a desire to change body composition, or where the athlete is suffering from fatigue, frequent illness, failure to grow at an appropriate rate, or other factors which can be linked to an energy imbalance or low energy availability.

Estimating the energy expenditure of athletes can be a complex task, even if you have tools by which you can measure some of the individual components—resting or basal metabolic rate (BMR), thermic effect of feeding (TEF), and the energy expenditure of exercise (EEE) (both planned exercise and non-sport related). Since measuring energy expenditure requires either expensive techniques (e.g. doubly-labelled water) or specialised equipment (indirect calorimetry), the practitioner generally relies on established prediction equations to estimate resting metabolic rate (RMR), then multiplies RMR by an appropriate activity factor to estimate total energy expenditure. Manore and Thompson (2010) determined that the prediction equations which best matched measured RMR for active males and females were the Cunningham (1980) equation (if a measure of lean body mass (LBM) is available) or the Harris-Benedict (1919) equation (when lean body mass cannot be directly measured).

Cunningham (1980): RMR = 500 + 22 (LBM in kg)
Harris-Benedict (1919):

Males: RMR = 66.47 + [13.75 × body mass in kg] +
[5 × height in cm] – [6.76 × age in y]

Females: RMR = 65.51 + [9.56 × body mass in kg] +
[1.85 × height in cm] – [4.68 × age in y]

Note: All equations estimate RMR in kcal/day, and hence need to be multiplied by 4.2 to provide kJ/day.

It is notable that these equations were determined from data derived from free-living, able-bodied, non-athletes—hence their applicability to athletes, individuals with spinal cord injuries, those with regular muscle spasm, and individuals whose body morphology (e.g. height and body mass) lies below the 5th or above the 95th percentile for age has not been determined.

Once RMR has been estimated, an activity factor (or factors) must then be applied to estimate total daily energy expenditure. Often, a single activity factor is selected (for example, 1.2 for bed rest or 1.5 for moderate exercise 3–5 days/week) and the RMR multiplied by this activity factor. The difficulty generally lies in determining how best to measure or estimate the energy expenditure of planned exercise. Attempting to separate out activities over a day and estimate expenditure within each component, from a compendium of exercise or similar (Ainsworth et al. 2000), is time consuming and relies on many assumptions. Recent technology has produced tools which simplify the process, including equipment that can directly measure power output during exercise and monitors such as Sensewear™, which assess daily energy expenditure through a complex collation of body temperature changes, heat flux and movement patterns. Nevertheless, in sports or activities with a complex range of movements (such as in stop-start sports with changes in direction, abnormal gait mechanics, high intensity exercise, or where muscle spasm is regularly occurring), the more difficult it becomes to accurately assess energy expenditure of activity.

Since no single tool is without measurement error (often in the order of 5–10%; Shephard and Aoyagi 2012), the outcome is inevitably going to be an approximation which should be interpreted accordingly. For example, if you estimate an athlete's daily energy expenditure to be approximately 10,000 kJ, their true energy expenditure may lie between 9000 and 11,000 kJ/d. Similarly, assessment of true energy intake in free-living individuals is complex, with underreporting being a common problem (Deakin 2010). At best, dietary records or dietary histories will provide qualitative information such as the nutrient density of the diet, food preferences, eating patterns over the day and in relation to training/exercise, and day-to-day variety. An experienced practitioner will also be able to recognise whether energy intake is within the ballpark of estimated energy expenditure, or whether there appears to be a substantial imbalance between the two.

Rather than rely on quantitative figures that may be imprecise, it is important for practitioners to recognise key clinical indicators of energy balance/imbalance to guide decisions around the adequacy of energy intake. It can generally be assumed that when an athlete is in energy balance (i.e. where energy consumed from the diet $[E_{in}]$ is equal to the energy expended over the day $[E_{out}]$), their body mass will be stable, ability to train is consistent without excessive fatigue, response to training is effective, and health and normal body functions (e.g. menstruation for females) are maintained. An athlete who is consistently in energy surplus ($E_{in} > E_{out}$) over time will gain body mass in the form of body fat and/or lean tissue, depending on the type and amount of activity being undertaken and how well trained they are. In contrast, while it might be logical to assume that an athlete who is consistently in energy deficit over time would lose body mass, this can often depend on how large the energy deficit is.

3.2.1.1 Energy Availability

Energy availability (EA) is defined as the energy that remains available to support the body's daily physiological needs after the energy expenditure of exercise has been accounted for and is quantified by the deduction of the energy cost of physical activity from daily energy intake:

Energy availability = Energy intake − Energy cost of training/competition

Evidence suggests that the body can cope with a small drop in energy availability, however if EA falls too low this will compromise the body's ability to maintain optimal health and function. Consequences of low EA include menstrual disturbances (females), lowered testosterone (males), reduced basal metabolic rate, compromised immunity, poor hormonal function, impaired bone density and fatigue (Loucks et al. 2011). For these reasons it is worth spending the additional time to undertake a more thorough assessment of cases of suspected low energy availability, including bone density, blood biochemistry, menstrual history in females, and more accurate estimations of both energy expenditure (assessing body composition, activity records including incidental activity, measurement of RMR if possible) and energy intake

TABLE 3.1
Assessment of Energy Availability

Energy Availability	Example
Adequate for weight maintenance ~190 kJ (~45 kcal) per kg fat-free mass (FFM)	Athlete: 65 kg and 15% body fat FFM = 85% × 65 kg = 55 kg Weekly training = 23.5 MJ (5600 kcal), averaging 3360 kJ/d Daily energy intake = 13.8 MJ (3285 kcal) Energy availability = (13,800 − 3360)/55 = 190 kJ/kg FFM
Low energy availability ~125 kJ (~30 kcal) per kg FFM	Athlete: 80 kg and 10% body fat FFM = 90% × 80 kg = 72 kg Weekly training = 21 MJ (5000 kcal), averaging 3000 kJ/d Daily energy intake = 12 MJ (2860 kcal) Energy availability = (12,000 − 3000)/72 = 125 kJ/kg FFM

(preferably through a 7 day weighed food record undertaken concurrently with activity records). Whereas energy availability associated with energy balance and healthy physiological function is generally around 190 kJ (45 kcal) per kilogram of fat-free mass ((FFM) = body mass minus kg of body fat), the threshold of low energy availability below which the consequences are particularly harmful is believed to be around 125 kJ (30 kcal)/kg FFM (Loucks 2003). Table 3.1 provides an example of the assessment of energy availability.

Low EA can occur inadvertently or via deliberate manipulation of energy intake and/or expenditure. The three main situations in which low EA is seen are restricted eating for loss of body fat or body mass, inadvertent failure to increase energy intake to match the training load (especially in high-volume training periods), and eating disorders or disordered eating behaviours (Loucks 2010). While energy availability hasn't been formally investigated in athletes with an impairment, some groups may be at higher risk of problems due to the chronic requirement to manage body mass/composition to promote mobility/mobilisation (for example, those with spinal cord injuries). It is not uncommon for these individuals to underestimate the energy expenditure of exercise and, as a consequence, fail to adequately increase energy intake in response to training. Regardless of the reason for low EA, reversal is necessary in order to improve the health, wellbeing and training capability of the athlete. Such treatment can be achieved by refeeding protocols in which daily energy intake is increased by approximately 1500 kJ (350 kcal), often via the consumption of one liquid meal supplement per day (Kopp-Woodroffe et al. 1999). The time required to see improvements in key indicators, such as the resumption of normal menses in females or improvements in bone density, is variable and may take a number of months to years (Kopp-Woodroffe et al. 1999), however training capabilities will often return more rapidly. Suspicion of disordered eating behaviour must also be addressed appropriately.

3.2.2 Changing Body Composition

During an athlete's lifetime, there will be periods where body composition changes as a result of growth and training responses. There may be other times where body composition is deliberately manipulated to optimise the athlete's physique characteristics for their sport—be that by increasing lean body mass (LBM) for greater strength/power, reducing body fat or absolute mass, or achieving a target weight in order to compete in weight category sports. Regardless of the desired change in body composition, it is important for the practitioner, athlete and coach to set realistic targets and provide optimal or at least adequate time to undertake the majority of changes so that the longer-term requirements of training are not compromised. It is also important that body composition is appropriately assessed (as will be described in Chapter 12) since body mass per se is not a sensitive marker of small but important changes in the components of body composition. The achievement of body composition goals often requires more than one season, especially when an athlete is still growing, is new to a sport, or there are other large changes being made to skill, fitness, or strength. Minimising the loss of conditioning that occurs during breaks in training (i.e. during the off-season or while injured) is also important to address.

The primary factors in changing body composition are the training stimulus and energy balance. Regardless of the macronutrient composition of the diet, long term changes in body composition and mass occur most effectively when there is an imbalance between E_{in} and E_{out} (Melby and Hill 1999; Manore and Thompson 2010). The principles of changing body composition are similar whether the goal is increased lean body mass or reduced body fat.

- The manipulation of energy intake should be relatively small (up to 2000 kJ or 500 kcal/day, or 10–20% of energy requirements) but consistent. Larger increases in energy intake in order to gain lean body mass are likely to also result in substantial increases in body fat which often then has to be lost at a later time. Greater deficits are likely to increase the risk of low EA and compromise training capacity.
- The regularity of food intake over the day should be maintained. When losing body fat, the preference should be to change portion sizes rather than frequency of feeding. This is particularly important for athletes who train more than once a day, since the removal of between-meal snacks could potentially compromise recovery between training sessions by failing to optimise the delivery of nutrients within the recovery period. When gaining LBM, it may be necessary to add eating occasions to the day to create additional opportunities to consume energy, since increasing the size of the meals may cause gastric discomfort. There is also evidence to suggest that consuming protein-rich foods/fluids (such as milk or cheese) before bed promotes muscle protein synthesis overnight (Res et al. 2012).
- An even spread of protein intake should be maintained over the day (i.e., each meal/snack should contain some protein) as this will help preserve muscle mass and help manage the appetite.

- Carbohydrate intake should be maintained at a level that is adequate for the training load. Manipulating the glycaemic index (GI) and fibre content of carbohydrate-rich foods can be useful to manage satiety, where lower-GI/higher-fibre choices help improve satiety for those losing body fat, and higher-GI/inclusion of some lower-fibre sources may help athletes who find it difficult to eat enough. Achieving adequate carbohydrate intake should take priority over the inclusion of other energy-dense macronutrients (e.g. fat, alcohol) in the diet, especially where body fat loss is the goal. However, this should not be to the detriment of the intake of essential fatty acids nor should an ad-libitum carbohydrate intake in excess of needs be promoted.
- Nutrient requirements should be met within the athlete's energy 'budget'. When energy intake is reduced to assist with loss of body fat it is important to focus on nutrient-dense foods and fluids and reduce the intake of energy-dense choices. This may mean increasing the priority of 'whole' foods which deliver a range of key nutrients and food factors before/during/after training in preference to specialised sports products which often contain only a few targeted nutrients. Although an increased energy intake may be required during periods of LBM gain, this doesn't mean that the athlete should consume lots of nutrient-poor foods. Rather, the athlete should focus their meals and snacks on compact forms of nutrients that manage their appetite and gastrointestinal comfort.

Table 3.2 provides an example of how a day's diet could be manipulated either by increasing or decreasing energy content by 2000 kJ in order to promote body composition changes without compromising the principles of training nutrition.

3.2.3   FUELLING TRAINING SESSIONS

The determinants of an athlete's need to consume fuel sources prior to and during training include their training status; the intensity, duration and type of session to be undertaken; the timing of subsequent training sessions; and the purpose of the training session. Most fuelling strategies target the body's carbohydrate reserves (muscle glycogen, liver glycogen and blood glucose), which are relatively small in comparison to the reserves of other body fuels (e.g. body fat), as well as to the heavy fuel demands of the training and competition schedules of some athletes. In many types of sport, reduced performance and fatigue are a consequence of the depletion of carbohydrate stores and our limited ability to convert other fuels (e.g. fat or amino acids) into the glucose desired by the muscle and central nervous system.

Table 3.3 presents current recommendations for the consumption of carbohydrate across the total day, and with respect to a training session. A recently formed message is that carbohydrate intakes should vary from day to day and across the training macrocycle in tune with the changing fuel requirements of the athlete's training load. Furthermore, it is unnecessary to undertake all training sessions with high carbohydrate availability and may even be beneficial in terms of promoting adaptations to

TABLE 3.2
Example of Modifying a Training Diet to Alter Body Composition

Daily Intake Example	Changes to Increase by 2000 kJ/d for Mass Gain	Changes to Reduce by 2000 kJ/d for Body Fat/Mass Loss
7:30 am: 1 cup cereal + 2 tablespoons muesli + 150 ml light milk; glass of juice		Remove muesli but add a serving of fruit (e.g. berries on top of cereal); omit juice
9–10 am: Gym		
10 am: After gym, 600 ml low-fat chocolate milk		
12:30 pm: 1 tuna and salad sandwich (light mayonnaise) with an apple	Add an extra sandwich	Add extra salad to sandwich
2:30 pm: 1 muesli bar		Change snack to 1 thick slice whole-grain toast with yeast extract spread
3–5 pm: Swim training		
5:15 pm: After training, 200 g low-fat flavoured yoghurt with 2 tablespoons nuts		Reduce nuts to 1 tablespoon
7 pm: 180 g grilled steak + 2 medium potatoes, carrots, broccoli, beans		Move dinner forward to 6.30 pm, reduce the size of the steak to 120 g and increase the amount of vegetables
9 pm: 1 bowl of berries + 2 scoops of ice cream	Add 1 cup hot chocolate (light milk)	Change ice cream to low fat custard or create a smoothie with berries and milk

Example based on a 60 kg female swimmer: 2 training sessions/d.
Nutritional targets: 10,500 kJ/d for weight maintenance, 360 g carbohydrate, 90 g protein with 20 g protein delivered within 60 min of finishing each training session and the rest distributed over the day.

the training stimulus, to undertake some sessions in a glycogen-depleted state (Philp et al. 2011; see Section 3.2.7). However, chronic periods of training with low carbohydrate availability may compromise both training capacity and mood state (Achten et al. 2004) or immune status (see Section 3.2.6).

During training sessions in which exercise capacity is likely to be limited by insufficient carbohydrate availability (for example, a single prolonged session, or a session undertaken within a phase of heavy training), it may be beneficial to consume carbohydrate during the session. Such benefits include improved concentration, maintenance of skill, improved endurance and high intensity exercise capacity (Burke et al. 2011), and attenuation of the decline in immune cell function post exercise (Braun and Von Duvillard 2004). Table 3.3 provides guidelines for carbohydrate intakes that can optimise performance during exercise of different duration; the science behind these recommendations will be discussed further in Section 3.3.5. Many options of everyday foods and specialised sports products (e.g. sports drinks, gels or bars) can contribute to these targets according to the practicality of consumption and

TABLE 3.3
Carbohydrate Needs for Training, Recovery and Fuelling

Training Load		Carbohydrate Intake Targets (g/kg of athlete's body mass or g/h during exercise)
Light	Low-intensity or skill-based activities	3–5g/kg/day
Moderate	Moderate exercise program (i.e. ~1 h/day)	5–7 g/kg/day
High	Endurance program (e.g. 1–3 h/day of mod-high-intensity exercise)	6–10 g/kg/day
Very high	Extreme commitment (i.e. at least 4–5 h/day of moderate to high-intensity exercise	8–12 g/kg/day
During Exercise		
During brief exercise	<45 min	Not needed
During sustained high-intensity exercise	45–75 min	Small amounts including mouth rinse
During endurance exercise including "stop and start" sports	1–2.5 h	30–60 g/h
During ultra-endurance exercise	>2.5–3 h	Up to 90 g/h
Post Exercise		
Rapid refuelling post exercise		1 g/kg/h for 4 h

Source: Adapted from Burke, L.M., et al., *Journal of Sports Sciences* 29(Suppl 1):S17–S27, 2011.

the need for other nutrients (including fluid). Figure 3.1 presents two case studies of athletes and their approximate carbohydrate needs, and how this might be distributed across the day and in relation to training. It is important to remember that these are recommendations only, and individual athletes will need to trial a few different strategies to understand how to best meet their own needs.

3.2.4 PRACTICING COMPETITION STRATEGIES OF FUELLING AND HYDRATION

Most athletes will have heard the phrase 'never try anything new on race day'. Training sessions not only drive the development of physiological capabilities and specific skills, but also can present opportunities to practice and refine competition nutrition strategies. Such practice is not only of practical importance (for example, developing the skills to drink while running, or to handle a bike while obtaining foods and fluids from a feed zone in a cycle race), but may also provide a physiological advantage. There is evidence, at least in endurance exercise, that the gut can be trained to absorb carbohydrate to be used as a fuel source during exercise

a. The case for a female adaptive rower

The following meal plan is based on a female adaptive rower who trains two to three times a day most days including a mix of low-intensity aerobic work, strength / resistance training, and high-intensity repeat effort work. Assuming body mass of 68 kg, approximate CHO requirements for this day are 6-8 g/kg BM (410-540 g).

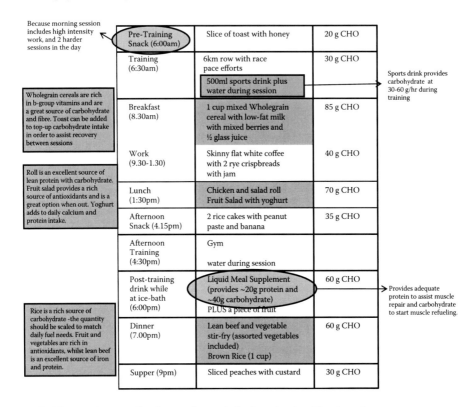

Because morning session includes high intensity work, and 2 harder sessions in the day	Pre-Training Snack (6:00am)	Slice of toast with honey	20 g CHO
	Training (6:30am)	6km row with race pace efforts	30 g CHO
		500ml sports drink plus water during session	Sports drink provides carbohydrate at 30-60 g/hr during training
Wholegrain cereals are rich in b-group vitamins and are a great source of carbohydrate and fibre. Toast can be added to top-up carbohydrate intake in order to assist recovery between sessions	Breakfast (8.30am)	1 cup mixed Wholegrain cereal with low-fat milk with mixed berries and ½ glass juice	85 g CHO
	Work (9.30-1.30)	Skinny flat white coffee with 2 rye crispbreads with jam	40 g CHO
Roll is an excellent source of lean protein with carbohydrate. Fruit salad provides a rich source of antioxidants and is a great option when out. Yoghurt adds to daily calcium and protein intake.	Lunch (1:30pm)	Chicken and salad roll Fruit Salad with yoghurt	70 g CHO
	Afternoon Snack (4.15pm)	2 rice cakes with peanut paste and banana	35 g CHO
	Afternoon Training (4:30pm)	Gym water during session	
	Post-training drink while at ice-bath (6:00pm)	Liquid Meal Supplement (provides ~20g protein and ~40g carbohydrate) PLUS a piece of fruit	60 g CHO
Rice is a rich source of carbohydrate -the quantity should be scaled to match daily fuel needs. Fruit and vegetables are rich in antioxidants, whilst lean beef is an excellent source of iron and protein.	Dinner (7.00pm)	Lean beef and vegetable stir-fry (assorted vegetables included) Brown Rice (1 cup)	60 g CHO
	Supper (9pm)	Sliced peaches with custard	30 g CHO

(6:00pm marked) Provides adequate protein to assist muscle repair and carbohydrate to start muscle refueling.

FIGURE 3.1   Case studies for varying carbohydrate intake. (Continued)

(Cox et al. 2010). It may not be necessary to consume carbohydrate in every training session, however certain sessions can be targeted for event practice, especially in the competition-specific phase of preparation.

Commencing exercise in a well-hydrated state is the first step towards optimising performance, especially in sessions undertaken in warm-hot environments. Due to restrictions on the availability or opportunity to consume fluids in comparison to rates of sweat loss during many types of exercise, it is not uncommon for athletes to develop a fluid deficit over a training session or competition event. In most instances, urine colour is a good indicator of chronic hydration status, and a variety of urine colour charts are available to assist the athlete in understanding this. Urine frequency is another indicator, although this can be influenced by nerves and some medications. For practitioners who can access a portable refractometer, the measurement of urine specific gravity (USG) on the first urine sample produced each morning can be a useful way of tracking individual hydration status

b. The case for a male track runner

The following meal plan is based on an 80kg male track athlete with cerebral palsy. Track athletes often train twice a day, and although one of these may be long the actual amount of work done is often quite small (2-3 minutes total of high intensity work). Approximate CHO requirements for this day are 5 g/kg BM (400 g).

Breakfast (7:00am)	2 slices wholegrain toast one with an egg, one with yeast spread	30 g CHO	Light breakfast due to high intensity work in track session. Doesn't want to feel sick during training
Training (9:00am)	Track session – warm up, 3 × 60m, 3 × 80m with 5 min break	10 g CHO	
	Sips of sports drink as CHO mouth rinse		Mouth rinse useful for high intensity work since lighter breakfast
Immediately post training (10.30am)	Large smoothee made with milk, yoghurt, honey and fruit	60 g CHO	Session does not require substantial refueling but does require protein and snack can be larger due to smaller breakfast
Lunch (1pm)	Large meat and salad roll Plus piece of fruit	90 g CHO	
Afternoon Training (3:00pm)	Gym session – core stability, stretch, form work		
Post-training snack (4:00pm)	200g flavoured yoghurt Muesli bar	50 g CHO	Recovery snack not strictly necessary however provides fuel and protein between lunch and dinner
Dinner (6.30pm)	Spaghetti bolognese with salad Garlic Bread - homemade	100 g CHO	
Supper	Bowl of fruit with custard or ice cream	40 g CHO	

FIGURE 3.1 (CONTINUED)   Case studies for varying carbohydrate intake.

over time and in response to different challenges (travel, altitude, heat, competition) (Maughan and Shirreffs 2008). Better attention to fluid intake over the day and around training sessions may be required if there is consistent evidence of dehydration. Over-hydration or over-zealous rehydration may also be problematic, particularly when this occurs late in the day and causes disruptions to sleep due to the need to urinate during the night. Advice should include planning appropriate fluid intake throughout the day to counter losses, drinking with meals (since the electrolytes and other meal components will assist in fluid retention), and the specific replacement of sweat electrolyte losses (via the use of sports drinks, specific electrolyte preparations or salt-rich foods) when addressing the restoration of large sweat losses (Maughan et al. 1997).

Recommendations for fluid intake before and during competition (see Section 3.3.4) revolve around an individualised fluid plan that is sympathetic to the athlete's expected sweat rates, the opportunity to consume fluids during their event, and the penalties associated with either too little or too much fluid intake. Training sessions can be used to collect this information and to develop and practice the individualised hydration plans. The strategy of consuming a bolus of fluid prior to exercise then topping up regularly during the session is likely to be more effective at achieving an appropriate pacing of fluid intake than commencing exercise without fluid and waiting until thirst dictates the need to drink. Indeed in many sports, practical factors such as restricted access to fluid or gastrointestinal discomfort may prevent an athlete from drinking a sufficient volume of fluid once they have become thirsty (see Section 3.3.4). In addition to these factors, some athletes with an impairment deliberately avoid consuming fluid prior to or during exercise due to the impracticalities of accessing a bathroom when required or for other reasons. Training sessions are therefore useful for trialling the timing, volume and type of drinks to be included in the fluid plan before and during exercise to suit the specific practical and physiological needs of the athlete.

To estimate dehydration and sweat rates incurred during an exercise bout:

1. Measure body mass both before and after at least one hour of exercise under conditions similar to competition or hard training (which may vary with environmental conditions, terrain, etc depending on the sport).
2. Measure body mass as accurately as possible by wearing minimal clothing, while barefoot, and preferably without prostheses, strapping, and other sporting equipment. In the case of post-exercise measurements, take as soon as possible after the session after having towel dried. For wheelchair-bound athletes, where possible use a set of seated or wheelchair scales.

Example:

$$\text{Pre-exercise mass} = 74 \text{ kg}$$

$$\text{Post-exercise mass} = 72.5 \text{ kg}$$

$$\text{Fluid deficit} = 1.5 \text{ kg}$$

To convert the fluid deficit to % body mass, divide the deficit by starting body mass and multiply by 100. For example, 1.5 kg/74 kg × 100 = 2%.

3. Estimate the weight of any fluid or foods consumed during the session (for example, 1 litre of fluid = 1 kg or 1000 g).
4. Calculate sweat loss by adding the weight of foods consumed during the session to the fluid deficit: Sweat loss (litres) = Body mass before exercise (in kg) – Body mass after exercise (kg) + Weight of fluids/foods consumed (kg).

Example:

$$74 \text{ kg} - 72.5 \text{ kg} = 1.5 \text{ kg fluid deficit} + 1 \text{ kg (fluid)}$$
$$= \text{sweat loss of 2.5 kg or 2500 mL}$$

To convert to a sweat rate per hour, divide by the exercise time in minutes and multiply by 60.

Use these calculations to assess how well the athlete hydrated during the session and how much they need to rehydrate afterwards. If they gained mass, fluid intake during the session was greater than required and they may need to reduce fluid intake. If they lost >2% BM, consider whether it is possible for the athlete to drink a greater volume during exercise.

3.2.5   RECOVERING BETWEEN WORKOUTS

The modern approach to recovery nutrition incorporates a holistic delivery of nutrients to support the responses of all body systems following the stressor of an exercise bout. The requirement for each component of recovery nutrition depends on the nature of the exercise bout itself—for example, not all exercise bouts will deplete muscle glycogen stores or create a large fluid deficit. Not all the sessions that are now regularly incorporated into an athlete's training plan require a proactive approach to recovery nutrition—for example, pilates or yoga, a stretching/recovery gym session, a skill session, a 30 min walk, or an "easy" swim may be undertaken without a specialised plan of recovery eating. The development of a recovery eating plan requires the understanding of the physiological stresses involved in each training session, the goals of each session and subsequent workouts, and the athlete's total training demands. It is also important to recognise that food and drinks consumed to promote recovery after a training session may not need to add extra kilojoules/energy to the day's intake. In many cases, larger meals may need to be reduced in size to create an opportunity to add a recovery snack into the day. Alternatively, the timing of training and/or the meal could be manipulated to coincide more effectively. Four key components of recovery nutrition, as summarised in Table 3.4, are refuelling, rehydration, repair/adaptation, and revitalisation.

3.2.5.1   Refuelling

The need for proactive refuelling between two training sessions depends on the glycogen demands of each session and period of time between them. Since glycogen storage occurs at a rate of about 5% per hour, it may take a day of carbohydrate-rich intake to fully restore or load glycogen between glycogen-depleting exercise bouts (Coyle 1991). When the program involves two bouts of glycogen-depleting exercise within 8–12 h, the athlete should promote effective refuelling by consuming carbohydrate-rich foods and drinks providing 1–1.2 g/kg/h soon after exercise towards their total daily carbohydrate requirements (as per Table 3.3). Such strategies will optimise the replenishment of muscle glycogen stores as well as promote the activity of many of the immune system white cells (Bishop et al. 2009).

3.2.5.2   Rehydration

Replacing the fluid and electrolytes lost as sweat is an important component of post-exercise recovery, especially when the losses are substantial, the environment is hot, and preparation time for the next session is relatively short. Since a rehydration plan

TABLE 3.4
Summary of Eating for Recovery

Issue	Key Sessions Requiring Proactive Strategies	Overview of Recommendations	Examples of Suitable Food Choices
Refuelling	High-intensity exercise or prolonged endurance activity (>60 min) where another training session is to be undertaken within 8–10 h	1 g carbohydrate/kg BM/h for 4 h	Bread, fruit, cereals, rice cakes, crackers Pasta, rice, potato, sweetened dairy products (flavoured milk, yoghurt, custard)
Rehydration	Activities which have induced a substantial (>2%) loss in body mass	120–150% of fluid losses consumed over the next few hours	Fluids containing electrolytes (especially sodium) such as sports drinks, milk, electrolyte solutions; or water consumed with food
Protein synthesis for repair and adaptation	Resistance exercise, high-intensity activity, prolonged-endurance exercise, high-impact activity where muscle damage is likely	20–25 g high-quality protein consumed soon after exercise, with evidence to support repeated small doses of protein every few hours through the day	Milk proteins (e.g. milk, yoghurt, custard) Meat, poultry, fish, eggs
General health and immune system support	Resistance exercise, high-intensity activity, prolonged-endurance exercise, high-impact activity where muscle damage is likely	Consume a range of whole foods wherever possible	Antioxidant nutrients (brightly coloured fruit and vegetables, whole grain cereals), omega-3 fatty acids (oily fish), probiotics (yoghurt)
Putting it all together		Protein + carbohydrate + electrolytes + micronutrients	Fruit smoothies, berries and sweetened yoghurt, tuna salad sandwiches, meat/ chicken and chicken stir fry with rice or noodles, iron-fortified cereals with milk and fruit toppings, omelette with mushrooms and parsley on toast

will also need to address ongoing sweat and urine losses, restoration of fluid balance in the hours after exercise will require the individual to consume a fluid volume equivalent to ~125–150% of the deficit created by the exercise bout. Replacement of sweat sodium losses contributes to rehydration goals by preserving thirst and minimising urine losses (Maughan et al. 1997). This can be achieved by choosing sodium-containing fluids (such as milk or sports drinks) or by eating a meal or snack that includes foods that are salt containing (such as bread, cheese, many breakfast cereals, yeast-extract spreads) or have salt added to them in preparation (such as eggs and most main meals).

3.2.5.3 Repair/Adaptation

In recent years there has been an increased appreciation that optimal adaptive responses to training represent an interaction between the exercise stimulus and the intake of protein, particularly of individual amino acids such as leucine. Research has provided strong evidence that the intake of moderate amounts of protein soon after training maximises muscle protein synthesis (Burd et al. 2011), not only for the development of muscle mass/strength but also for the synthesis of muscle proteins involved in endurance exercise (e.g. enzymes) and hormones which regulate metabolism and immune function. Combining protein with carbohydrate-rich meals and snacks consumed after exercise is also advantageous in optimising glycogen synthesis in situations where muscle damage has occurred or where carbohydrate intake is sub-optimal (Betts and Williams 2010).

While the daily protein intakes recommended to athletes may be elevated to 1.2–1.6 g/kg BM/day, it appears that the timing and frequency of this intake are of most importance to capitalise on the increased rates of muscle protein synthesis that occur for at least 24 h after an exercise bout. To optimise the immediate post-exercise response, it appears that athletes should consume 20–25 g of high quality protein sources containing 2–3 g leucine (e.g. dairy, meat products, eggs) soon after exercise. This can be provided as a fluid (such as milk), a snack or as components of a meal, depending on the timing of the exercise and the athlete's total energy budget. While these protein targets can be easily obtained through food sources, there is also a range of protein powders (such as whey protein) and liquid meal supplements based on dairy which can be useful after exercise as a compact, easily transportable source of protein. As outlined in Chapter 11, care must be taken with using any nutritional supplement to thoroughly check ingredients, especially where athletes may be subject to anti-doping regulations.

3.2.5.4 Revitalisation

Many micronutrients (vitamins, minerals, antioxidants, phytochemicals) are important co-factors in metabolism and may contribute favourably to the recovery processes after exercise. Although we are uncertain about the effects of regular exercise on micronutrient requirements, it is prudent for athletes to take advantage of opportunities to increase their intake of micronutrients and phytochemicals by consuming a wide range of nutrient-rich foods whenever possible. Balanced against the practicality offered by specially manufactured sports foods and supplements in meeting targets for isolated macronutrients such as protein and carbohydrate, whole foods are likely to offer the advantages of a greater range and quantity of micronutrients. Furthermore, the combination of foods within a meal or snack can strategically optimise the absorption of nutrients (e.g. combining vitamin C-containing foods/ fluids such as citrus fruits, tomatoes or peppers with iron-rich plant products such as iron-fortified breakfast cereals, green leafy vegetables and legumes to enhance iron absorption). Focussing on nutrient-dense foods is particularly important for those who are on a relatively low energy budget since achieving all of the micronutrients requirements is more difficult when total food intake is restricted.

3.2.6 MINIMISING ILLNESS AND INJURY

During periods of heavy training and competition, athletes can be at increased risk of infectious illnesses, especially of the upper respiratory tract (Davison and Simpson 2011), and of injuries related to their sport (Rogalski et al. 2013). Injury and illness result in the loss or modification of training sessions, which interrupts the optimal accumulation of the adaptive training response. If this occurs at a crucial time in race preparation, or immediately prior to competition, the consequences can undo months, if not years, of progress towards an athlete's goals. Infection can also place fellow athletes/team members at risk of illness. There are a number of dietary factors which have been linked to the immune system and may require consideration in the athlete's eating plans.

3.2.6.1 Carbohydrate and Total Energy Intake

Maintaining adequate energy and carbohydrate intake, especially during periods of heavy training, is an important component in reducing the degree of detrimental immune disturbances which result from exercise (Walsh et al. 2011). Negative energy balance and/or low energy availability may result in the inability to supply all dietary nutrients required to support immune function. Decreased substrate availability (i.e. total energy deficit, muscle glycogen depletion, reduced blood glucose concentrations) acts indirectly by exacerbating the stress response of exercise, increasing the degree of immune disturbances, and limiting the full function of immune cells which require glucose as an energy substrate (Davison and Simpson 2011). Some injuries may result from fatigue or poor concentration due to poor energy or carbohydrate availability.

3.2.6.2 Protein and Amino Acids

Protein has an important role in many aspects of immune function. While it is uncommon for athletes to consume insufficient amounts of protein, there are some individuals who may be at risk due to their energy budget or their dietary preferences (for example, vegetarians). Sports scientists have been interested in the role of the nonessential amino acid glutamine in immune function related to exercise. Glutamine can be used as an energy substrate by a number of immune cells, and low blood concentrations of glutamine have been found to coincide with immunodepression (Castell 2003). Since plasma glutamine concentrations are decreased following prolonged or strenuous exercise, both acutely and more chronically, there has been interest in supplementing with glutamine to improve immune function.

Although supplementing with glutamine has been shown to prevent the exercise-induced fall in plasma glutamine, this has had no effect on immune cell number and function after exercise, and inconsistent effects on symptoms of illness (Hiscock and Pedersen 2002; Castell 2003). Therefore to date there is no evidence to support supplementation with glutamine, other than to ensure adequate overall dietary protein from a range of food sources in order to ensure an appropriate balance of individual amino acids.

3.2.6.3 Antioxidants

It is well recognised that exercise induces oxidative stress—indeed, this appears to be one of the mechanisms driving the adaptations to training (Power et al. 2011). Oxidative stress can also lead to the damage or modification to immune cells and tissues resulting in an impairment of function (Gleeson et al. 2004), hence a number of antioxidant nutrients have been investigated for the purpose of improving immune status. Vitamin A deficiency is associated with T-cell function (Ross 2012) and is therefore an important antioxidant nutrient. Very low fat or low animal protein diets can result in reduced vitamin A intakes, therefore it is important to ensure athletes consume adequate sources of vitamin A and its precursors.

There has been a long history of research on vitamin C in relation to preventing upper respiratory tract infections ("colds") and boosting immune function. Indeed, there is some evidence that supplementation with vitamin C (together with zinc) at the onset of cold symptoms can reduce the duration and impact of a cold (Hemila and Chalker 2013). In addition, megadoses of vitamin C taken after an ultra-endurance competition have been shown to reduce the incidence of infection in the post competition phase (Peters et al. 1993). However, there is limited evidence to support daily vitamin C, vitamin E or zinc supplementation in athletes. While megadoses of these nutrients may suppress cortisol and interleukin-6 responses to exercise (Fischer et al. 2004), they appear to have minimal effects on most aspects of immunity and incidence of upper respiratory tract illnesses in well-nourished individuals.

The bioflavonoid quercetin is another antioxidant which has received a great deal of recent interest in the sports nutrition literature as an immune stimulator with antimicrobial and antiviral properties, and as an anti-inflammatory agent (Davis et al. 2009). Quercetin is found naturally in many foods including onions, berries, apples, cherries, teas and green leafy vegetables. Despite promising research in rodents, the benefits of quercetin have not translated well into the human literature, with no evidence to suggest an impact on immune cells and very limited evidence to support changes in immune function following supplementation (Walsh et al. 2011). While further research is necessary, it may be prudent to focus on ensuring high intakes of quercetin- and other polyphenol-rich foods.

The potential benefits of supplementing with antioxidants for immune function need to be counterbalanced by emerging evidence of the potential for antioxidant supplements to diminish the adaptive response to exercise (Ristow et al. 2009) and slow the recovery of muscle function after eccentric exercise (such as has been found with high-dose vitamin C supplements; Close et al. 2006). Therefore the preference is to promote an increased intake of antioxidant-rich foods, especially in periods of heavy training, over supplementation with high doses of antioxidants.

3.2.6.4 Probiotics

Probiotics have been associated with improvements in gut barrier function, an important first line of defence in the immune system. There is evidence that pro-biotic intake can enhance the immune system, improve intestinal tract health and reduce prevalence of allergy in susceptible individuals (West et al. 2009). Several large studies in athletes have provided evidence of reduced illness symptom days (Cox et al. 2008; West et al. 2011), reduced severity of gastrointestinal symptoms (West et al. 2011) and improved symptoms in fatigued athletes with an identifiable immune deficiency (Clancy et al. 2006). Since there is a synergistic effect between food compounds and probiotic cultures, dairy products such as yoghurt and aci-dophilus milk are a good avenue for the consumption of probiotics. Alternatively, probiotic supplements may be useful in athletes.

3.2.6.5 Calcium

Injury and chronic leg pain related to the chronic bone microtrauma known as stress fractures is common in many sports (Sanborn et al. 2011). While the aetiology of stress fractures is complex and multifactorial, low bone density is considered a major contributing factor (Scofield and Hecht 2012). While weight-bearing and high-impact exercise can promote bone strength, there is increasing evidence of inad-equate bone density in a range of athlete populations, including cyclists (Scofield and Hecht 2012). While low energy availability is an important risk factor in impaired bone health (see Section 3.2.1.1), a key nutrient in optimising bone density is cal-cium. Although recommended dietary intakes of calcium vary between countries, it is well recognised that the richest and most well absorbed sources of calcium are dairy products. Unfortunately, many athletes reduce or limit their dairy intake due to their concerns regarding weight (body fat) gain and/or lactose intolerance. However, there is now a large body of information that supports a positive role for dairy prod-ucts in both body composition management and the achievement of sports nutrition goals. Therefore it is important for athletes to include sufficient dairy products (and other calcium-rich food sources) in their diet to achieve calcium requirements, using low-lactose variants where lactose intolerance has been diagnosed.

3.2.6.6 Vitamin D

Vitamin D is a nutrient classified as a fat-soluble vitamin, which acts functionally as a hormone. Our primary source of vitamin D is ultraviolet B (UVB) radiation from sunlight, and recent studies have found vitamin D deficiency and sub-optimal status in many populations, with athletes being no less susceptible (Willis et al. 2008). Of particular concern are athletes who train predominantly indoors, have dark skin pigmentation, live at latitudes > 35 degrees north or south of the equator, and/or who expose relatively small skin surface area to sunlight. Vitamin D has many roles within the body, the most well recognised being in optimising bone strength through its integral role in the uptake of calcium into bone. In addition, insufficient vitamin D status has been shown to reduce immune function and muscle strength (Cannell et al. 2009). While vitamin D is a dietary nutrient, dietary sources are generally unable to alter vitamin D status substantially enough to reverse a clinical deficiency.

Instead, safe sun exposure as advised by most national cancer councils or public health authorities is promoted, with regular checks of vitamin D status being undertaken in all athletes, particularly at the end of summer and more often in those at risk of inadequate exposure. Appropriate supplementation should be organised in those found to have insufficient (<32 ng/ml) or deficient (<20 ng/ml) vitamin D levels (see Chapter 10).

3.2.7 SPECIAL ISSUES AND CONTROVERSIES IN TRAINING NUTRITION

Technological advances have allowed a more in-depth perspective on the metabolic response to exercise and nutrition. As is often the case, this can raise more questions than it answers, but it also initiates new insights into the complex interactions that occur within the human body in response to various manipulations of exercise and diet. Currently, there are a number of areas of research that may further refine and individualise the practice of sports nutrition, which have been summarised in Table 3.5.

Although performance is maximised when training is undertaken with high carbohydrate availability (i.e. glycogen stores that are matched to the fuel cost of the event), recent studies of the signalling pathways which promote the adaptations to training show greater increases in cellular transcription factors and protein expression when the same exercise is undertaken in a low-glycogen environment (Philp et al. 2011). This has led to training studies in which subjects have completed chronic periods (3–10 w) in which some (e.g. 50%) or all of their workouts have been done with low carbohydrate availability achieved either by scheduling two training sessions close together without opportunity for refuelling before the second one, or by undertaking sessions in a fasted state and without further carbohydrate intake (see Burke 2010a). While the "train low" condition has typically been associated with enhancements of the cellular response to exercise, such as greater increases in glycogen stores and enzymes associated with fat utilisation, to date only the study undertaken in previously untrained subjects has observed a larger increase in the performance improvements achieved by training (Hansen et al. 2005). Furthermore, there have been observations of a reduced capacity to train at high intensity/power which may be counterproductive to performance gains (Yeo et al. 2008). Therefore further study is needed and may require a more sophisticated periodisation of train low strategies into the training macrocycle and microcycle. Indeed, in real life, it is observed that athletes periodise their nutrition strategies for training sessions, by both accident and design, so that some are undertaken with high fuel availability and others in a depleted fuel status. Therefore, optimal practice may require some simple tweaking of this mix.

3.3 COMPETITION NUTRITION

Competition nutrition presents a different range and level of issues to the athlete than encountered in the training phase. Additional challenges include the overlay of pressure to achieve success, the presence of rules or a competition timetable that interferes with desirable nutrition practices, issues related to travel, an unfamiliar

TABLE 3.5
New Issues in Sports Nutrition

Issue	Theme	Overview	Current Recommendations
Optimising adaptation to training	"Training low" with carbohydrate may enhance training adaptations	Undertaking exercise with low carbohydrate availability (either muscle glycogen or blood glucose) may amplify the training stimulus and increase the expression of enzymes that promote fat metabolism	Consider targeting some training sessions during the base phase of training for lowered carbohydrate state, by either training fasted first thing in the morning or consuming minimal carbohydrate between two sessions undertaken on the same day
	Anti-oxidant supplements may block training adaptations	Oxidative stress may be important as a signal that promotes adaptation to the training stimulus. Antioxidant supplements may block this signal and reduce the adaptation to an exercise bout	Choose a diet rich in sources of a range of antioxidants during most training periods. Consider anti-oxidant supplements only if there is an additional stressor (such as altitude, heat) or in periods of frequent competition (e.g. tournaments) where the need for recovery outweighs the need to drive training response
Periodising nutritional goals to phase of training	Off season	Minimise changes in body composition, training usually very light and non-specific	Be aware of energy-dense foods and fluids (including alcohol) and modify energy intake to meet reduced energy needs
	Base phase	High-volume training, best opportunity to manipulate body composition	Target specific body composition changes through manipulation of energy intake
	Specific competition preparation	Training increases in intensity, often with specialised periods in different environments (e.g. heat, altitude) Increase in skills and tactical training in team sports	Increase carbohydrate intake to match intensity in training. Consume a source of high quality protein and carbohydrate soon after training to promote refuelling and adaptation Consider the use of supplements carefully. Practice competition fuelling and hydration strategies

Taper for competition	Intensity usually remains higher while volume decreases Energy requirements usually fall Opportunities to eat increase, but appetite may not fall in line with reduced training load	Be aware of lowered energy expenditure and increased opportunities/time to eat (including boredom eating) to prevent any body fat gains during this time Consider carbohydrate loading for events > 2.5 h duration
Individualising goals to special needs of sport		
Endurance sports	Maintenance of high power-to-weight ratios creates interest in achieving low body mass and body fat levels Carbohydrate availability during event promotes performance and needs to be practised during training	Choose a suitable competition weight that can be achieved safely and without chronic low energy availability Periodise nutrition according to microcycles and macrocycles of training Practice race day nutrition strategies to promote physiological and behavioural characteristics that enable them
Team sports	Differences in activity patterns and game roles among team members may require different nutrition programs Competition formats may include weekly fixture or tournament formats Team athletes are at greater risk of poor alcohol practices than other athletes, particularly after the match or during the off season	Individualise nutritional programs to the needs of each player as well as the period of the sporting calendar Promote recovery after matches whether in tournament or weekly fixture Promote sound nutrition practices after matches and during the off season, particularly with regard to alcohol intake
Weight category sports	Emphasis on low body fat levels for weight class Culture within sport to train above weight division Emphasis on weight creates an increased risk of low energy availability/issues with eating and body image	Choose a weight division that can be achieved safely and with minimal stress Choose nutrient-dense foods, sufficient carbohydrate to support high-intensity training, and a good spread of high-quality protein over the day to meet nutritional goals Rehydrate/refuel immediately after weigh-in according to the techniques used to make weight

(Continued)

TABLE 3.5 (CONTINUED)
New Issues in Sports Nutrition

Issue	Theme	Overview	Current Recommendations
	Power/strength sports	Goals are to enhance power and strength and possibly muscle hypertrophy	Consume a diet high in energy to support high lean mass
		Culture of interest in supplements and high protein intakes	Enable adequate carbohydrate intake to fuel resistance training sessions
		Competitive events often involve multiple throws, lifts or rounds	Consume adequate but not excessive protein and spread protein intake over the day
			Consume a source of high-quality protein (20–25 g) soon after resistance workouts
	Skill sports	Heavy reliance on concentration and fine motor skills, often over extended periods of time	Consume a nutritionally balanced diet to optimise health, wellbeing and body composition
		Culture within sport to consider impact of nutrition on performance to be minimal	Commence training and competition in a hydrated state
		Often avoid eating/drinking pre competition due to potential impact on gut comfort and heart rate	Consume a pre-training/competition meal which ensures stable blood glucose concentrations and achieves gut comfort

---

COMMENTARY BOX 3.1

ATHLETE INSIGHT: To upcoming sports nutritionists.

Get your athletes to write down what they eat over a typical fortnight and see if they are getting what nutrition they need. Talk with them so they understand the need for good "fuel" and what "fuel" they need for their sport. Be a pain in the butt! They will thank you when they achieve PBs or stand on the podium!

**—Richard Nicholson, track and field athlete
and ex-powerlifter, multiple Paralympian**

---

environment and communal living, and a limited number of opportunities to undertake high-level practice for specific competition scenarios. On the other hand, the competition environment can support good nutritional practices in terms of presenting a large incentive to get things right, or providing an infrastructure of aid stations, feedzones or other mechanisms of making nutrition support available before, during and after events. Sporting competitions vary according to a range of factors—the intensity, duration and type of exercise, the environment in which it is performed, whether it is an individual event or a team effort, and the number and frequency of times that the athlete must perform to decide the eventual winner. Despite the diversity of features, competition involves a common theme: athletes desire to perform at their best or, at least, better than their rivals. Therefore the starting point is to understand the factors that will cause the athlete to fatigue or experience a downturn in their performance.

3.3.1 LIMITATIONS TO PERFORMANCE DURING COMPETITION

At some point during most sporting events, athletes experience deterioration in exercise outputs such as speed, power output, time spent in high-intensity activities, or skill and concentration. This failure to maintain a desired or optimal exercise level is commonly termed fatigue, and may occur intermittently throughout the event, but particularly towards the end. Typically, success in competitive events is achieved by reducing or delaying the onset of such fatigue.

There are a variety of ways in which fatigue can occur during a sports competition, with nutrition playing a role in many of these (see Table 3.6). Their risk of occurrence depends on factors such as the duration and intensity of the event, environmental conditions (e.g. temperature and humidity), an athlete's training status and individual characteristics, and the opportunity to undertake nutrition strategies before, during and in the recovery between events. Whatever the sport or event, sports scientists try to pinpoint the likely risk that various factors will cause fatigue, based on the available applied sports research, as well as accounts of the past competition experiences of the athletes involved. With this knowledge, athletes can then be guided to undertake specific competition nutrition strategies that will minimize or delay the onset of these problems.

TABLE 3.6
Factors Related to Nutrition That Could Produce Fatigue or Suboptimal Performance during Sports Competition

Factor	Description	Examples of High-Risk/Common Occurrence in Sports	Nutritional Strategies to Address Issue
Dehydration	Failure to drink enough fluid to replace sweat losses during an event. May be exacerbated if the athlete begins the event in fluid deficit.	Events undertaken in hot conditions, particularly for athletes with high-intensity activity patterns and/or heavy protective garments. Repeated competitions (e.g. tournaments) may increase risk of compounding dehydration from one event to the next. **Risk in para-sports:** It is difficult to obtain and consume fluids during the wheelchair marathon and ultra-endurance sports.	The athlete should try to drink well in the period before the event so that they start well hydrated. Drinking during the event should track sweat rates to prevent a large fluid deficit from occurring.
Muscle glycogen depletion	Depletion of important muscle fuel due to high utilization in a single event and/or poor recovery of stores from previous activity/event. Generally thought to occur in events longer than 90 min.	Generally occurs in events lasting longer than 90 min such as marathon, road cycling and Ironman triathlons. May occur in some team sports in "running" players with large total distances covered at high intensities (e.g. midfield players in football). Repeated competitions (e.g. tournament) may increase risk of poor refuelling from one match to the next. **Risk in para-sports:** Although few events are >90 min, many are dependent on smaller muscle groups (arms) with smaller glycogen stores that may benefit from loading (e.g. wheelchair marathon, wheelchair basketball or tennis tournaments).	Carbohydrate loading—achieved by tapering exercise and eating a high-carbohydrate diet (10 g/kg BM/d) for 24–48 h can supercompensate muscle glycogen stores and prolong the time before they become depleted.

Hypoglycemia and depletion of central nervous system fuels	Reduction in blood glucose concentrations due to poor carbohydrate availability. Note that some athletes do not experience fatigue even when blood glucose concentrations become low. New research shows that even when the central nervous system is not depleted, the intake of carbohydrate can promote a "happy brain" that will allow the muscles to work at a higher power output.	Depletion of blood glucose may occur in athletes with high carbohydrate requirements (see above) who fail to consume carbohydrate during their event. **Risk in para-sports:** Team sport tournaments where more than one game is played per day. Events of 45–75 min duration may benefit from carbohydrate intake to promote a happy brain. **Risk in para-sports:** Some skill-based athletes (e.g. shooting, archery) will avoid fluid and food prior to competition to help control heart rate, avoid the need to use bathroom facilities, and for gut comfort.	Intake of carbohydrate during an event will prevent hypoglycaemia and provide fuel for the central nervous system. In shorter events, even tasting carbohydrate can promote a brain response. Regular tasting or intake of carbohydrate during the event enhances brain activity leading to better performance.
Disturbance of muscle acid-base balance	High rates of H+ production via anaerobic glycolytic power system.	Prolonged high-intensity activities lasting 1–8 min (e.g. rowing events, middle distance running, 200–800 m swimming, track cycling team pursuit). May also occur in events with repeated sustained periods of high-intensity activity—perhaps in some team games, racquet sports. **Risk in para-sports:** Athletes with an impairment compete in many events listed above.	An increase in extracellular (plasma) buffering capacity can be achieved via acute loading with sodium bicarbonate (300 mg/kg), 90–120 min prior to an event. Increase in the stores of intracellular buffer carnosine can be achieved by chronic (6–14 weeks) supplementation with β-alanine.

(Continued)

TABLE 3.6 (CONTINUED)
Factors Related to Nutrition That Could Produce Fatigue or Suboptimal Performance during Sports Competition

Factor	Description	Examples of High-Risk/Common Occurrence in Sports	Nutritional Strategies to Address Issue
Depletion of phosphocreatine stores	Inadequate recovery of phosphocreatine system of power production leading to gradual decline in power output in subsequent efforts.	Occurs in events with repeated efforts of high-intensity activity with short recovery internals—perhaps in some team games, racquet sports. **Risk in para-sports:** May be a factor in wheelchair basketball, tennis and rugby.	Creatine supplementation (loading with 5 days @ 20–30 g/day and maintenance with 3–5 g/day) can increase muscle phosphocreatine content and enhance recovery from repeated high-intensity sprints.
Gastrointestinal disturbances	GI disturbances including vomiting and diarrhea may directly reduce performance as well as interfere with nutritional strategies aimed at managing fluid and fuel status.	Poorly chosen intake of food and fluid before and/or during event. Risks include consuming a large amount of fat or fibre in pre-event meal, consuming excessive amounts of single carbohydrates during the event, or becoming significantly dehydrated. **Risk in para-sports:** Many athletes with an impairment have predisposing gut problems which are exacerbated by exercise. Tight positioning in wheelchairs can also increase the risk of gastrointestinal disturbance.	The athlete should seek expert advice to identify the foods or eating practices which cause gut disturbances. Intake of food and fluids before and during events should be chosen, based on practice, to minimise these disturbances.
Salt depletion	Inadequate replacement of sodium lost in sweat. There is anecdotal evidence that salt depletion may increase the risk of a specific type of whole-body muscle cramp.	Salty sweaters—individuals with high sweat rates and high sweat sodium concentrations who may acutely or chronically deplete exchangeable sodium pools. **Risk in para-sports:** Athletes with cystic fibrosis.	This is a controversial area. While most cramps are caused by local muscle fatigue, there is anecdotal evidence that a subset of cramps occurs in salty sweaters and is reduced by appropriate salt replacement during and after exercise.

| Water intoxication/hyponatremia (low blood sodium) | Excessive intake of fluids can lead to hyponatremia ranging from mild (often asymptomatic) to severe (can be fatal). While this problem is more of a medical concern than a cause of fatigue, symptoms can include headache and disorientation, which can be mistaken as signs of dehydration. | Athletes with low sweat losses (e.g. low-intensity exercise in cool weather) who overzealously consume fluid before and during the event. This has most often been seen during marathons, ultra-endurance sports and hiking. **Risk in para-sports:** Spinal cord athletes may have low sweat losses yet perceive the need to drink due to heat load. Some intellectually impaired athletes may lack the understanding required to manage fluid intake effectively. | Practice in training will identify a fluid plan that does not allow the athlete to drink excessively during their event. |

Source: Adapted from Burke, L.M., in *Sport and Exercise Nutrition*, ed. S.A. Lanham-New et al., London: Wiley-Blackwell, 2011, pp. 200–209.

The range of competition strategies available to athletes to combat such fatigue factors includes practices of fluid and food intake before, during and in the interval between events, as well as the acute or chronic use of supplements with ergogenic effects such as caffeine, creatine and the buffering agents (i.e. extracellular buffering with bicarbonate supplementation, intracellular cellular buffering via beta-alanine supplementation). The role of ergogenic aids is covered in other areas of this text (see Chapter 11) and in other resources (Burke et al. 2010). Meanwhile, many of the following dietary strategies which form the basis of competition eating should also be integrated into some training sessions. This will allow the athlete to experiment with, and fine-tune, a personalized competition plan, including learning the habits or developing the gastrointestinal tolerance needed to carry it out successfully. These strategies may also help to support training sessions and allow the athlete to train well.

3.3.2 Precompetition Fuelling

An important goal of pre-competition eating is to store sufficient muscle glycogen to meet the anticipated fuel needs of the event. Training typically enhances the muscle's capacity for glycogen storage such that the elevated "resting" values seen in endurance athletes are generally sufficient to meet the needs of events of <90 min duration (Hawley et al. 1997). Unless there is muscle damage, the athlete should be able to achieve such levels with as little as a day of a carbohydrate-rich diet in combination with rest or light training (Bussau et al. 2002). The amount of dietary carbohydrate needed to restore glycogen will vary according to the level of depletion, but somewhere in the range of 5–10 g/kg of the athlete's body mass will generally be sufficient to normalise muscle glycogen content (Burke et al. 2011).

The fuel demands of some events, such as an ultra-endurance Ironman triathlon, are greater than the muscle's normal glycogen stores. Muscle glycogen depletion, causing a fatigue commonly known as "hitting the wall," can occur during events of greater than ~90 min duration, of both continuous or intermittent high-intensity nature. In such events, athletes should try to "carbohydrate load" or supercompensate glycogen stores prior to competition. Although the first protocols involved a week to implement via separate phases of glycogen depletion then supercompensation (Bergstrom et al. 1967), more recent work has shown that a well-trained athlete can achieve the same outcomes simply by combining as little as 24–36 h of high-carbohydrate intake and rest/exercise taper (Bussau et al. 2002). Therefore the modern version of carbohydrate loading is a practical option for a large range of athletes who compete in fuel-demanding events. While some athletes may simply have to taper their training volume to allow glycogen to store, others may need to increase their intake of carbohydrate-rich foods and drinks above habitual levels to achieve the targets provided in Table 3.3. In addition, some athletes like to combine carbohydrate loading with a low-residue/low-fibre dietary plan that reduces gastrointestinal contents over the day(s) before competition (Burke 2011). This provides the advantage of reducing body mass by 0.5–2 kg (providing a small but useful advantage in sports where the athlete carries their own body mass over distances) or removing the likelihood for a bowel movement on the day of the event (sometimes impractical in the field of play).

A practical consideration in competition preparation is the effect and the environment of the competition taper. In many sports, the achievement of a competition peak is preceded by a distinct training taper in which the volume of training is dramatically reduced for a period of 1–3 weeks. This reduces the athlete's energy expenditure, but ironically, also increases their amount of leisure time, which encourages "boredom eating." Energy intake can also be mismatched during this period because of the food environment frequently encountered in the competition phase. Athletes who travel away from home and dietary supervision are frequently exposed to "all you can eat" catering in athlete villages or hotels. Unless the athlete is sufficiently knowledgeable and committed, it can be easy to overeat. On the other hand, many athletes find themselves in a location or with a catering plan that fails to provide them with their usual or important foods and drinks, or without access to snacks between meals. This may interfere with their ability to consume sufficient energy and nutrients, or to cater to their special competition or recovery eating plans. Athletes should think ahead to bring their special food needs on their travels (customs regulations allowing) and to adapt their eating habits to their real needs rather than opportunities to eat.

3.3.3 The Pre-Event Meal

Foods and drinks consumed in the 4 h before an event have a role in fine-tuning competition preparation in meeting the following goals (Burke 2011):

- To enhance muscle glycogen stores if they have not been fully restored or loaded since the last exercise session. This is often an issue in sports where the athlete competes in heats and finals, or several matches in a tournament.
- If events are undertaken in the morning, to restore liver glycogen stores (important for maintaining blood glucose concentrations) after an overnight fast.
- To ensure that the athlete is well hydrated, especially where a fluid deficit is likely to occur during the event and/or the athlete may be dehydrated from a hot environment or previous exercise.
- To achieve gut comfort throughout the event, not letting the athlete become hungry or suffer gastrointestinal distress or upset.
- To include foods and eating practices that are important to the athlete's psychology or superstition.

There is no single routine that will suit the array of events, environments, timetables and food options in which competition is undertaken or the individual preferences of each athlete. Instead, each athlete should develop a personalised eating plan, guided by their specific circumstances, personal preferences and past experiences. Some general principles include the consumption of substantial amounts of carbohydrate-rich foods or drinks prior to endurance events (Sherman et al. 1989), and the avoidance of large amounts of fibre or fat by athletes who are at risk of gut problems. Pre-event hydration should involve drinking a comfortable amount of fluid sufficiently ahead of the event so that there is time for the urination of excess fluids. Athletes who suffer from pre-event nerves or undertake events scheduled in the early morning, where it is difficult to eat a substantial amount of food beforehand, often find it useful to choose a liquid version of the pre-event meal such as specially formulated liquid meal replacement products or milk/fruit smoothies. For some athletes, such as wheelchair racers who fit very compactly into their chairs, it is physically difficult to consume a large volume of food/fluid within 2–3 h of an event, hence very compact but easily digestible forms of fuel (such as gels) may be most useful.

Special attention has been focussed on the possible disadvantages of consuming carbohydrate in the hours prior to exercise. Although pre-event intake of carbohydrate can enhance body carbohydrate stores, it also increases the rate at which carbohydrate is utilised as a fuel during subsequent exercise due to alterations in prevailing hormone (i.e. insulin) concentrations (Coyle et al. 1985). Early sports nutrition guidelines warned against the intake of carbohydrate in the hour before exercise in case the increased rates of carbohydrate utilisation impaired performance via a rebound hypoglycaemia or an earlier depletion of muscle glycogen stores (Foster et al. 1979). This may be the case for some individual athletes, especially in situations where the amount of carbohydrate consumed pre-event is small and unable to counter the increase in exercise carbohydrate use (Kuipers et al. 1999). However, in the majority of cases, the risk of a detrimental effect on performance is low, and in fact, performance is unaltered or enhanced by the additional carbohydrate availability (Jeukendrup and Killer 2010).

Several options are possible to minimize the potential problems associated with pre-exercise carbohydrate intake: these include consuming adequate carbohydrate (>1 g/kg BM) to offset the increased reliance on carbohydrate fuel use and choosing carbohydrate-rich sources that are low in glycaemic index (GI) (Burke 2011). Indeed, low-GI carbohydrate-rich foods have been promoted as a superior choice for the pre-event meal, offering a source of sustained release carbohydrate with less perturbation to the hormonal environment (Thomas et al. 1991). This may provide a benefit for particular scenarios or individuals but outcomes of superior endurance compared with the intake of high-GI carbohydrate choices (Thomas et al. 1991) have not been found to be universal (Burke 2010b). Of course, the most effective strategy to maintain carbohydrate availability during the event is to continue to consume it throughout exercise; this offers a number of benefits to the muscle and central nervous system that will be subsequently discussed.

3.3.4 FLUID INTAKE DURING EXERCISE

In events lasting longer than ~45 min there may be opportunities and advantages to consuming fuel and fluids during the session. Sweat is lost during exercise as a means to dissipate the heat generated by muscular work or absorbed from the environment, and when it can be evaporated it provides an effective strategy to maintain body temperature within its homeostatic range. As the resulting fluid deficit increases, however, it gradually increases the stress associated with exercise. Typically, it is noted that when dehydration increases above 2% BM, there is an increasing effect on work rates and skills during prolonged exercise (ACSM et al. 2007). Critics of this view argue that it is almost entirely based on laboratory studies which can't incorporate the cooling effects of wind and air resistance (Dugas et al. 2009) or the motivating effects of the competition atmosphere. As such, the presently available studies might overestimate the true effect of dehydration on performance in real-life conditions. But a counter-argument is that the statistical interpretation of most studies is weighted against finding small but potentially important effects of dehydration on performance. Combining probability statistics with small sample sizes generally means that sports research is only capable of detecting substantial reductions or differences in performance (Hopkins et al. 1999). Such analyses may fail to recognise performance changes that would affect the outcomes of real-life sport, where events are decided by milliseconds and millimetres. Indeed, in studies where the same exercise is undertaken in a hot environment with incrementally increasing fluid deficits from 0 to 4% body mass, there is a parallel increase in thermoregulatory strain, cardiovascular drift and perception of effort (Montain and Coyle 1992). Intuitively, a similar subtle decrease in performance and/or increase in the effort required to perform is also happening, but we find it hard to draw the line in the sand where we consider it important. Indeed, the point at which this becomes noticeable or significant will depend on the individual, the environment (effects are greater in the heat or at altitude) and perhaps the focus of the exercise (recreational exercisers may stop exercising if it becomes uncomfortable; elite athletes may be prepared to tolerate greater discomfort but equally, may have a greater incentive to perform well given the small margins between winning and losing).

In general, it is suggested that athletes develop a personalised hydration plan that utilises the opportunities that are specific to their event to keep the fluid deficit below 2% of body mass in stressful environments, or where this is not possible, to replace as much of their sweat loss as is practical. Table 3.7 summarises the main issues with fluid intake across a range of types of sports. Depending on the event, there may be opportunities to drink during breaks in play (i.e. half time, substitutions or time-outs in team games) or during the exercise itself (from aid stations, handlers or self-carried supplies). As discussed in Section 3.2.7, athletes can get a feel for their typical sweat losses during an event by conducting periodic checks of hydration during training sessions or events as is practical.

Fluid mismatches during competitive events mostly err on the side of a fluid deficit which the athlete may then judge as being tolerable or needing to be addressed within the logistics of their sport and the availability of fluids (Garth and Burke, 2013). However, it is possible for some athletes to overhydrate if they drink excessively during events in which sweat rates are low. Risk factors for this situation include being female, being small, exercising at low intensities (Almond et al. 2005) and having a spinal cord injury (see Chapter 4). This situation is generally unnecessary and may even be dangerous if it leads to the potentially fatal condition of hyponatremia (low blood sodium concentration; often known as water intoxication) (Hew-Butler et al. 2008). Good drink choices will depend on the sport and on other nutritional goals that might be important. First, a fluid needs to be palatable and available to encourage intake. However other characteristics include temperature (Burdon et al. 2010, 2012), which can be manipulated both to enhance palatability in the specific environment and to contribute to body temperature regulation (cold fluids and ice slurries can reduce core temperature in hot conditions while warm fluids may increase body temperature losses in cold environments). Second, there is the opportunity for a drink to contain other nutrients that might enhance performance,

TABLE 3.7
Summary of Key Issues Involved in Developing Individual Hydration and Fuelling Plans for Various Types of Sporting Activities

Type of Sports	Key Issues to Consider in Devising Specific Plan for Competition Fluid/Fuel Replacement
Continuous endurance events (e.g. distance running, road cycling, triathlon)	• Fluids and foods must be consumed during the race while athlete is "on the move" • Access to supplies is enhanced in events where drinks are provided by aid stations or handlers • Access to drinks/foods is reduced in events where athlete must carry their own supplies • Opportunity to drink/eat is limited by consideration of the time lost in obtaining and consuming fluid • Opportunity to drink/eat is limited by gastrointestinal discomfort associated with drinking while exercising • Ability to consume fluid/foods during races may be enhanced by practising during training to develop gastrointestinal tolerance and the skills that allow drinking on the move • Creative devices such as fluid backpacks and spill-proof bottles may enhance access to fluid and the ease of drinking on the move **Special issues regarding para-sports:** It is less easy to obtain and consume drinks in wheelchair or arm-cranked activities since the arms are needed for propulsion. Cerebral palsy and some other disabilities may reduce fine motor control, increasing the likelihood of spillage/difficulty opening vessels.
Team and racquet sports (rugby, tennis, basketball)	• Fluids/foods can be consumed during breaks in game or pauses in play that are specific to the sport (e.g., time-outs, change of ends, half-time, substitutions) • Opportunities to drink/eat are increased in sports in which there are a number of formal and informal breaks, and where there is free player rotation • Access to fluid is increased by having a team drink supply close to the field of play and, where rules permit, having trainers take drinks to players • Access to fluid is reduced in sports in which rules prevent carriage of fluid onto field of play • In some team sports there is a culture that dehydration during training can "toughen" players • Individual drink bottles may enhance hydration practices by increasing awareness of total fluid intake **Special issues regarding para-sports:** In spinal cord injuries, the heat load induced by the inability to sweat effectively can drive a greater fluid intake than needed.

(Continued)

TABLE 3.7 (CONTINUED)

Summary of Key Issues Involved in Developing Individual Hydration and Fuelling Plans for Various Types of Sporting Activities

Type of Sports	Key Issues to Consider in Devising Specific Plan for Competition Fluid/Fuel Replacement
Sprint, strength and power events—brief high-intensity sports (e.g. track and field events, track cycling)	• No need or opportunity to hydrate/fuel during brief events, but athletes may need to rehydrate/refuel between events, especially in multiple-event competition. **Special issues regarding para-sports:** Gastrointestinal comfort may be impacted by body positioning (for example, wheelchair athletes) which influences pre event/training food and fluid intake.
Weight-making sports (judo, boxing, martial arts, powerlifting)	• Education is needed to minimise reliance on dehydration to make weight for competition • Weight-making practices may also involve poor fuelling in the days leading into the event • Depending on the rules of the competition, the recovery period between weigh-in and competition varies from an hour to a day; aggressive refuelling and rehydration may be needed, but caution may be needed to reduce risk of gut upsets during the event **Special issues regarding para-sports:** The nature of some disabilities can make it more difficult to use traditional techniques (such as dehydration) to reduce body mass acutely, meaning a smaller margin between training and competition weight is necessary.
Skill sports (shooting, archery, boccia)	• Access to fluid is reduced when sessions are undertaken in remote environment
Aquatic sports (swimming)	• Fluid needs are likely to be lower than equivalent land-based sports activities due to opportunity to dissipate heat through convection/conduction in water rather than sweating • Drink bottles on pool deck are suitable
Winter sports (alpine and Nordic skiing, snowboarding)	• Access to fluid and food is reduced when session is undertaken in remote environment or subzero temperatures (food and drinks freeze) Fluid needs (sweat losses) altered by cold environment or altitude • Voluntary fluid intake may be enhanced by provision of warm fluids **Special issues regarding para-sports:** In addition to reduced access to food and fluid, the impracticality of removing tight ski suits and more limited mobility also mean reduced access to bathroom facilities, increasing the likelihood of limiting fluid and food intake before and during training/competition.

Source: Adapted from Burke, L.M., in *Sport and Exercise Nutrition*, ed. S.A. Lanham-New et al., London: Wiley-Blackwell, 2011, pp. 200–209.

such as carbohydrate (Jeukendrup 2010; Jeukendrup and Chambers 2010) or caffeine (Burke 2008). Sports drinks which are formulated to meet a range of needs provide carbohydrate and electrolytes, with the latter encouraging fluid intake by maintaining thirst.

3.3.5 FUEL INTAKE DURING COMPETITION

The muscle and central nervous system can both benefit from the intake of carbohydrate during exercise (Karelis et al. 2010). A range of mechanisms is possible including providing a source of substrate to the muscle (Coyle et al. 1986) and enhancing the reward centres of the central nervous system (Chambers et al. 2009); these may occur singly or in combination according to the intensity and duration of the event and the athlete's nutritional preparation. Until recently, guidelines for the intake of carbohydrate during exercise stated that it would only be valuable during events longer than 1 h in duration and recommended an intake of 30–60 g/h, fine-tuned with individual experience (ACSM et al. 2007). Again, the specific characteristics of a sport such as the scheduling of breaks, competition rules, logistics and culture will determine the opportunities for consuming a sports drink or other carbohydrate-containing sources such as gels, bars or confectionery during the event (see Table 3.7). Some new research, however, has suggested ways in which fuelling guidelines need to be updated for shorter sustained-intensity events, and for longer or ultra-endurance sports.

In longer events such as Ironman triathlons or stage races in road cycling, it has been curious to observe that top athletes self-select carbohydrate intakes that are much higher than recommended by sports nutrition guidelines—often around 80–90 g/h (Kimber et al. 2002). This poses the question of who is wrong—the guidelines or the athletes? The answer has been answered in several ways. The first piece of information is emerging evidence of a dose-response relationship between carbohydrate intake and performance of sports lasting 3 or more hours—in other words, the greater the carbohydrate dose, the better the performance (up to a point, of course) (Smith et al. 2013). The limiting factor to the supply of exogenous carbohydrate to the muscle is the amount of carbohydrate that can be absorbed from the gut. However, this can be enhanced if the athlete consumes a blend of different types of carbohydrates that are transported across the intestine in different ways; the maximum absorption of glucose appears to be about 60 g/h, but if a blend of glucose and fructose is consumed, it can be increased to 90 g/h (Jeukendrup 2010). Thus the new guidelines continue to recommend intakes of 30–60 g/h in endurance events of 1–3 h, but for longer events, intake of up to 80–90 g/h are likely to contribute to the special fuel needs (Burke et al. 2011). It appears also that the gut can be "trained" to increase its absorption rates of carbohydrate by regularly training with carbohydrate intake (Cox et al. 2010).

The new insight into carbohydrate intake during events of intermittent or sustained high intensity lasting ~1 h is just as intriguing (Jeukendrup and Chambers 2010). In such events, muscle glycogen stores are adequate for fuel needs so theoretically there should be no advantage to consuming carbohydrate during the event. Yet a number of studies involving continuous cycling or running have recorded benefits from intake of carbohydrate just before and during exercise (Below et al. 1995; Jeukendrup et al. 1997), even if the carbohydrate is simply swilled around the mouth and spat out (Carter et al. 2004). The emerging theory is that there are receptors in the mouth that sense the presence of carbohydrate, allowing the brain to feel energised and pace at a higher level (Chambers et al. 2009). Thus new guidelines recommend that athletes in shorter events should also consider the benefits of consuming or tasting even a small amount of carbohydrate at regular intervals throughout the event (Burke et al. 2010).

3.3.6 RECOVERY BETWEEN EVENTS

In many sports, competition involves a series of events or matches before the final winner is decided, and the athlete will need to recover as quickly or as effectively as possible for the next round. The period between events may be less than an hour (e.g. races in a swimming program or track meet), 3–4 hours (e.g. singles and doubles matches on the same day of a tennis tournament) or 1–2 days (e.g. team sports in a tournament format). The principles of eating to promote rehydration, refuelling, repair, and adaptation, covered in the previous section on training nutrition, may be more challenging to achieve in the competition environment due to issues such as poor access to food supplies or interference from post-event activities such as drug testing, media commitments and performance debriefs. With good planning, however, the athlete should aim to recover as well as possible—or at least better than his or her competitors.

3.4 SUMMARY

Research over the past three decades has produced a large amount of information that can now be shaped at an individualised level to maximise adaptations to chronic exercise (i.e. training) and to optimise performance on a specific occasion (i.e. competition). The evolution of the science and practice of sports nutrition now allows athletes to develop specific eating practices for the demands of their sport to achieve a suitable physique, to reduce the risk of illness and injury, and to support the demands

---

COMMENTARY BOX 3.2

ATHLETE INSIGHT: The value of a sports nutrition practitioner.

Teaching me about nutrition and how to maximise my energy levels to allow me to do the training is an important part. Also to be the voice in my head and make me accountable to myself as well as being the voice that helps me make good choices against all the bad voices of my peers who can eat and drink whatever they want.

**—Michael Milton, five-time Winter Paralympian
and medallist, Summer Paralympic cyclist**

of training and recovery. In the competition arena, well-practiced nutrition strategies undertaken before, during and in the interval between events can contribute to personal best performances. Although the demands of para-sports may be unique, most of the principles of sports nutrition that have been developed from studies of able-bodied athletes also apply to these special populations. The remainder of this book will endeavour to further investigate the application of sports nutrition to the specialised needs of para-sports.

APPENDIX: SPECIAL COMMENTARY: WEIGHT CATEGORY SPORTS

At the Paralympic level, there are two weight category sports in which athletes with an impairment can compete: powerlifting (for those whose lower limbs are most affected by their impairment) and judo (for visually impaired athletes only). At a non-elite level, athletes with an impairment may be involved in a wider range of weight category sports.

Each weight category sport has different rules regarding weigh-in requirements, including the time of weigh-in prior to competition. In para-sports, there may also be different rules applied and these may be modified for smaller competitions. For example in powerlifting, where two lifters lift the same weight, their final ranking can be decided according to their actual body mass (i.e. the lighter of the two will be ranked higher). In smaller competitions where there are only one or two individuals per weight class, this ruling may be applied to rank all competitors regardless of their weight division. It is important for the practitioner to be aware of variations in rules in order to best support the athlete's body mass management.

Athletes in some weight category sports compete regularly throughout the competition season, sometimes on a weekly basis. Therefore they will be required to "make weight" repeatedly throughout this period of time. Other weight category sports only compete three or four times over a year due to more limited opportunities for competition. The key to consistent success in weight category sports is achieving a sustainable weight early in the pre-competition period, then minimising weight fluctuations throughout the competition period. There is a competitive advantage to training above competition weight (rather than *at* competition weight) in most weight category sports, since this allows for a taller and more muscular physique which can provide greater strength, power, and leverage. By the same token, the closer an athlete is to their competition weight through the training period, the easier it will be to both make weight and effectively control body mass over a competitive season, minimising both the physical and psychological stress of making weight. The practitioner must work with the athlete and coach to determine what this training weight should be, and how best to achieve it. The principles of body mass control in athletes with an impairment in weight category sports are no different to those for able-bodied athletes, however the means to achieve acute weight loss may be less effective or have greater impact on the health and performance of these athletes, and so require extra care. The key principles, strategies and recommendations are summarised in Table 3.8.

TABLE 3.8
Body Composition Control in Weight Category Sports

Outcome	Suggested Strategies	Considerations for Athletes with an Impairment
Setting a realistic weight category	• Assess body composition (DXA, surface anthropometry) in a hydrated state at start of training phase • Set lowest possible weight category based on minimum % body fat of 5% (males) or 12% (females) • Allow for maximal weight loss of 0.5 kg/week over training phase	Accurate assessment of body composition via surface anthropometry may not be possible DXA scans may not be easy to repeat frequently, and hence may be best used in combination with another method Higher body fat levels may be necessary for SCI athletes to prevent pressure wounds Smaller weight loss targets may be necessary Consider impact of weight change on prostheses fitting It may be better to set a higher weight category than what might be considered achievable
Set preferred training weight	• Training weight (hydrated) should be no more than 5% above competition weight • Goal is to achieve this in pre-competition phase, then maintain throughout competition season • Checks for hydration status can be useful to reinforce the importance of adequate hydration on health and performance	If safe acute weight loss strategies are limited, training weight should be closer to competition weight
Advise athlete regarding strategies to achieve chronic body mass loss progressively	• Energy restriction (~2000–4000 kJ/day or 500–1000 kcal/day) • Avoid low energy availability • Optimise fuel for training • Adequate protein and even distribution over the day with timing post-exercise prioritised	The degree of energy deficit should be proportional to current energy requirements, which may be lower (for example in spinal cord injured)

(Continued)

TABLE 3.8 (CONTINUED)
Body Composition Control in Weight Category Sports

Outcome	Suggested Strategies	Considerations for Athletes with an Impairment
Use safe acute weight-making strategies that can be recovered from in time to compete (ensure these are trialled in training)	• Small energy deficit (if not already in place) • 2–3 days low fibre/residue diet • Salt restriction if habitually consume a high-sodium diet • 24 h fluid restriction and/or sweat loss without fluid replacement (sauna, hot bath, light exercise)	Athletes who have very controlled bowel management programs will be more resistant to using a low-fibre/residue diet Sweat loss capability may be limited in some athletes Dehydration can increase the risk of urinary tract infections, which some athletes are more prone to
Recover between weigh-in and competition "bout"	• Rehydrate with fluid including electrolytes (150% of weight lost through fluid restriction) • Carbohydrate to restore blood glucose and liver glycogen	Rapid rehydration requires good access to bathroom facilities and must be trialled in training period
Prevent weight rebound post-competition	• Manage alcohol intake • Control food volume and type	

Some excellent resources are available to guide sports nutrition practitioners working with weight category sports, including:

O'Connor, H., and Slater, G. 2011. Losing, gaining and making weight for athletes. In *Sport and exercise nutrition*, ed. S.A. Lanham-New, S.J. Stear, S.M. Shirreffs, and A.L. Collins, 210–232. West Sussex, UK: Wiley-Blackwell.
Walberg Rankin, J. 2010. Making weight in sports. In *Clinical sports nutrition*, ed. L. Burke and V. Deakin, 149–168. 4th ed. Sydney: McGraw-Hill.

RECOMMENDED READINGS

Burke, L.M., and Cox, G. 2010. *The complete guide to food for sports performance*. Sydney: Allen & Unwin.
Burke, L.M., and Deakin, V. 2010. *Clinical sports nutrition*. 4th ed. Sydney: McGraw Hill.
Lanham-New, S.A., Stear, S.J., Shirreffs, S.M., and Collins, A.L. 2011. *Sport and exercise nutrition*. London: Wiley-Blackwell.
Maughan, R.J., and Burke, L.M. 2011. *Sports nutrition: more than just calories—triggers for adaptation*. Nestle Nutrition Institute Workshop Series, vol. 69. Basel: S. Karger AG.

SCIENTIFIC PAPERS PRESENTED AT THE IOC CONSENSUS CONFERENCE ON NUTRITION FOR SPORT HELD AT THE IOC OFFICES IN LAUSANNE IN OCTOBER 2010

Loucks, A.B., Kiens, B., and Wright, H.H. 2011. Energy availability in athletes. *Journal of Sports Sciences* 29(S1):S7–S15.

Burke, L.M., Hawley, J.A., Wong, S.H., and Jeukendrup, A.E. 2011. Carbohydrates for training and competition. *Journal of Sports Sciences* 29(S1):S17–S27.

Phillips, S.M., and van Loon, L.J.C. 2011. Dietary protein for athletes: from requirements to optimum adaptation. *Journal of Sports Sciences* 29(S1):S29–S38.

Shirreffs, S.M., and Sawka, M.N. 2011. Fluid and electrolyte needs for training, competition and recovery. *Journal of Sports Sciences* 29(S1):S39–S46.

Powers, S., Nelson, W.B., and Larson-Meyer, E. 2011. Antioxidant and vitamin D supplements for athletes: sense or nonsense? *Journal of Sports Sciences* 29(S1):S47–S55.

Maughan, R.J., Greenhaff, P.L., and P. Hespel. 2011. Dietary supplements for athletes: emerging trends and recurring themes. *Journal of Sports Sciences* 29(S1):S57–S66.

Slater, G., and Phillips, S.M. 2011. Strength sports: weightlifting, throwing events, body building, sprints. *Journal of Sports Sciences* 29(S1):S67–S77.

Stellingwerff, T., Maughan, R.J., and Burke, L.M. 2011. Nutrition for power sports: middle-distance running, track cycling, rowing, canoeing/kayaking, and swimming. *Journal of Sports Sciences* 29(S1):S79–S89.

Jeukendrup, A.E. 2011. Endurance sports: marathon, triathlon, road cycling. *Journal of Sports Sciences* 29(S1):S91–S99.

Sundgot-Borgen, J., and Garthe, I. 2011. Elite athletes in aesthetic and Olympic weight-class sports and the challenge of weight and body composition. *Journal of Sports Sciences* 29(S1):S101–S114.

Holway, F., and Spriet, L.L. 2011. Practical strategies for team sports. *Journal of Sports Sciences* 29(S1):S115–S125.

Meyer, N.L., Manore, M., and Helle, C. 2011. Winter sports. *Journal of Sports Sciences* 29(S1):S127–S136.

REFERENCES

Achten, J., Halson, S.L., Moseley, L., Rayson, M.P., Casey, A., and Jeukendrup, A.E. 2004. Higher dietary carbohydrate content during intensified running training results in better maintenance of performance and mood state. *Journal of Applied Physiology* 96:1331–1140.

Ainsworth, B.E., Haskell, W.L., Whitt, M.C., et al. 2000. Compendium of physical activities: an update of activity codes and MET intensities. *Medicine and Science in Sports and Exercise* 32(Suppl 9):S498–504.

Almond, C.S., Shin, A.Y., Fortescue, E.B., et al. 2005. Hyponatremia among runners in the Boston marathon. *New England Journal of Medicine* 352:1550–1556.

American College of Sports Medicine (ACSM), Sawka, M.N., Burke, L.M., et al. 2007. American College of Sports Medicine position stand. Exercise and fluid replacement. *Medicine and Science in Sports and Exercise* 39:377–390.

Below, P.R., Mora-Rodriguez, R., Gonzalez-Alonso, J., and Coyle, E.F. 1995. Fluid and carbohydrate ingestion independently improve performance during 1 h of intense exercise. *Medicine and Science in Sports and Exercise* 27:200–210.

Bergstrom, J., Hermansen, L., Hultman, E., and Saltin, B. 1967. Diet, muscle glycogen and physical performance. *Acta Physiologica Scandinavica* 71:140–150.

Betts, J.A., and Williams, C. 2010. Short-term recovery from prolonged exercise: exploring the potential for protein ingestion to accentuate the benefits of carbohydrate supplements. *Sports Medicine* 40:941–959.

Bishop, N.C., Walker, G.J., Gleeson, M., Wallace, F.A., and Hewitt, C.R. 2009. Human T lymphocyte migration towards the supernatants of human rhinovirus infected airway epithelial cells: influence of exercise and carbohydrate intake. *Exercise Immunology Review* 15:127–144.

Braun, W.A., and Von Duvillard, S.P. 2004. Influence of carbohydrate delivery on the immune response during exercise and recovery from exercise. *Nutrition* 20:645–650.

Burd, N.A., West, D.W., Moore, D.R., et al. 2011. Enhanced amino acid sensitivity of myofibrillar protein synthesis persists for up to 24 h after resistance exercise in young men. *Journal of Nutrition* 141:568–573.

Burdon, C.A., Johnson, N.A., Chapman, P.G., and O'Connor, H.T. 2012. Influence of beverage temperature on palatability and fluid ingestion during endurance exercise: a systematic review. *International Journal of Sport Nutrition and Exercise Metabolism* 22:199–211.

Burdon, C.A., O'Connor, H.T., Gifford, J.A., and Shirreffs, S.M. 2010. Influence of beverage temperature on exercise performance in the heat: a systematic review. *International Journal of Sport Nutrition and Exercise Metabolism* 20:166–174.

Burke, L.M. 2010a. Fueling strategies to optimize performance: training high or training low? *Scandinavian Journal of Medicine and Science in Sports* 20(Suppl 2):11–21.

Burke, L. 2010b. Preparation for competition. In *Clinical sports nutrition*, ed. L. Burke and V. Deakin, 304–327. 4th ed. Sydney: McGraw-Hill.

Burke, L., Cort, M., Cox, G., et al. 2010. Supplements and sports foods. In *Clinical sports nutrition*, ed. L. Burke and V. Deakin, 419–500. 4th ed. Sydney: McGraw-Hill.

Burke, L.M. 2008. Caffeine and sports performance. *Applied Physiology Nutrition and Metabolism* 33:1319–1334.

Burke, L.M. 2011. Competition nutrition. In *Sport and exercise nutrition*, ed. S.A. Lanham-New, S.J. Stear, S.M. Shirreffs, and A.L. Collins, 200–209. London: Wiley-Blackwell.

Burke, L.M., Hawley, J.A., Wong, S.H., and Jeukendrup, A.E. 2011. Carbohydrates for training and competition. *Journal of Sports Sciences* 29(Suppl 1):S17–S27.

Bussau, V.A., Fairchild, T.J., Rao, A., Steele, P.D., and Fournier, P.A. 2002. Carbohydrate loading in human muscle: an improved 1 day protocol. *European Journal of Applied Physiology* 87:290–95.

Cannell, J.J., Hollis, B.W., Sorenson, M.B., Taft, T.N., and Anderson, J.J.B. 2009. Athletic performance and vitamin D. *Medicine and Science in Sports and Exercise* 41:1102–1110.

Carter, J.M., Jeukendrup, A.E., and Jones, D.A. 2004. The effect of carbohydrate mouth rinse on 1-h cycle time trial performance. *Medicine and Science in Sports and Exercise* 36:2107–2111.

Castell, L. 2003. Glutamine supplementation in vitro and in vivo, in exercise and in immunodepression. *Sports Medicine* 33:323–345.

Chambers, E.S., Bridge, M.W., and Jones, D.A. 2009. Carbohydrate sensing in the human mouth: effects on exercise performance and brain activity. *Journal of Physiology* 587:1779–1794.

Clancy, R.L., Gleeson, M., Cox, A., et al. 2006. Reversal in fatigued athletes of a defect in interferon gamma secretion after administration of *Lactobacillus acidophilus*. *British Journal of Sports Medicine* 40:351–354.

Close, G.L., Ashton, T., Cable, T., et al. 2006. Ascorbic acid supplementation does not attenuate post-exercise muscle soreness following muscle-damaging exercise but may delay the recovery process. *British Journal of Nutrition* 95:976–981.

Cox, A.J., Pyne, D.B., Saunders, P.U., and Fricker, P.A. 2008. Oral administration of the pro-biotic *Lactobaccillus fermentum* VRI-003 and mucosal immunity in endurance athletes. *British Journal of Sports Medicine* 44:222–226.

Cox, G.R., Clark, S.A., Cox, A.J., et al. 2010. Daily training with high carbohydrate avail-ability increases exogenous carbohydrate oxidation during endurance cycling. *Journal of Applied Physiology* 109:126–34.

Coyle, E.F. 1991. Timing and method of increased carbohydrate intake to cope with heavy training, competition and recovery. *Journal of Sports Sciences* 9(Suppl):29–51.

Coyle, E.F., Coggan, A.R., Hemmert, M.K., and Ivy, J.L. 1986. Muscle glycogen utilisa-tion during prolonged strenuous exercise when fed carbohydrate. *Journal of Applied Physiology* 61:165–172.

Coyle, E.F., Coggan, A.R., Hemmert, M.K., Lowe, R.C., and Walters, T.J. 1985. Substrate usage during prolonged exercise following a preexercise meal. *Journal of Applied Physiology* 59:429–433.

Cunningham, J.J. 1980. A reanalysis of the factors influencing basal metabolic rate in normal adults. *American Journal of Clinical Nutrition* 33:2372–2374.

Davis, J.M., Murphy, E.A., and Charmichael, M.D. 2009. Effects of the dietary flavonoid quercetin upon performance and health. *Current Sports Medicine Reports* 8:206–213.

Davison, G., and Simpson, R.J. 2011. Immunity. In *Sport and exercise nutrition*, ed. S.A. Lanham-New, S.J. Stear, S.M. Shirreffs, and A.L. Collins, 281–303. Oxford: Wiley-Blackwell.

Deakin, V. 2010. Measuring nutritional status of athletes: clinical and research perspectives. In *Clinical sports nutrition*, ed. L. Burke and V. Deakin, 19–43. 4th ed. Sydney: McGraw-Hill.

Dugas, J.P., Oosthuizen, U., Tucker, R., and Noakes, T.D. 2009. Rates of fluid ingestion alter pacing but not thermoregulatory responses during prolonged exercise in hot and humid conditions with appropriate convective cooling. *European Journal of Applied Physiology* 105:69–80.

Fischer, C.P., Hiscock, N.J., Penkowa, M., et al. 2004. Supplementation with vitamins C and E inhibits the release of interleukin-6 from contracting human skeletal muscle. *Journal of Physiology* 558 (Pt 2):633–645.

Foster, C., Costill, D.L., and Fink, W.J. 1979. Effects of preexercise feedings on endurance performance. *Medicine and Science in Sports and Exercise* 11:1–5.

Garth, A.K., and Burke, L.M. 2013. What do athletes drink during competitive sporting activi-ties? *Sports Medicine*, 47:539-564.

Gleeson, M., Nieman, D.C., and Pedersen, B.K. 2004. Exercise, nutrition and immune func-tion. *Journal of Sports Sciences* 22:115–125.

Hansen, A.K., Fischer, C.P., Plomgaard, P., Andersen, J.L., Saltin, B., and Pedersen, B.K. 2005. Skeletal muscle adaptation: training twice every second day vs. training once daily. *Journal of Applied Physiology* 98:93–99.

Harris, J.A., and Benedict, F.G. 1919. *A biometric study of basal metabolism in man.* Carnegie Institute Washington Publication 279. Philadelphia: FB Lippincott Co.

Hawley, J.A., Schabort, E.J., Noakes, T.D., and Dennis, S.C. 1997. Carbohydrate-loading and exercise performance: an update. *Sports Medicine* 24:73–81.

Hemila, H., and Chalker, E. 2013. Vitamin C for preventing and treating the common cold. *Cochrane Database Systematic Reviews*, doi: 10.1002/14651858.CD000980.pub4.

Hew-Butler, T., Ayus, J.C., Kipps, C., et al. 2008. Statement of the Second International Exercise-Associated Hyponatremia Consensus Development Conference, New Zealand, 2007. *Clinical Journal of Sport Medicine* 18:111–121.

Hiscock, N., and Pedersen, B.K. 2002. Exercise-induced immunodepression—plasma gluta-mine is not the link. *Journal of Applied Physiology* 93:813–822.

Hopkins, W.G., Hawley, J.A., and Burke, L.M. 1999. Design and analysis of research on sport performance enhancement. *Medicine and Science in Sports and Exercise* 31:472–485.

Jeukendrup, A.E. 2010. Carbohydrate and exercise performance: the role of multiple transportable carbohydrates. *Current Opinion in Clinical Nutrition and Metabolic Care* 13:452–457.

Jeukendrup, A., Brouns, F., Wagenmakers, A.J.M., and Saris, W.H.M. 1997. Carbohydrate-electrolyte feedings improve 1 h time trial cycling performance. *International Journal of Sports Medicine* 18:125–129.

Jeukendrup, A.E., and Chambers, E.S. 2010. Oral carbohydrate sensing and exercise performance. *Current Opinion in Clinical Nutrition and Metabolic Care* 13:447–451.

Jeukendrup, A.E., and Killer, S.C. 2010. The myths surrounding pre-exercise carbohydrate feeding. *Annals of Nutrition and Metabolism* 57(Suppl 2):18–25.

Karelis, A.D., Smith, J.W., Passe, D.H., and Péronnet, F. 2010. Carbohydrate administration and exercise performance: what are the potential mechanisms involved? *Sports Medicine* 40:747–763.

Kimber, N.E., Ross, J.J., Mason, S.L., and Speedy, D.B. 2002. Energy balance during an Ironman triathlon in male and female triathletes. *International Journal of Sport Nutrition and Exercise Metabolism* 12:47–62.

Kopp-Woodroffe, S.A., Manore, M.M., Dueck, C.A., Skinner, J.S, and Matt, K.S. 1999. Energy and nutrient status of amenorrheic athletes participating in a diet and exercise training intervention program. *International Journal of Sport Nutrition and Exercise Metabolism* 9:70–88.

Kuipers, H., Fransen, E.J., and Keizer, H.A. 1999. Pre-exercise ingestion of carbohydrate and transient hypoglycemia during exercise. *International Journal of Sports Medicine* 20:227–231.

Loucks, A. 2010. The evolution of the female athlete triad. In *Clinical sports nutrition*, ed. L. Burke and V. Deakin, 193–199. 4th ed. Sydney: McGraw-Hill.

Loucks, A.B. 2003. Energy availability, not body fatness, regulates reproductive function in women. *Exercise and Sports Science Reviews* 31:144–148.

Loucks, A.B., Kiens, B., and Wright, H.H. 2011. Energy availability in athletes. *Journal of Sports Sciences* 29(Suppl 1):S7–S15.

Manore, M.M., and Thompson, J.L. 2010. Energy requirements of the athlete: assessment and evidence of energy efficiency. In *Clinical sports nutrition*, ed. L. Burke and V. Deakin, 95–115. 4th ed. Sydney: McGraw-Hill.

Maughan, R.J., Leiper, J.B., and Shirreffs, S.M. 1997. Factors influencing the restoration of fluid and electrolyte balance after exercise in the heat. *British Journal of Sports Medicine* 31:175–182.

Maughan, R.J., and Shirreffs, S.M. 2008. Development of individual hydration strategies for athletes. *International Journal of Sports Nutrition and Exercise Metabolism* 18:457–472.

Melby, C.L., and Hill, J.O. 1999. Exercise, macronutrient balance, and body weight regulation. *Sports Science Exchange* 112:1–6.

Montain, S.J., and Coyle, E.F. 1992. Influence of graded dehydration on hyperthermia and cardiovascular drift during exercise. *Journal of Applied Physiology* 73:1340–1350.

Peters, E.M., Goetzsche, J.M., Grobbelaar, B., and Noakes, T.D. 1993. Vitamin C supplementation reduces the incidence of postrace symptoms of upper-respiratory-tract infection in ultramarathon runners. *American Journal of Clinical Nutrition* 57:170–174.

Philp, A., Burke, L.M., and Baar, K. 2011. Altering endogenous carbohydrate availability to support training adaptations. *Nestle Nutrition Institute Workshop Series* 69:19–37.

Powers, S., Nelson, W.B., and Larson-Meyer, E. 2011. Antioxidant and vitamin D supplements for athletes: sense or nonsense? *Journal of Sports Sciences* 29(S1):S47–S55.

Res, P.T., Groen, B., Pennings, B., et al. 2012. Protein ingestion before sleep improves postexercise overnight recovery. *Medicine and Science in Sports and Exercise* 44:1560–1569.

Ristow, M., Zarse, K., Oberbach, A., et al. 2009. Antioxidants prevent health-promoting effects of physical exercise in humans. *Proceedings of the National Academy of Science USA* 106:8665–8670.

Rogalski, B., Dawson, B., Heasman, J., and Gabbett, T.J. 2013. Training and game loads and injury risk in elite Australian footballers. *Journal of Science and Medicine in Sport* [epub ahead of print].

Ross, A.C. 2012. Vitamin A and retinoic acid in T-cell related immunity. *American Journal of Clinical Nutrition* 96:1166S–1172S.

Sanborn, C., Nichols, D.L., and DiMarco, N.M. 2011. In *Sport and exercise nutrition*, ed. S.A. Lanham-New, S.J. Stear, S.M. Shirreffs, and A.L. Collins, 244–263. Oxford: Wiley-Blackwell.

Scofield, K.L., and Hecht, S. 2012. Bone health in endurance athletes: runners, cyclists and swimmers. *Current Sports Medicine Reports* 11:328–334.

Shephard, R.J., and Aoyagi, Y. 2012. Measurement of human energy expenditure, with particular reference to field studies: an historical perspective. *European Journal of Applied Physiology* 112:2785–2815.

Sherman, W.M., Brodowicz, G., Wright, D.A., Allen, W.K., Simonsen, J., and Dernbach, A. 1989. Effects of 4 h preexercise carbohydrate feedings on cycling performance. *Medicine and Science in Sports and Exercise* 21:598–604.

Smith, J.W., Pascoe, D.D., Passe, D.H., et al. 2013. Curvilinear dose-response relationship of carbohydrate (0–120 g•h^{-1}) and performance. *Medicine and Science in Sports and Exercise* 45:336–341.

Thomas, D.E., Brotherhood, J.R., and Brand, J.C. 1991. Carbohydrate feeding before exercise: effect of glycemic index. *International Journal of Sports Medicine* 12:180–186.

Walsh, N.P., Gleeson, M., Pyne, D.B., et al. 2011. Position statement. Part two: maintaining immune health. *Exercise Immunology Review* 17:64–103.

West, N.P., Pyne, D.B., Cripps, A.W., et al. 2011. *Lactobaccilus fermentum* (PCC®) supplementation and gastrointestinal and respiratory-tract illness symptoms: a randomised control trial in athletes. *Nutrition Journal*, doi: 10.1186/1475-2891-10-30.

West, N.P., Pyne, D.B., Peake, J.M., and Cripps, A.W. 2009. Probiotics, immunity and exercise: a review. *Exercise Immunology Reviews* 15:107–126.

Willis, K.S., Peterson, N.J., and Larson-Meyer, D.E. 2008. Should we be concerned about the vitamin D status of athletes? *International Journal of Sports Nutrition and Exercise Metabolism* 18:204–224.

Yeo, W.K., Paton, C., Garnham, A.P., Burke, L.M., Carey, A.L., and Hawley, J.A. 2008. Skeletal muscle adaptation and performance responses to once a day versus twice every second day endurance training regimens. *Journal of Applied Physiology* 105:1462–1470.

4 Spinal Cord Injuries

Victoria Goosey-Tolfrey,
Jennifer Krempien and Mike Price

CONTENTS

4.1 INTRODUCTION

Nutrition recommendations currently used in sport for those with an impairment are primarily based upon data from able-bodied athletes (as outlined in Chapter 3), but these are almost certainly not directly transferable to athletes with a spinal cord injury (SCI). As an example, the smaller working muscle mass used by an athlete with SCI during wheelchair propulsion will lead to lower energy requirements during training than those of able-bodied (AB) athletes (Glaser 1985) in equivalent sports (Price 2010). Furthermore, there may be considerable muscle atrophy in the lower limbs, leading to a lower resting metabolic rate and, in turn, a further reduction in daily energy expenditure (EE). To prevent unwanted weight gain, energy intake must be correspondingly reduced. Consequently, a number of intriguing questions centre on the physiology of individuals with SCI particularly in relation to EE, energy requirements and performance, all of which will be discussed in this chapter. For the purposes of this chapter, spinal cord injuries include spina bifida and traumatic and nontraumatic spinal cord lesions.

4.2 SPINAL CORD INJURY

The spine has two main components: the spinal column and the spinal cord. To understand the classification system for athletes with a SCI sport the anatomy of different regions of the column and any resultant loss of function must be understood. There are 33 vertebrae which are divided into five types: 7 cervical, 12 thoracic, 5 lumbar, 5 sacral, and 4 coccygeal, and referred to by a letter and numerical code (e.g. T1–T12 for the thoracic vertebrae). The spinal cord, which is divided into 31 segments, determines the main muscles that are innervated through the motor nerves. In brief, thoracic or lumbar spinal cord injuries cause functional loss in the legs and trunk muscles/organs innervated below the level of lesion (paraplegic athletes), while cervical spinal cord injuries cause functional loss in all four extremities (athletes with quadriplegia), with the degree of dysfunction approximately proportional to the level of lesion (Janssen and Hopman 2005). Paraplegia and quadriplegia are typically caused by an injury to the spinal cord with the resultant level of the injury determining the extent of the motor loss, which can vary from impaired function to complete muscle group or limb paralysis. The SCI may also be complete or incomplete. A complete injury will mean loss of all function, motor and sensory, below the level of the injury. An incomplete lesion is one where there is neurological function below the level of the injury whereby there may be complete motor loss but incomplete sensory loss, or vice versa. There may also be a combination of sensory impairments where, for example, the spinothalamic tracts are injured resulting in loss of pain and temperature sensation but the dorsal columns are preserved with normal light touch and position sense. Figure 4.1, taken from the American Spinal Injury Association (ASIA) classification manual, details the sensory and motor impairments likely to occur along the spinal cord.

4.2.1 Physiological Adaptations Following a Spinal Cord Injury

Spinal cord injury results in a reduction of physical work capacity as shown by variables such as peak oxygen uptake ($\dot{V}O_{2peak}$), synonymous with maximal oxygen uptake ($\dot{V}O_{2max}$) in AB athletes, and maximal power output. The reduction in functional capacity is generally considered to be due to the reduced muscle mass as a result of paralysis and the reduced sympathetic nervous system (SNS) activity below the level of lesion. Indeed, measures from standard laboratory-based tests for

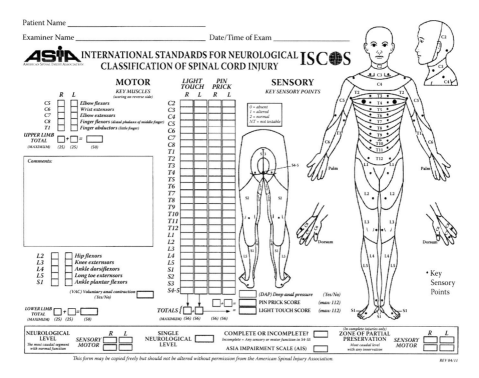

FIGURE 4.1 The American Spinal Injury Association (ASIA) standards for neurological classification of SCI worksheet. (From American Spinal Injury Association, *International Standards for Neurological Classification of Spinal Cord Injury*, Atlanta, GA, 2011.)

aerobic capacity are reduced in proportion to the lesion level. For example, athletes with quadriplegia demonstrate the lowest values for $\dot{V}O_{2peak}$ (1.67 ± 0.38 vs. 2.47 ± 0.33 L/min) and peak heart rate (129 ± 12 vs. 184 ± 10 beats/min) when compared to athletes with paraplegia (Leicht et al. 2012), the latter being due to the complete loss of SNS activity in quadriplegia and subsequently the cardioaccelerator nerves innervated between T1 and T4. For athletes with low level paraplegia (T7 and below) peak heart rate can be similar to that observed for upper body trained AB and non-SCI wheelchair athletes (~180–190 beats/min) but with lower $\dot{V}O_{2peak}$ values (2.47 L/min vs. 3.35 L/min, for SCI and non-SCI wheelchair athletes respectively; Leicht et al. 2012). Although laboratory-based measures can be obtained for athletes with SCI, those athletes with a reduced range of heart rate values (i.e. athletes with quadriplegia) may find that the use of heart rate as a measure of exercise intensity may be inappropriate. Here, other intensity indicators such as ratings of perceived exertion may be more practical (Goosey-Tolfrey and Price 2010; Paulson et al. 2013).

As a result of a spinal cord injury there are considerable changes in body composition due to muscle wastage below the level of lesion, alongside bone demineralisation and joint deterioration (Jacobs and Nash 2004). Several researchers have used AB age-matched reference values for comparative purposes and noted lower lean mass in the SCI groups. Longitudinal work using segmental body composition analysis has shown that lean mass in the upper body increases by up to 15% during the first year after onset of a SCI due to intensive rehabilitation (Wilmet et al. 1995). Although the absolute lean mass in the upper limbs of sedentary individuals with paraplegia is similar to that in the AB population (Spungen et al. 2000, 2003), in a wheelchair sporting context, lean mass of the upper body is actually greater than that of an AB cohort (Sutton et al. 2009). Figure 4.2a and b shows an example of the body composition taken from a dual-energy x-ray absorptiometry (DXA) scan for a female athlete with SCI. The scan highlights that:

- Wheelchair use combined with high-level sport participation results in an improved lean tissue component of the upper body.
- Whole-body DXA values mask regional differences, suggesting that the superior composition of the upper body in SCI athletes 'compensates' for the poorer lower-body composition when looking at the body as a whole.

When compared to an age-matched control, the lower bone mineral density (BMD) and lean mass, and corresponding high percentage fat evident in the lower limbs reflect bone demineralisation and atrophy of the lower-limb musculature. Please refer to Section 4.4.2 for further discussion on BMD and vitamin D.

4.2.2 Gastric Emptying

Among the multitude of factors contributing to successful absorption and assimilation of nutrients is gastric emptying. If gastric emptying is affected by SCI then the ability to take up nutrients along the intestine may also be affected. Clinically, gastric emptying is slower in patients with high level SCI when compared to those with low level SCI (Kao et al. 1999; Lin et al. 2002) with many SCI patients tested (53–58%) demonstrating abnormal indices of gastric function after solid meals (Kao et al. 1998, 1999). This is especially true for those with quadriplegia (Fealey et al. 1984; Kao et al. 1998, 1999; Rajendran et al. 1992), although a number of studies have shown no differences in gastric emptying for both persons with quadriplegia and those with paraplegia when compared to AB persons (Lu et al. 1998; Zhang et al. 1994). It is known from exercise studies of AB individuals that moderate exercise intensities (15 minutes duration, five-a-side soccer) are sufficient to slow gastric emptying, as does brief high-intensity exercise (interval training at 66 and 75% $\dot{V}O_{2max}$) (Leiper et al. 2001a, 2001b, 2005). As many wheelchair sports are intermittent in nature and of moderate to high intensity, an already slowed gastric emptying as a result of SCI may be accentuated, although this as yet has not been investigated. Since sympathetic nervous system and other limiting factors for gastric function are affected by SCI, future work should be undertaken to examine the combined effects of SCI and exercise on gastric emptying and nutrient absorption.

4.2.3 Energy Expenditure

The EE and metabolism of athletes with spinal cord injury have recently been reviewed (Price 2010). Here it was noted that the EE of athletes competing in

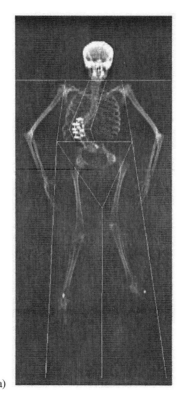

(a)

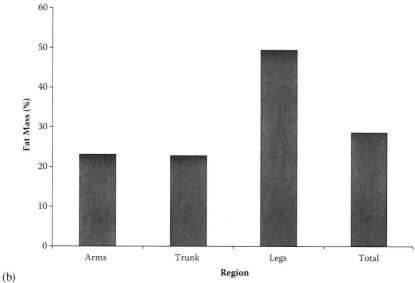

(b)

FIGURE 4.2 (a) Dual-energy x-ray absorptiometry (DXA) scan of female athlete aged 33 with a spinal cord injury, with (b) an illustration of the segmental and total body measures of percent fat. (Permission obtained from the athlete and image courtesy of Laura Sutton.)

COMMENTARY BOX 4.1

EXPERT COMMENTARY: Muscle atrophy and the risk of insulin resistance in spinal cord injured individuals
Dr. Luc van Loon, Maastricht University

When you perform muscle biopsies on denervated muscle (vastus lateralis) in paraplegics, you find a few interesting things:

- Although there is muscle atrophy in both type 1 and 2 muscle fibres, there remain ample satellite cells to allow skeletal muscle hypertrophy. So if you find ways to stimulate the muscle, you should be able to initiate muscle reconditioning.
- Intramuscular triglyceride (IMTG) stores in denervated muscle of paraplegics are similar to able-bodied individuals—so there seems to be little excess accumulation of IMTG in the denervated muscle of healthy, active SCI individuals, despite a reduced muscle fibre oxidative capacity.
- The changes in muscle oxidative capacity and mitochondrial function occur mostly in the sub-sarcolemmal region rather than the inter-myofibrillar regions.
- There is a shift in muscle fibre type distribution, with reduced type 1 muscle fibres and increased type 2 fibres in the paraplegic individuals compared to able-bodied controls.

Overall, this means that the change in muscle fibre composition induced by denervation was different from that seen in insulin resistance or type 2 diabetes.

wheelchair sports varied depending upon the mode of exercise and nature of the activity undertaken. As expected the EE for athletes with a SCI was lower than that for the equivalent AB sports and, depending on the sport, was in the range of 26–85% of AB values. More specifically, the lowest EE values were noted for table tennis and fencing, which may be considered as more static versions of the AB sports, and for wheelchair rugby, due to the participants being predominantly those with quadriplegia and demonstrating the lowest available muscle mass for movement. Both wheelchair tennis and basketball exhibited greater EEs than table tennis and fencing with the basketball data being lower than predicted values from McArdle et al. (2000) for full on-court competition. However, recent data from Croft et al. (2010) reported that elite wheelchair tennis and basketball players demonstrated much greater EE values than for recreational or national level players (Figure 4.3).

One of the most important factors contributing to the difference in energy requirements of AB and athletes with SCI is the fact that a smaller working muscle mass is used during everyday and sporting movements (Glaser 1985). A second factor

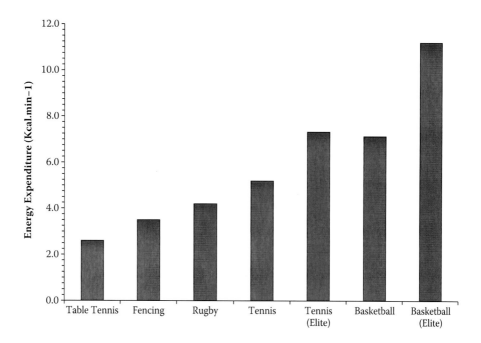

FIGURE 4.3 Energy expenditure for a range of wheelchair sports. Elite data represent international standard athletes for tennis and basketball, respectively (Croft et al. 2010). Basketball data (nonelite) are averages for data during a practice session (Burke et al. 1985), competition (Bernardi et al. 1988), and basketball (endurance) training (Abel et al. 2008). Tennis data is the average of competitive match play (Roy et al. 2006) and training sessions (Abel et al. 2008). Rugby data is from Abel et al. (2008) whereas fencing and table tennis data are from Bernardi et al. (1988).

generally accepted to be of importance to EE is the amount of SNS available for exercise. The sympathetic nervous system relates to the 'fight or flight' responses of the body to stressful situations, particularly the use of carbohydrate and fat in metabolism. With respect to the SNS, physiologically we are concerned with the amount of adrenaline (epinephrine) and noradrenaline (norepinephrine) released. It is well known that, when compared to AB persons, those with SCI can have a reduced production of these catecholamines (Schmid et al. 1998; Steinberg et al. 2000). More specifically, those with quadriplegia and high level paraplegia (T1–T5) often have a reduced response, especially for adrenaline, when compared to those with low-level paraplegia (T5 and below). Furthermore, there is likely to be a wide range of energy requirements in athletes with SCI based on the onset and nature of the spinal cord injury (i.e. the level and completeness of the lesion level). In cases where a wheelchair is used for daily mobility, there may be considerable muscle atrophy in the lower limbs and consequently it would seem reasonable to assume that the daily EE would be lower in persons with SCI.

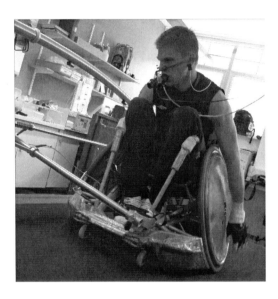

FIGURE 4.4 Expired air collection during wheelchair locomotion on a motorised treadmill.

4.2.4 MEASURING ENERGY EXPENDITURE

When determining the EE of an activity, metabolic rate can be measured using expired gasses during incremental exercise tests (Figure 4.4) to determine the responses to a range of exercise intensities. However, for many activities, especially competitions, using this technique is impractical due to the requirements of using a mouthpiece or wearing a face mask to collect the expired gas. Energy expenditure can also be predicted from laboratory-based incremental exercise tests of heart rate and oxygen consumption with the latter enabling EE to be calculated. In this instance, the heart rate during an actual activity can be matched to that obtained in the laboratory and an equivalent EE value obtained. Predictive methods such as those highlighted above do have potential errors as values are not obtained from the actual event. However, there are a range of normative values available for AB sports from which EE can be predicted (e.g. McArdle et al. 2000). Although there are fewer predictive values available for wheelchair sports and activities, these normative values are becoming more specific as more research is undertaken in this area. For example Ainsworth et al. (2000) and Collins et al. (2010) provided a range of EE values for wheelchair-based activities in a non-athlete population with the latter determining that the standard metabolic equivalent of task (MET) value for SCI wheelchair users should be reduced to 2.7 ml/kg/min rather than the accepted values of 3.5 ml/kg/min. These developments are welcomed but there is still a need for values relating to elite athletes and young athletes to be derived.

4.2.5   DAILY LIVING VS. SPORTING ENERGY EXPENDITURE

The available literature which has examined wheelchair-dependent patients performing activities of daily living (ADL) has suggested that during ADL the basal metabolic rate (BMR) and total EE are significantly correlated with lesion level (Mollinger et al. 1985). Although this information has helped dietitians to establish the average energy needs of this patient population, it must be borne in mind that many studies are limited by the hospital environment, where activities such as travel outside the hospital are restricted and where there is limited physical therapy. In addition, the majority of data is collected from non-athletic populations. Hence, for the individual athlete with SCI within their own environment there may well be significantly different demands of wheelchair locomotion and the reported EE values may well be exceeded.

Within the context of Paralympic sport performance only a small body of literature exists regarding EE during sports performance or sport training. Previous studies have focused mainly upon men's wheelchair basketball and there has recently been descriptive literature produced on hand cycling, wheelchair tennis, and wheelchair rugby (Abel et al. 2003). For example, Burke et al. (1985) demonstrated an EE of 6.5 METs, or 2160 kJ/h (516 kcal/h) during wheelchair basketball. Other relevant work includes that of Bernardi et al. (1988), who described the EE of five Paralympic sports (including wheelchair fencing and table tennis). Unfortunately, this work has never really been followed up by the broader research community, and in the context of the increasingly professionalised arena of Paralympic sport, the findings are now dated. Historically it would seem that the more active sports for athletes with an impairment have attracted a higher degree of interest in terms of research. However, from the practitioner perspective, the athletes in the less active sports present an equal and continuing challenge in terms of weight loss and weight maintenance. Consequently information regarding nutritional advice for all athletes with SCI would help guide the practices of those working with athletes with an impairment.

A number of wheelchair sports are not played (or classified) solely on the basis of spinal cord injury. For example, basketball, tennis and fencing involve athletes competing with or against athletes with other impairments. Being able to determine EE's of a large number of athletes with SCI (or indeed other impairments) is therefore often difficult within a squad of athletes. To illustrate this point Figure 4.5 demonstrates the differences in EE for wheelchair or seated fencing when compared to conventional fencing and between wheelchair fencers with and without SCI. The seated and conventional fencing EEs were obtained using AB fencers experienced in playing and coaching wheelchair fencing thus representing a consistent level of skill (unpublished data courtesy of Iglesias, Rodríguez, Vallejo, Rodríguez-Zamora and Price). The data for the athletes with SCI is taken from Bernardi et al. (1988). Figure 4.5 clearly shows that within a sport involving different impairments (i.e. seated athletes with SCI vs. those without SCI and likely full or greater muscle mass available) the potential for a wide range of EE values exists.

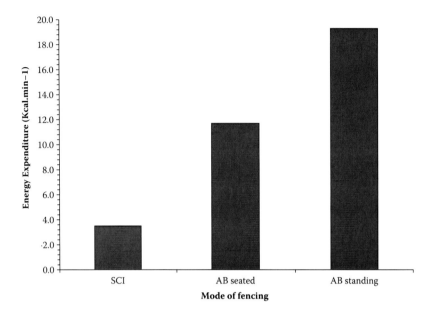

FIGURE 4.5 Energy expenditure for seated and standing fencing compared to wheelchair fencing in athletes with SCI. (Unpublished data courtesy of Iglesias, Rodríguez, Vallejo, Rodríguez-Zamora and Price.)

4.3   SWEAT LOSSES AND FLUID REPLACEMENT

It is well known that appropriate fluid replacement is vital to good performance in AB athletes. For example, when water is consumed during exercise, performance at exercise intensities of up to ~70% $\dot{V}O_{2max}$ has been shown to be improved when compared to no fluid replacement (Barr et al. 1991; Coyle and Montain 1992; Fallowfield et al. 1996), whereas that at greater exercise intensities (85% $\dot{V}O_{2max}$) has been shown not to improve (Deschamps et al. 1989). The latter is most likely due to performance at greater exercise intensities being limited by factors other than hydration. Within the literature pertaining to athletes with a spinal cord injury no studies have reported a direct comparison between fluid consumption and no fluid consumption and the effects on performance. The main data available concerning fluid intake has been reported through studies of thermoregulation where ad libitum drinking was allowed during prolonged bouts of exercise in cool and hot conditions (Price and Campbell 1997, 1999, 2003). Price (2006) noted that from such studies it was clear that those athletes with low level thoracic spinal cord injuries lost more sweat than those with high level thoracic spinal cord injuries, who in turn lost more than athletes with quadriplegia. Such responses demonstrated the proportional loss of sympathetic nervous system innervation in relation to the level of spinal cord injury and the subsequent ability to sweat in athletes with paraplegia and the loss of sweating capacity in athletes with quadriplegia (Hopman et al. 1993). Fluid losses for the high level (T1–T5) and low level (T6 and below) paraplegic groups in warm conditions (31°C) were similar at approximately 0.71 and 0.69 L/h, respectively (Price and Campbell 2003).

When compared to upper body trained AB athletes sweat loss values were ~1.3 L/h whereas the athletes with quadriplegia lost 0.31 L/h (Price and Campbell 2003).

Athletes with paraplegia have demonstrated voluntary fluid intakes similar to those in AB athletes (i.e. 50–55% of fluid losses). However, athletes with quadriplegia have been shown to drink much greater volumes of fluid (0.764 L/h) than athletes with paraplegia (~0.430 L/h) under the same conditions of exercise intensity (60% $\dot{V}O_{2peak}$) and duration (60 min) in hot conditions (31°C). Such a response is presumably due to their inability to sweat effectively, resulting in their body temperature increasing more than the athletes with paraplegia thus voluntarily drinking more fluid (Price and Campbell 2003). This fact has since been noted anecdotally by athletes with quadriplegia playing rugby and tennis and is highlighted in the practical case studies at the end of this chapter (Section 4.6). Here athletes will either drink a lot of fluid in response to large increases in body temperature or conversely they will restrict fluid intake to avoid gains in body mass from drinking (but not losing fluid through sweating) which athletes consider will affect their on-court performance. Drinking large amounts of fluid may have serious negative effects for athletes with quadriplegia or high level thoracic injuries with respect to inducing autonomic dysreflexia (an acute condition where an exaggerated release of norepinephrine results in a large increase in blood pressure) (Price et al. 2010), which can be triggered by a range of factors including a full bladder. Athletes who are prone to such conditions should take medical advice.

Another scenario where fluid replacement may be of importance is for sports where protective clothing is worn, such as fencing. Although such competitions are usually undertaken in sports halls rather than outside in more extreme environments, the potential increases in body temperature and sweat losses should not be underestimated. Unfortunately there are no data available at this time to provide guidelines for fluid replacement in these instances but athletes should become aware of how to measure body mass changes pre and post exercise and determine their own sweat rate to help guide their fluid replacement needs (see Chapter 3 for further details).

4.4   NUTRITIONAL REQUIREMENTS

The standards for nutritional requirements used in para-sport are generally based upon recommendations for AB athletes. As discussed previously in this chapter, a number of differences between the two groups do exist. Caution should be exhibited when adapting or accepting nutritional recommendations developed for AB athletes. Within a group of athletes with SCI, EE, and thus energy intake, is variable but smaller in magnitude than for AB athletes. Differences in EE have been illustrated based on severity of SCI, lean mass and sport requirements. The potential role of macronutrients to support training and performance in athletes with SCI is less well understood with many assumptions that the preferred fuel sources and metabolism of macronutrients are similar to those of AB athletes. Athletes with SCI do have some altered nutrient requirements related to bone health and wound healing.

4.4.1 MACRONUTRIENT REQUIREMENTS

In AB athletes, the predominant muscle fuel source in lower intensity exercise is intramuscular triglyceride and free fatty acids. When exercise intensity increases, muscle glycogen and blood glucose become increasingly important fuel sources. As humans have a limited capacity to store muscle and liver glycogen, dietary carbohydrate intake is recommended for athletes to ensure a sufficient availability of glucose for training and competition. In contrast to the limited glycogen stores, fat stores are abundant and a training goal of athletes is to promote the adaption of working muscles to increase the capacity to use fat as a fuel source during training.

There is no strong evidence that the functional muscle of athletes with SCI will respond in a profoundly different manner than that which has been observed in AB athletes.

4.4.1.1 Carbohydrate Ingestion before or during Exercise in Athletes with SCI

The ingestion of carbohydrate (CHO) prior to exercise can significantly improve endurance performance (Tsintzas et al. 1995; Wilber and Moffatt 1992; Wright et al. 1991) and the performance of intermittent exercise akin to many team sports (Patterson and Gray 2007; Nicholas et al. 1995; Sugiura and Kobayashi 1998). However, there is surprisingly little literature regarding this aspect in athletes with SCI.

Spendiff and Campbell (2002) examined ingestion of an 8% CHO solution prior to one hour of arm crank ergometry followed by a subsequent 20 minute performance trial. Performance in the time trial was improved by 1 km (12.5 vs. 11.5 km) when consuming the CHO solution compared to placebo. Although the athletes tested were upper body trained AB individuals, the results were similar to those which may be expected for lower body exercise. In a subsequent study using the same methods, but with wheelchair athletes (predominantly with SCI) Spendiff and Campbell (2003) again observed that the athletes performed significantly better following ingestion of CHO (10.8 km) when compared to the placebo trial (10.2 km). A third study of wheelchair athletes involved a comparison of two different CHO drinks, a 4 vs. 11% solution on performance during wheelchair ergometry (Spendiff and Campbell 2005). Both drinks raised blood glucose to similar levels pre-exercise but there was no difference in wheelchair performance over 20 min (5.1 vs. 5.0 km, respectively) following 60 min of submaximal exercise. However there was a tendency for the average power output during the time trial to be greater in the 11% CHO trials along with greater blood glucose and respiratory exchange ratio and lower blood fatty acids. Based on these results the authors suggested that the 11% solution may be more beneficial for the athletes. Although the evidence suggests that ingestion of CHO 20 minutes prior to exercise is beneficial to endurance performance, no data has been reported regarding the effects on intermittent sports such as basketball or tennis. Preliminary studies suggest that the ingestion of a CHO-containing drink prior to endurance events provides a beneficial energy source with the potential to improve performance. Future work is needed to better understand both the physiological and performance effects of CHO ingestion before and during exercise in individuals with SCI.

COMMENTARY BOX 4.2

EXPERT COMMENTARY: Muscle protein synthesis in spinal cord injured individuals

Dr. Luc van Loon, Maastricht University, and Professor Kevin Tipton, Stirling University

Question: Do you believe the protein requirements for optimising muscle protein synthesis (i.e. 20–25 g post exercise) are the same in athletes with spinal cord injuries compared to able-bodied individuals?

Answer: Yes. If anything, they may even be a little higher. Although the amount of 'active' or functional muscle mass is lower in athletes with spinal cord injuries, there is still muscle turnover occurring in the denervated areas and this muscle will still take up amino acids. Furthermore, muscle inactivity is known to reduce the protein synthetic response to protein intake, which could be at least partly compensated for by ingesting more protein.

Although the absolute EE's of most wheelchair activities in athletes with SCI are lower than for AB athletes the relative proportions of CHO and fat metabolism appear to be similar, at least in athletes with low level spinal cord injuries (Price 2010; Jung and Yamasaki 2009). However, little data is available regarding athletes with high level lesions where the sympathetic nervous system is often absent and where increases in adrenaline and noradrenaline are potentially lower than for athletes with low level spinal cord injuries (Schmid et al. 1998; Steinberg et al. 2000). For example, Stallknecht et al. (2001) observed not only lower increases in adrenaline and noradrenaline during 60 minutes of exercise in persons with spinal cord injury (T1–T5) but also that adipose tissue lipolysis was lower in those with SCI.

The concept and evidence for the benefit of recovery nutrition with the ingestion of carbohydrate-rich foods/fluids along with a moderate amount of protein is well established in AB athletes (as outlined in Chapter 3). At this time, there remains no evidence to suggest that athletes with a SCI would not benefit from a recovery nutrition regime. What remains to be determined are the optimal amounts of carbohydrate and protein to support an efficient recovery without any undesirable side effects.

4.4.1.2   Protein and Amino Acids

The optimal amount of dietary protein, amino acid composition and timing of ingestion to best support recovery from training continues to be an area of great debate amongst clinicians and researchers working with AB athletes. At the present time there is a dearth of reported literature assessing the protein or amino acid requirements for athletes with SCI. Given this lack of impairment-specific evidence, clinicians and sport scientists continue with the assumption that protein utilization and requirements to optimize post-exercise recovery are similar to current recommendations for AB athletes. Total requirements may be slightly higher if the athlete has a pressure ulcer or wound to support and promote healing (Lee et al. 2006; Reddy et al. 2008). If the athlete has chronic renal insufficiency, the total protein intake should be carefully evaluated to find the balance between what is required to best support training and recovery while not placing any unnecessary burden on the kidneys.

4.4.1.3 Arginine for Wound Healing

Pressure ulcers can be devastating for an athlete with SCI resulting in a significant loss of training time, as the athlete spends more time out of the wheelchair to reduce pressure and promote healing. Prevention is the key and frequent monitoring of skin integrity to ensure any breakdown is identified early. Many nutrients play a key role in the inflammatory, proliferative and remodelling phases of wound healing with arginine supplementation showing some promise to improve the rate of wound healing (Sherman and Barkley 2011). During wound healing, arginine becomes a conditionally essential nutrient as a substrate for nitric oxide, ornithine and proline encouraging vasodilation, collagen synthesis and deposition along with cytokine response (Curran et al. 2006; Witte and Barbul 2003). In a small group of individuals with SCI with a pressure ulcer, daily supplementation with 9 grams of arginine reduced healing times (10.5 ± 1.3 vs. 21 ± 3.7 weeks, $p < 0.05$) as compared to a historical control group (Brewer et al. 2010). This reduced healing time could positively affect the training potential of an athlete.

4.4.2 MICRONUTRIENT REQUIREMENTS

There is no evidence at this time to determine whether athletes with a SCI have increased micronutrient requirements to support the demands of training and competition. Given this lack of information, the assumption remains that intakes determined for AB data are adequate. The one exception to this is the knowledge that a high incidence of vitamin D insufficiency and deficiency has been observed in those with SCI, with some evidence that poor vitamin D status is prevalent in many athletes with an impairment.

Low BMD associated with acute and chronic SCI is well established (Bauman et al. 1999). While physical activity and weight-bearing activity have been shown to maintain or slightly increase bone mineral density above the injury level (Goktepe et al. 2004), reduced BMD, osteoporosis and fracture risk in the lower limbs remain significant risks (Dauty et al. 2000; de Bruin et al. 2000). One strategy to slow the progression of osteoporosis is to optimize vitamin D status and ensure dietary calcium is adequate. For athletes, a vitamin D receptor in skeletal muscle has been identified, suggesting a role of vitamin D in muscle function and overall strength (Hamilton 2011).

Optimal serum 25(OH) vitamin D concentrations remain somewhat controversial with the following ranges agreed upon for athletes and those with SCI: <25 nmol/L, deficient; 25–50 nmol/L, insufficient; 50–75 nmol/L, suboptimal; and >75 nmol/L, sufficient (Hamilton 2011; Nemunaitis et al. 2010; Oleson et al. 2010), as outlined in Chapter 10. However, Heaney (1999) suggests 25(OH) vitamin D concentrations below 80 nmol/L are insufficient as parathyroid hormone remains upregulated and calcium absorption is somewhat inhibited.

Those with SCI are at a considerable risk of suboptimal vitamin D concentrations. Prevalence of vitamin D inadequacy (<75 nmol/L) was measured in 93% of a sample of individuals with acute and chronic SCI (Nemunaitis et al. 2010) and 96% of those with chronic SCI in winter months (Oleson et al. 2010). A recent surveillance study of Australian Paralympic athletes found a similarly high incidence of vitamin D deficiency and insufficiency (Broad 2012). Only 9% ($n = 1/11$) of athletes had 25(OH) vitamin D concentrations greater than 75 nmol/L when blood status was measured at the end of winter with a slight increase to 20% ($n = 5/25$) of athletes having normal vitamin D concentrations when assessments were undertaken at the end of summer. Of the athletes with SCI ($n = 7$), none had a normal vitamin D concentration. Overall results for the study found that 17% of all athletes with an impairment tested had a normal vitamin D concentration. In a small study of seven adults with SCI, Bauman et al. (2011) showed that a 90-day trial of oral supplementation with 2000 IU of cholecalciferol (vitamin D3) and 1300 mg of elemental calcium was shown to increase vitamin D concentrations to above 75 nmol/L with concurrent decreases in parathyroid hormone and no changes to urinary calcium excretion or serum calcium concentrations. It is recommended that all athletes with SCI should have their serum 25(OH) vitamin D concentrations monitored yearly (ideally at the end of summer) and oral supplementation of vitamin D3 as needed to maintain a sufficient vitamin D status (see Chapter 10).

4.4.3 ADDITIONAL NUTRIENTS

Dietary fibre intake is consistently reported to be low in both athletes and nonathletes with SCI (Goosey-Tolfrey and Crosland 2010; Krempien and Barr 2011; Levine et al. 1992; Walters et al. 2009). Typically, a high fibre diet with adequate fluid intake is recommended as a strategy for managing bowel routines and function, but depending on the autonomic dysfunction/control of the gastrointestinal tract this may not be the best approach (Chung and Emmanuel 2006). In one study, increasing dietary fibre by the addition of bran further increased the colonic transit time, suggesting that SCI bowel function may not respond well to additional dietary fibre (Cameron et al. 1996). Recent use of SmartPill technology in adults with SCI has confirmed the safety of this diagnostic tool and could be used with athletes who struggle with bowel function (Williams et al. 2012). Bowel habits and function are unique to the athlete, and the risk of stool incontinence has the potential to negatively impact performance during sporting events.

4.5 PATTERNS OF NUTRIENT INTAKE IN ATHLETES WITH SCI

As outlined in the previous section, athletes with SCI have relatively modest energy requirements. As the level of impairment increases from incomplete paraplegia to complete quadriplegia, the energy requirements are reduced given that the amount of available active muscle mass is known to be a key determinant of EE. Reduced energy intakes have been observed in non-athletes (Groah et al. 2009; Levine et al. 1992; Tomey et al. 2005; Walters et al. 2009), semi-competitive or recreational athletes (Potvin et al. 1996; Ribeiro et al. 2005) and elite athletes (Goosey-Tolfrey and Crosland 2010; Krempien and Barr 2011). The daily diets from a variety of elite athletes with

SCI report an average energy intake of 6275 to 12,550 kJ (1500 to 2300 kcal) (Goosey-Tolfrey and Crosland 2010; Krempien and Barr 2011). In these studies, carbohydrate intake contributed 3.4–4.4 g carbohydrate per kg bodyweight, or ~46–53% of total calories. Protein intake was assessed at 1.0–1.5 g/kg or 15–20% of calories with the remaining 28–37% of calories resulting from dietary fat intake. The macronutrient intakes generally fell within the broad recommendations for the general population but fell short of what would be considered to be the optimal fuel intake to support the training of an elite athlete (as outlined in Chapter 3), in particular the carbohydrate intake.

The adequacy of vitamins and minerals has also been assessed and a high prevalence of inadequacy reported for calcium, magnesium, zinc, riboflavin, folate and vitamin D. Krempien and Barr (2011) compared the micronutrient adequacy from food alone and food with the additional nutrients provided by vitamin/mineral supplements and found that although the mean intakes improved for many nutrients, the prevalence of inadequacy did not decrease. In other words, almost half (44%) of the participants consumed some form of vitamin or mineral supplement but the additional nutrients did not improve the mean intake of a given micronutrient to change their status from inadequate to adequate. Of primary concern were poor intakes of calcium and vitamin D given the increased prevalence of poor bone mineralization and increased risk of fractures (Eser et al. 2005; Jiang et al. 2006).

4.6 PRACTICAL ASPECTS

4.6.1 CAN AN ATHLETE WITH SCI USE BODY MASS FOR AN INDEX OF HYDRATION STATUS?

The suggestion that a change in body mass is often used as an index of changes in body water content and thus hydration (McArdle et al. 2000) has been used by several practitioners in the past. For the athlete with SCI this requires that an individual know their normal body weight which often presents a problem for those who require accessible platform or seated scales. Moreover, for the AB athlete it has been suggested that morning body weight must be maintained within 1% of the normal baseline from day to day (Armstrong 2007). Cheuvront et al. (2004) also found that a valid, average baseline body mass (with daily variability of 0.51 ± 0.20 kg; mean ± SD) can be determined by measuring body mass on three consecutive days. The application of this to an individual with SCI is problematic as colonic transit time can be extended up to 80 hrs. When compared to the AB population, an extended transit time in the colon can lead to an increased likelihood of constipation (Geders et al. 1995). An example of this can be seen in Figure 4.6, where morning body mass and hydration status were measured at a 7-day training camp; whilst an ideal (consistent) level of hydration was achieved, the athlete's body mass increased by almost 2 kg over the camp duration.

4.6.2 WHY DO SOME ATHLETES WITH SCI GAIN WEIGHT FOLLOWING EXERCISE?

As previously outlined, sweat rates for athletes with SCI depend upon the completeness of the SCI and are generally proportional to the level of lesion. Below is an

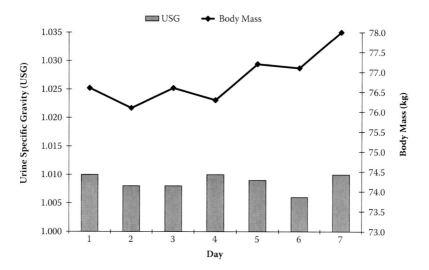

FIGURE 4.6 Body mass and hydration status of a wheelchair rugby player over the course of a 7-day training camp. USG, urine specific gravity.

example of the hourly fluid balance of seven wheelchair rugby players following an intense scrimmage session in a neutral environment (Figure 4.7). This case study highlights the variability in individual sweat rates within this population, as well as supporting what has been noted in the literature, where the ad libitum drinking volumes (0.4 to 2.5 L) matched and in some cases were greater than the total sweat losses (Goosey-Tolfrey et al. 2008; Moran and Broad 2012).

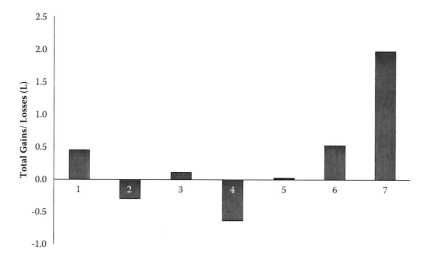

FIGURE 4.7 Fluid balance in wheelchair rugby players following a 60 min scrimmage session. Each number represents an individual athlete.

COMMENTARY BOX 4.3

EXPERT COMMENTARY: Influencing the brain
  Professor Romain Meeussen, Vrije University

Question: In reference to data presented regarding low sweat rates and higher
           core temperatures in some spinal cord injured athletes, from the
           research you've done, do you believe there are some strategies these
           athletes could use to improve performance in the heat?
Answer: There are a few strategies which may be worthwhile investigating,
           other than the obvious one of matching their fluid intake to their
           sweat losses. Certainly, we know the feedback to the brain is com-
           plex and comes from many areas—the carbohydrate mouth rinse is
           a good example of this (see Chapter 3). Some thoughts are:

- Using a cooling vest/neckpiece, although the weight and size of
  the vest may impact performance in some athletes. See further
  discussion in Section 4.6.3.
- A mouth rinse containing ethanol. As the ethanol evaporates, it
  can create a cool sensation in the mouth.
- An ice slurry. We know that ingesting ice slurries reduces core
  temperature. There may be some possibility that exposing the
  mouth to an ice slurry may create a sensation of coolness that
  could help maintain performance for longer.

COMMENTARY BOX 4.4

EXPERT COMMENTARY: Risk of hyponatremia (low plasma sodium concentrations) in high level spinal cord injuries
  Professor Ron Maughan, Loughborough University

Question: Looking at the data presented in Figure 4.7 indicating body mass
           gains during exercise due to relatively low sweat rates being over-
           compensated by fluid intake, do you believe there is any cause for
           concern about hyponatremia in this population?
Answer: I have not read or heard of any reports of hyponatremia in a spinal
           cord injured athlete. I don't think these values would cause any con-
           cerns. If you do the sums, you need to drink a lot to drop plasma
           sodium levels, and this usually involves drinking more than you
           sweat over an extended period of time, which is not the conditions
           under which these athletes are exercising.

4.6.3   CAN ATHLETES WITH SCI BENEFIT BY ADOPTING A COOLING STRATEGY DURING EXERCISE?

Wheelchair tennis players competing in hot and humid environments are faced with an increased risk of heat-related illness and impaired performance. Interestingly, when wheelchair tennis players wore a cooling hat/neck band whilst completing a 60 min laboratory-based protocol of intermittent sprinting at $30.4 \pm 0.6°C$ they felt cooler, even when the body's temperature (aural and mean skin temperature) was in fact similar between trials (Goosey-Tolfrey et al. 2008). This finding could be seen as positive in the competitive tennis environment, where a lower thermal sensation may provide the player a psychological edge. A similar protocol undertaken by athletes with quadriplegia resulted in improved time to exhaustion, improved ability to undertake repeated sprint exercise and reduced core temperatures without any significant change in rating of perceived exertion (Webborn et al. 2010). Goosey-Tolfrey and colleagues (2008) noted a counterproductive effect of wearing the head/neck cooling garments on water consumption, as players consumed 42% less water $(0.70 \pm 0.39$ vs. 1.20 ± 0.66 L) when wearing these cooling aids, with no change in their mean sweat rate (0.69 ± 0.35 vs. 0.65 ± 0.36 L/h for the control and cooling aid conditions, respectively). For some individuals this means that fluid intake better matched their sweat losses, while in others it may result in some degree of dehydration, so individual responses must be assessed in practice.

There is also recent evidence that athletes with a SCI can achieve partial heat acclimation by exposure to hot conditions despite their reduced sweat response. Castle and colleagues (2013) exposed Paralympic shooters to seven consecutive days of heat exposure of 60 minutes duration and found an increased plasma volume, reduced resting aural temperature, and a more dampened increase in aural temperature upon exposure to heat. Therefore it would be worthwhile trialling a combination of heat acclimation and active cooling in SCI athletes.

4.7   TAKE-HOME MESSAGES

1. Energy expenditure, and thus energy intake, for athletes with SCI is less than AB athletes, making it more challenging to meet some of the recommended micronutrient intakes. This reduced energy intake highlights the importance of incorporating nutrient-dense foods into the athlete's diet to meet micronutrient intakes.

2. Sweat losses are generally proportional to the level of SCI with those athletes with quadriplegia generally having an absent or much reduced ability to sweat. Therefore a thorough needs analysis is essential to determine the nature and level of SCI. Sweat rates must be determined for each individual athlete under different environmental conditions to understand the hydration strategy needed.

3. Ingestion of water and/or carbohydrate (8% solution) is likely to improve endurance performance. However, athletes should be cautioned not to drink too much fluid if they are susceptible to autonomic dysreflexia

while remembering to include this CHO consumption in daily energy intake calculations.

4. Gastric emptying is often slower in persons with SCI compared to able-bodied persons. If concerns around gastric motility exist, a physician should be consulted.

5. Vitamin D status should be measured in all athletes with SCI with appropriate repletion with oral vitamin D supplements where necessary.

6. Body mass may appear to be a simple marker for coaches and athletes to use, but for some athletes with SCI a stable daily body mass is not always achieved. It is important that a health screening check-list noting bowel management programmes be recorded to assist data interpretation.

7. Heat acclimation together with localised head and neck cooling for athletes with SCI may be a good strategy to manage body temperature and perception of effort and better match fluid intake to actual sweat losses in hot temperatures, especially for athletes with quadriplegia. Conversely, athletes with quadriplegia may also suffer from hypothermia in cool conditions and may require additional clothing or warm fluids if training/competition conditions are cool.

REFERENCES

Abel, T., Kroner, M., Rojas Vega, S., Peters, C., Klose, C., and Platen, P. 2003. Energy expenditure in wheelchair racing and handbiking, a basis for prevention of cardiovascular diseases in those with disabilities. *European Journal of Cardiovascular Prevention and Rehabilitation* 10:371–376.

Abel, T., Platen, P., Rojas Vega, S., Schneider, S., and Strüder, H.K. 2008. Energy expenditure in ball games for wheelchair users. *Spinal Cord* 46:785–790.

Ainsworth, B.E., Haskell, W.L., Whitt, M.C., et al. 2000. Compendium of Physical Activities: an update of activity codes and MET intensities. *Medicine and Science in Sports and Exercise* 32(Suppl 9):S498–S504.

Armstrong, L.E. 2007. Assessing hydration status: the elusive gold standard. *Journal of the American College of Nutrition* 26(Suppl 5):575S–584S.

Barr, S.I., Costill, D.L., and Fink, W.J. 1991. Fluid replacement during prolonged exercise: effects of water, saline, or no fluid. *Medicine and Science in Sports and Exercise* 23:811–817.

Bauman, W.A., Emmons, R.R., Cirnigliaro, C.M., Kirshblum, S.C., and Spungen, A.M. 2011. An effective oral vitamin D replacement therapy in persons with spinal cord injury. *Journal of Spinal Cord Medicine* 34:455–460.

Bauman, W.A., Spungen, A.M., Wang, J., Pierson, R.N., Jr., and Schwartz, E. 1999. Continuous loss of bone during chronic immobilization: a monozygotic twin study. *Osteoporosis International* 10:123–127.

Bernardi, M., Canale, I., Felici, F., and Marchettoni, P. 1988. Field evaluation of the energy cost of different wheelchair sports. *International Journal of Sports Cardiology* 5:58–61.

Brewer, S., Desneves, K., Pearce, L., et al. 2010. Effect of an arginine-containing nutritional supplement on pressure ulcer healing in community spinal patients. *Journal of Wound Care* 19:311–316.

Broad, E. 2012. Vitamin D status of Paralympic athletes. *Medicine and Science in Sport and Exercise* 44(Suppl 1):S137.

Burke, E.J., Auchinachie, J.A., Hayden, R., and Loftin, J.M. 1985. Energy cost of wheelchair basketball. *Physician and Sports Medicine* 13:99–102.

Cameron, K.J., Nyulasi, I.B., Collier, G.R., and Brown, D.J. 1996. Assessment of the effect of increased dietary fibre intake on bowel function in patients with spinal cord injury. *Spinal Cord* 34:277–283.

Castle, P.C., Kularatne, B.P., Brewer, J., et al. 2013. Partial heat acclimation of athletes with spinal cord lesion. *European Journal of Applied Physiology* 113:109–115.

Cheuvront, S.N., Carter, R., Montain, S.J., and Sawka, M.N. 2004. Daily body mass variability and stability in active men undergoing exercise-heat stress. *International Journal of Sport Nutrition and Exercise Metabolism* 14:532–540.

Chung, E.A., and Emmanuel, A.V. 2006. Gastrointestinal symptoms related to autonomic dysfunction following spinal cord injury. *Progress in Brain Research* 152:317–333.

Collins, E.G., Gater, D., Kiratli, J., Butler, J., Hanson, K., and Langbein, W.E. 2010. Energy cost of physical activities in persons with spinal cord injury. *Medicine and Science in Sports and Exercise* 42:691–700.

Coyle, E.F., and Montain, S.J. 1992. Benefits of fluid replacement with carbohydrate during exercise. *Medicine and Science in Sports and Exercise* 24(Suppl 9):S324–S30.

Croft, L., Dybrus, S., Lenton, J., and Goosey-Tolfrey, V. 2010. A comparison of the physiological demands of wheelchair basketball and wheelchair tennis. *International Journal of Sports Physiology and Performance* 5:301–315.

Curran, J.N., Winter, D.C., and Bouchier-Hayes, D. 2006. Biological fate and clinical implications of arginine metabolism in tissue healing. *Wound Repair and Regeneration* 14:376–386.

Dauty, M., Perrouin Verbe, B., Maugars, Y., Dubois, C., and Mathe, J.F. 2000. Supralesional and sublesional bone mineral density in spinal cord injured patients. *Bone* 27:305–309.

de Bruin, E.D., Dietz, V., Dambacher, M.A., and Stussi, E. 2000. Longitudinal changes in bone in men with spinal cord injury. *Clinical Rehabilitation* 14:145–152.

Deschamps, A., Levy, R.D., Cosio, M.G., Marliss, E.B., and Magder, S. 1989. Effect of saline infusion on body temperature and endurance during heavy exercise. *Journal of Applied Physiology* 66:2799–2804.

Eser, P., Frotzler, A., Zehnder, Y., and Denoth, J. 2005. Fracture threshold in the femur and tibia of people with spinal cord injury as determined by peripheral quantitative computed tomography. *Archives in Physical Medicine and Rehabilitation* 86:498–504.

Fallowfield, J.L., Williams, C., Booth, J., Choo, B.H., and Growns, S. 1996. Effect of water ingestion on endurance capacity during prolonged running. *Journal of Sports Sciences* 14:497–502.

Fealey, R.D., Szurszewski, J.H., Merritt, J.L., and DiMagno, E.P. 1984. Effect of traumatic spinal cord transection on human upper gastrointestinal motility and gastric emptying. *Gastroenterology* 87:69–75.

Geders, J.M., Gaing, A., Bauman, W.A., and Korsten, M.A. 1995. The effect of cisapride on segmental colonic transit time in patients with spinal cord injury. *American Journal of Gastroenterology* 90:285–289.

Glaser, R.M. 1985. Exercise and locomotion for the spinal cord injured. *Exercise and Sport Science Reviews* 13:263–303.

Goktepe, A.S., Yilmaz, B., Alaca, R., Yazicioglu, K., Mohur, H., and Gunduz, S. 2004. Bone density loss after spinal cord injury: elite paraplegic basketball players vs. paraplegic sedentary persons. *American Journal of Physical Medicine and Rehabilitation* 83:279–283.

Goosey-Tolfrey, V.L., and Crosland, J. 2010. Nutritional practices of competitive British wheelchair games players. *Adapted Physical Activity Quarterly* 27:47–59.

Goosey-Tolfrey, V.L., Diaper, N., Crosland, J., and Tolfrey, K. 2008. Fluid intake during wheelchair exercise in the heat: effects of localized cooling garments. *International Journal of Sports Physiology and Performance* 3:145–156.

Goosey-Tolfrey, V.L., and Price, M.J. 2010. Physiology of wheelchair athletes. In *Wheelchair Sport*, ed. V. Goosey-Tolfrey, 47–62. Champaign, IL: Human Kinetics.

Groah, S.L., Nash, M.S., Ljungberg, I.H., et al. 2009. Nutrient intake and body habitus after spinal cord injury: an analysis by sex and level of injury. *Journal of Spinal Cord Medicine* 32:25–33.

Hamilton, B. 2011. Vitamin D and athletic performance: the potential role of muscle. *Asian Journal of Sports Medicine* 2:211–219.

Heaney, R.P. 1999. Lessons for nutritional science from vitamin D. *American Journal of Clinical Nutrition* 69:825–826.

Hopman, M.T.E., Oeseburg, B., and Binkhorst, R.A. 1993. Circulatory responses in persons with paraplegia to prolonged arm exercise and thermal stress. *Medicine and Science in Sports and Exercise* 25:577–583.

Jacobs, P.L., and Nash, M.S. 2004. Exercise recommendations for individuals with spinal cord injury. *Sports Medicine* 34:727–751.

Janssen, T.W.J., and Hopman, M.T.E. 2005. Spinal cord injury. In *Exercise testing and exercise prescription for special cases*, ed. J.S. Skinner, 203–219. 3rd ed. Baltimore: Lippincott Williams and Wilkins.

Jiang, S.D., Jiang, L.S., and Dai, L.Y. 2006. Mechanisms of osteoporosis in spinal cord injury. *Clinical Endocrinology* 65:555–565.

Jung, W., and Yamasaki, M. 2009. Effect of pre-exercise carbohydrate ingestion on substrate consumption in persons with spinal cord injury. *Spinal Cord* 47:464–469.

Kao, C.H., ChangLai, S.P., Chieng, P.U., and Yen, T.C. 1998. Gastric emptying in male neurologic trauma. *Journal of Nuclear Medicine* 39:1798–1801.

Kao, C.H., Ho, Y.J., Changlai, S.P., and Ding, H.J. 1999. Gastric emptying in spinal cord injury patients. *Digestive Diseases and Sciences* 44:1512–1515.

Krempien, J.L., and Barr, S.I. 2011. Risk of nutrient inadequacies in elite Canadian athletes with spinal cord injury. *International Journal of Sport Nutrition and Exercise Metabolism* 21:417–425.

Lee, S., Posthauer, M., Dorner, B., Redovian, V., and Maloney, M. 2006. Pressure ulcer healing with a concentrated, fortified, collagen protein hydrolysate supplement: a randomized controlled trial. *Advances in Skin Wound Care* 19:92–96.

Leicht, C., Bishop, N.C., and Goosey-Tolfrey, V.L. 2012. Submaximal exercise responses in tetraplegic, paraplegic and non spinal cord injured elite wheelchair athletes. *Scandinavian Journal of Medicine and Science in Sport* 22:729–736.

Leiper, J.B., Broad, N.P., and Maughan, R.J. 2001a. Effect of intermittent high-intensity exercise on gastric emptying in man. *Medicine and Science in Sports and Exercise* 33:1270–1278.

Leiper, J.B., Nicholas, C.W., Ali, A., Williams, C., and Maughan, R.J. 2005. The effect of intermittent high-intensity running on gastric emptying of fluids in man. *Medicine and Science in Sports and Exercise* 37:240–247.

Leiper, J.B., Prentice, A.S., Wrightson, C., and Maughan, R.J. 2001b. Gastric emptying of a carbohydrate-electrolyte drink during a soccer match. *Medicine and Science in Sports and Exercise* 33:1932–1938.

Levine, A.M., Nash, M.S., Green, B.A., Shea, J.D., and Aronica, M.J. 1992. An examination of dietary intakes and nutritional status of chronic healthy spinal cord injured individuals. *Paraplegia* 30:880–889.

Lin, V.W., Kim, K.H., Hsiao, I., and Brown, W. 2002. Functional magnetic stimulation facilitates gastric emptying. *Archives of Physical Medicine and Rehabilitation* 83:806–810.

Lu, C.L., Montgomery, P., Zou, X., Orr, W.C., and Chen, J.D. 1998. Gastric myoelectrical activity in patients with cervical spinal cord injury. *American Journal of Gastroenterology* 93:2391–2396.

McArdle, W.D., Katch, F.I., and Katch, V.L. 2000. *Exercise physiology; energy, nutrition and human performance*. Philadelphia: Lea and Febiger.

Mollinger, L.A., Spurr, G.B., Ghatit, E.I., Barboriak, J.J., Rooney, C.B., and Davidoff, D.D. 1985. Daily energy expenditure and basal metabolic rates in patients with spinal cord injury. *Archives of Physical Medicine and Rehabilitation* 66:420–426.

Moran, S.T., and Broad, E.M. 2012. Fluid balance in Australian wheelchair rugby athletes. *Medicine and Science in Sport and Exercise* 44(Suppl 1):S138.

Nemunaitis, G.A., Mejia, M., Nagy, J.A., Johnson, T., Chae, J., and Roach, M.J. 2010. A descriptive study on vitamin D levels in individuals with spinal cord injury in an acute inpatient rehabilitation setting. *Physical Medicine and Rehabilitation* 2:202–208.

Nicholas, C.W., Williams, C., Lakomy, H.K., Phillips, G., and Nowitz, A. 1995. Influence of ingesting a carbohydrate-electrolyte solution on endurance capacity during intermittent, high-intensity shuttle running. *Journal of Sports Sciences* 13:283–290.

Oleson, C.V., Patel, P.H., and Wuermser, L.A. 2010. Influence of season, ethnicity, and chronicity on vitamin D deficiency in traumatic spinal cord injury. *Journal of Spinal Cord Medicine* 33:202–213.

Patterson, S.D., and Gray, S.C. 2007. Carbohydrate-gel supplementation and endurance performance during intermittent high-intensity shuttle running. *International Journal of Sports Nutrition and Exercise Metabolism* 17:445–455.

Paulson, T., Leicht, C., Bishop, N., and Goosey-Tolfrey, V.L. 2013. Perceived exertion as a tool to self-regulate exercise in individuals with tetraplegia. *European Journal of Applied Physiology* 113:201–209.

Potvin, A., Nadon, R., Royer, D., and Farrar, D. 1996. The diet of the disabled athlete. *Science and Sports* 11:152–156.

Price, M.J. 2006.Thermoregulation during exercise in individuals with spinal cord injuries. *Sports Medicine* 20:457–463.

Price, M.J. 2010. Energy expenditure and metabolism during exercise in persons with a spinal cord injury. *Sports Medicine* 40:681–696.

Price, M.J., and Campbell, I.G. 1997. Thermoregulatory responses of able-bodied and paraplegic athletes to prolonged upper body exercise. *European Journal of Applied Physiology* 76:552–560.

Price, M.J., and Campbell, I.G. 1999. Thermoregulatory responses of able-bodied, paraplegic and a tetraplegic athlete at rest, during prolonged upper body exercise and during passive recovery. *Spinal Cord* 37:772–779.

Price, M.J., and Campbell, I.G. 2003. Effects of spinal cord lesion level upon thermoregulation during exercise in the heat. *Medicine and Science in Sports and Exercise* 35:1100–1107.

Price, M.J., Crosland, J., and Webborn, N. 2010. The travelling athlete. In *Wheelchair sport*, ed. V. Goosey-Tolfrey, 87–98. Champaign, IL: Human Kinetics.

Rajendran, S.K., Reiser, J.R., Bauman, W., Zhang, R.L., Gordon, S.K., and Korsten, M.A. 1992. Gastrointestinal transit after spinal cord injury: effect of cisapride. *American Journal of Gastroenterology* 87:1614–1617.

Reddy, M., Gill, S.S., Kalkar, S.R., Wu, W., Anderson, P.J., and Rochon, P.A. 2008. Treatment of pressure ulcers: a systematic review. *Journal of the American Medical Association* 300:2647–2662.

Ribeiro, S.M., Da Silva, R.C., De Castro, I.A., and Tirapegui, J. 2005. Assessment of nutritional status of active handicapped individuals. *Nutrition Research* 25:239–249.

Roy, J.L., Menear, K.S., Schmid, M.M., Hunter, G.R., and L.A. Malone. 2006. Physiological responses of skilled players during a competitive wheelchair tennis match. *Journal of Strength and Conditioning Research* 20:665–671.

Schmid, A., Huonker, M., Barturen, J.M., et al. 1998. Catecholamines, heart rate, and oxygen uptake during exercise in persons with spinal cord injury. *Journal of Applied Physiology* 85:635–641.

Sherman, A.R., and Barkley, M. 2011. Nutrition and wound healing. *Journal of Wound Care* 20:357–367.

Spendiff, O., and Campbell, I.G. 2002. The effect of glucose ingestion on endurance upper-body exercise and performance. *International Journal of Sports Medicine* 23:142–147.

Spendiff, O., and Campbell, I.G. 2003. Influence of glucose ingestion prior to prolonged exercise on selected responses of wheelchair athletes. *Adapted Physical Activity Quarterly* 20:80–90.

Spendiff, O., and Campbell, I.G. 2005. Influence of pre-exercise glucose ingestion of two concentrations on paraplegic athletes. *Journal of Sports Science* 23:21–30.

Spungen, A.M., Adkins, R.H., Stewart, C.A., et al. 2003. Factors influencing body composition in persons with spinal cord injury: a cross-sectional study. *Journal of Applied Physiology* 95:2398–2407.

Spungen, A.M., Wang, J., Pierson, R.N., and Bauman, W.A. 2000. Soft tissue body composition differences in monozygotic twins discordant for spinal cord injury. *Journal of Applied Physiology* 88:1310–1315.

Stallknecht, B., Lorentsen, J., Enevoldsen, L.H., Bülow, J., Biering-Sørensen, F., Galbo, H., and Kjaer, M. 2001. Role of the sympathoadrenergic system in adipose tissue metabolism during exercise in humans. *Journal of Physiology* 536:283–294.

Steinberg, L.L., Lauro, F.A., Sposito, M.M., et al. 2000. Catecholamine response to exercise in individuals with different levels of paraplegia. *Brazilian Journal of Medical and Biological Research* 33:913–918.

Sugiura, K., and Kobayashi, K. 1998. Effect of carbohydrate ingestion on sprint performance following continuous and intermittent exercise. *Medicine and Science in Sports and Exercise* 30:1624–1630.

Sutton, L., Wallace, J., Goosey-Tolfrey, V.L., Scott, M., and Reilly, T. 2009. Body composition of female wheelchair athletes. *International Journal of Sports Medicine* 30:259–265.

Tomey, K.M., Chen, D.M., Wang, X., and Braunschweig, C.L. 2005. Dietary intake and nutritional status of urban community-dwelling mean with paraplegia. *Archives in Physical Medicine and Rehabilitation* 86:664–671.

Tsintzas, O.K., Williams, C., Singh, R., Wilson, W., and Burrin, J. 1995. Influence of carbohydrate-electrolyte drinks on marathon running performance. *European Journal of Applied Physiology* 70:154–160.

Walters, J.L., Buchholz, A.C., and Martin Ginis, K.A. 2009. Evidence of dietary inadequacy in adults with chronic spinal cord injury. *Spinal Cord* 47:318–322.

Webborn, N., Price, M.J., Castle, P., and Goosey-Tolfrey, V.L. 2010. Cooling strategies improve intermittent sprint performance in the heat of athletes with tetraplegia. *British Journal of Sports Medicine* 44:455–460.

Wilber, R.L., and Moffatt, R.J. 1992. Influence of carbohydrate ingestion on blood glucose and performance in runners. *International Journal of Sports Nutrition* 2:317–327.

Williams, R.E., 3rd, Bauman, W.A., Spungen, A.M., et al. 2012. SmartPill technology provides safe and effective assessment of gastrointestinal function in persons with spinal cord injury. *Spinal Cord* 50:81–84.

Wilmet, E., Ismail, A.A., Heilporn, A., Welreads, D., and Bergmann, P. 1995. Longitudinal study of bone mineral content and soft tissue composition after spinal cord section. *Paraplegia* 33:674–677.

Witte, M.B., and Barbul, A. 2003. Arginine physiology and its implication for wound healing. *Wound Repair and Regeneration* 11:419–423.

Wright, D.A., Sherman, W.M., and Dernbach, A.R. 1991. Carbohydrate feedings before, during, or in combination improve cycling endurance performance. *Journal of Applied Physiology* 71:1082–1088.

Zhang, R.L., Chayes, Z., Korsten, M.A., and Bauman, W.A. 1994. Gastric emptying rates to liquid or solid meals appear to be unaffected by spinal cord injury. *American Journal of Gastroenterology* 89:1856–1858.

5 Cerebral Palsy and Acquired Brain Injuries

Jeanette Crosland and Craig Boyd

CONTENTS

5.1 INTRODUCTION

Cerebral palsy (CP) is the term used to describe several conditions of posture and motor impairment that result from an insult to the developing brain, in turn affecting central nervous system function (Bax et al. 2005). It is documented as the most common paediatric physical impairment (Odding et al. 2006), with symptoms varying widely between individuals. There are a number of other neurological conditions that can result in similar functional disturbances. Strokes and acute head trauma accidents are known antecedents to CP-like impairments. In sport for athletes with an impairment these conditions are classified alongside CP and many of the issues discussed here apply to athletes with these conditions. The level of functional ability of the individual athlete will determine which information is applicable. For the purposes of this chapter and for brevity, it should be assumed that associated neurological disorders as a consequence of acute trauma such as stroke and head injury are inferred when discussing CP.

The motor disorders of CP and related neurological dysfunction are often accompanied by disturbances of sensation, cognition, communication, perception, and/or behaviour, and/or by a seizure disorder (Rosenbaum et al. 2007). CP usually occurs before, during or after birth, or in the early years of childhood, and affects around one in every 400 children. The majority of research conducted in this area is largely clinical and based on children. Research with adult populations is less common. Consequently, very little is known about how the condition specifically affects sports performance variables in adult athletes with CP. Various studies have regularly reported that children with CP have delayed motor skill acquisition in comparison to similar-aged children without the condition (Rose et al. 2002). Delays in independent stance and walking control are often linked to poor postural balance associated with muscle coordinative asymmetry (Bleck 1994) and this can adversely affect movement economy. Severe forms of CP lead to a permanent wheelchair-bound state for the individual, where spasticity and involuntary movements such as shakes, twitches and elevated muscle tone expend energy in activities often deemed as sedentary in able-bodied (AB) counterparts.

It is clear that CP can have an adverse effect on physical development and maturation and, in turn, movement economy through childhood and adolescence. Moreover, it leads to a range of psycho-sociological issues that need to be considered in order to address appropriate energy demands and eating behaviours for an individual suffering with CP. There is also an increased incidence of epilepsy in individuals with CP which may require medication to manage.

This chapter explores the key aspects of understanding the nutritional issues associated with individuals with CP taking part in sport and exercise. It highlights the physical impairments associated with CP, outlining the role sporting classification can play in the evaluation of nutritional needs while underlining the necessity to individualise any nutritional strategy. In addition, it provides insight into the applied practice considerations for individuals with CP who take part in sport and exercise.

5.2   THE PHYSIOLOGY OF CEREBRAL PALSY

5.2.1   TERMINOLOGY AND SYMPTOMS

A striking feature of CP is the variability in its clinical presentation as a consequence of the complexities of dysfunction it manifests (Dobson et al. 2006). Motor control of an action depends upon visual, vestibular (inner ear) and somatosensory feedback (i.e. from soft tissues associated with joints) and the recruitment of various postural muscles as and when needed. However, individuals with CP have upper motor neuron damage (Sheean 2002). This in turn affects motor control by decreasing the number of effective motor units, theoretically reducing proprioception, kinaesthetic senses and resulting in abnormal muscle control (Damiano and Abel 1998). This reduces somatosensory feedback, consequently disproportionately increasing muscle activity in order to maintain balance and coordination (Burtner et al. 1998). Increased muscle activity for a given movement requires increased energy expenditure due to the inefficient ambulation of the individual. These neuromuscular factors are often accompanied by mechanical changes in posture resulting from bone deformities developed during maturation and severe spasticity in some muscle groups, which are suggested to contribute to the lack of control in these individuals (Burtner et al. 1998). In essence what we see is an individual exhibiting signs of poor coordination and increased effort to complete a given physical task or action.

The degree of impairment as a consequence of CP has been generally defined by descriptions that pertain to the number of limbs or region of the body that the condition affects. Minor impairments caused by CP may only affect one limb (monoplegia). More commonly, one side of the individual's body can be impaired resulting in hemiplegia, affecting lower limbs, trunk and upper limbs. Finally, diplegia is an observed impairment to the lower limbs more than the upper, sometimes with a degree of asymmetry (CPISRA 2011).

There are a number of symptoms associated with CP that are associated with each topography. The three broad symptoms affecting muscle control in athletes with CP are spastic, athetoid and ataxic cerebral palsy. In certain cases individuals may have a combination of all three types of CP. Spastic cerebral palsy refers to an exhibition of shortened muscles and a decreased range of motion around the joints and is present in most individuals who have CP. Individuals exhibiting this symptom often suffer from enforced flexion of the wrist or plantar flexion of the ankle, leading to difficulties in handling skills or an inability to heel strike and thus often walk with a pronounced asymmetrical gait.

Less commonly found in around 10–20% of CP sufferers is dyskinetic or athetoid cerebral palsy, where sufferers experience uncontrolled involuntary muscle contractions, which often occur all over the body. This manifests itself in the form of shakes and twitches, which can make fine motor skills challenging for the sufferer. Elevated energy expenditure is likely to be an outcome of athetoid symptoms since it has been found that there are elevated levels of co-contractions in muscle groups of children with hemiplegia (Feltham et al. 2010). The third and least common type of CP affecting around 5–10% of CP sufferers is ataxic cerebral palsy. Defined as an inability to activate the correct muscle patterns, sufferers of this particular symptom may also have poor spatial awareness and have trouble walking. All of the aforementioned conditions can be seen with a range of severity in ambulatory and those with non-ambulatory CP.

5.2.2 MUSCULOSKELETAL ISSUES AND SPORTING CLASSIFICATION

In sports competition for those with an impairment, it is important to ascertain the effect CP has upon an individual's performance. The determination of the degree to which impairment affects performance is a central component to the ethos of fair competition.

For equality in international competition, athletes are placed into classification categories for participation determined by the severity of their impairment. Classification seeks to fairly assess athletes in an attempt not to penalise those who enhance their physical attributes through training and diet. Furthermore, physical adaptations through training and diet should not promote changes to their classification (Tweedy and Vanlandewijck 2011). Classification aims to equate impairments of various types to permit fair competition.

The Cerebral Palsy International Sports and Recreation Association (CPISRA) and the International Paralympic Committee (IPC) classify all non-ambulatory

TABLE 5.1
Cerebral Palsy Classification Spectrum
Relative to Participation in Sports

Archery	CP 3, 4, 5, 6, 7, 8
Alpine skiing	CP 3, 4, 5, 6, 7, 8
Athletics	CP 3, 4, 5, 6, 7, 8
Basketball (wheelchair)	CP 4, 5, 6, 7, 8
Boccia	CP 1, 2
Curling	CP 3, 4, 5
Cycling	CP 3, 4, 5, 6, 7, 8
Equestrian	CP 3, 4, 5, 6, 7, 8
Fencing (wheelchair)	CP 3, 4, 5, 6, 7, 8
Nordic skiing	CP 3, 4, 5, 6, 7, 8
Powerlifting	CP 3, 4, 5, 6, 7, 8
Rowing	CP 3, 4, 5, 6, 7, 8
Sailing	CP 3, 4, 5, 6, 7, 8
Shooting	CP 3, 4, 5, 6, 7, 8
Sledge hockey (ice)	CP 4, 5, 6
Soccer (or football)	CP 5, 6, 7, 8
Swimming	CP 1, 2, 3, 4, 5, 6, 7, 8
Table tennis (wheelchair)	CP 3, 4, 5, 6, 7, 8
Tennis (wheelchair)	CP 3, 4, 5, 6

Source: Adapted from information derived from www.para-sport.org.uk.

and ambulatory athletes with CP. Each individual sport may possess classification nuances that are unique but in more general terms CP athletes are principally classed from CP1 (most affected by CP or related condition) to CP8 (least affected by CP or related brain trauma condition) for sports such as boccia, 7-a-side soccer, swimming, cycling and athletics. Some sports, for the purpose of IPC events, prefix the classification number with another number to distinguish between other disabilities competing in the same sporting event following a similar classification numbering system. For example, in track athletics, athletes with CP are classed as T32–T38 while wheelchair-bound athletes would range from T51 to T54, where T represents "track," the first number represents the form of impairment, and the second number represents the degree of impairment. Table 5.1 outlines the classifications of CP that participate in each of the Paralympic sports.

Within individual sports there may be events where the number of competitors is small and so different classes have to compete directly against each other. In these circumstances, there is often an adjustment factor points system employed to create parity across the classes. In athletics, for example, it is sometimes necessary for events to utilise the RAZA points scoring system (www.paralympic.org). RAZA is a mathematical algorithm based upon a database of previous performances across the

TABLE 5.2
Cerebral Palsy Classification Categories for Non-Ambulatory Athletes

Class 1	The most severely disabled. Individuals who have to use an electric chair for independent mobility and who will need assistance with daily living skills. All four limbs will be severely affected.
Class 2	CP2 athletes often use an electric chair for preference, as whilst they can propel a manual wheelchair, slopes, uneven ground and distance will present problems. Again, all four limbs will be affected, but some limited function will be evident.
Class 3	CP3 athletes can manipulate a wheelchair but will usually have some difficulty in trunk range of movement and balance, affecting their wheelchair mobility. At least one upper limb will be significantly affected.
Class 4	The athlete presents with no functional limitation of upper limbs, excellent wheelchair control and good trunk mobility.

Source: Adapted from information derived from www.cpisra.org.

classes for a given event. For example, in field events such as shot put, the distance thrown in metres is converted into a points score to account for the severity of the impairment. The overall competition places are then decided by ranking the points scored rather than the absolute distance thrown. In the case of team sports, there is often a competition rule whereby each team must field a given ratio of athletes from across the class range. In football, a modified 7-a-side game is played. Rules state that each team must field at least one CP5 or CP6 and can only field two CP8 (associated neurological disorder impaired athletes). In both cases this allows for a range of athletes with CP to participate on an equal standing.

Although there are occasions where athletes from different classes compete directly with each other, there still exists a series of descriptors specifically for each class (CP1–CP8). Tables 5.2 and 5.3 illustrate the general descriptors associated with both non-ambulatory (CP1–CP4) and ambulatory (CP5–CP8) cerebral palsy classes across sports.

It is noteworthy that CP1–CP4 (Table 5.2) are a continuum of impairments, whereas CP5–CP8 (Table 5.3) are based upon different topographical impairments where more discrete regions of the body are affected. This means that there is not necessarily a clear progression of impairment descending from CP8–CP5, but different types of impairment.

What is apparent from the descriptors in Tables 5.2 and 5.3 is the qualitative nature of the classes which encompass all aspects of the symptoms associated with CP. Like all classification systems in para-sport the evaluation of an athlete undergoing classification includes clinical and functional assessments and in some cases, performance-based observations. The descriptors permit a case-by-case approach to classify each individual athlete fairly. Classes are not devised to segregate specific symptoms but aim to collate similar levels of impairment across symptoms. What is clear across the classifications is that, to varying degrees, the spectrum of impairments associated with CP often lead to musculoskeletal asymmetry and thus over- and underdevelopment of the musculoskeletal system in terms of bony structures, muscle development, neuromuscular coordination and balance. In cases of severe

TABLE 5.3
Cerebral Palsy Classification Categories for Ambulatory Athletes

Class 5[a]	These athletes are diplegic but are fully ambulatory without assistance. They have a noticeable hip and shoulder rotation when walking, inwardly rotated hips, knees and feet in standing/walking. There is only minimal difficulty with upper limbs. Exertion will increase tone and decrease function. The athletes will have difficulty in turning, pivoting and stopping, usually running only short distances due to involvement in both lower limbs. Stride length is reduced/decreased with exertion.
Class 6	These athletes also walk without any assistive devices, but have involvement in all four limbs. They have particular problems in trying to control their movements. Walking is laboured and uncoordinated, often rolling head movement during running. CP6 athletes will have trouble stopping and changing direction quickly. Coordination and timing problems will be seen in more complex movements. Explosive movements are difficult to perform.
Class 7	CP7 athletes are generally hemiplegic, but walking with a marked limp is often noticed. The dominant upper limb should have normal strength and movement. The affected upper limb is usually more apparent during activity, possibly flat footed on affected side when running, or conversely does not have a heel strike. Often head tilting to one side can be observed. The athlete will walk with a noticeable limp, but may appear to have a smoother stride when running but will not have a heel strike. The athlete has difficulty when pivoting and balancing on the impaired side, and therefore often pivots on the unaffected side. The athlete's affected arm muscles will have an increase in tone when running and appear bent when walking. There are many patterns in the lower limb demonstrating spasticity in the hemiplegic limb. Training does not change these patterns; it only changes the quality of the movement of functional ability.
Class 8	These athletes are minimally affected diplegic, hemiplegic, monoplegic or have minimal movement control problems. They will run without noticeable limp, but impairment is more evident on exertion; must demonstrate evidence of a functional impairment during testing. Athletes with minimal involvement may appear to have near normal function when running, but the athlete must demonstrate a limitation in function to classifiers based on evidence of spasticity (increased tone), ataxic, athetoid or dystonic movements while performing in competition or in training.

Source: Adapted from information derived from www.cpisra.org.
[a] CP5–CP8 are different impairments and are not a continuum.

spasticity, the stress placed upon bony features and sites of muscle attachments may be greater than that in a normal functioning musculoskeletal system. Hemiplegic and non-ambulatory sufferers of CP may also experience abnormalities in bone mineral density due to asymmetrical or limited loading on bone tissue. Those working in para-sport should be aware of this possibility. Dual x-ray absorptiometry (DXA) scans are useful to identify the issue and there could be an issue of duty of care for sports staff to ensure referral for medical treatment if the individual is being encouraged to take part in any sports where there is an increased risk of bone damage. Consequently, body composition and skeletal integrity, movement economy and physical capacity are all implicated for the CP athlete. As such, the impact upon

---

COMMENTARY BOX 5.1

EXPERT COMMENTARY: Muscle strength development in CP
 Dr. Keith Baar, University of California, Davis

Question: Do you think that athletes with cerebral palsy can improve muscle
 function in their affected limbs?
Answer: The decreased electrical signal to the muscle due to impaired motor
 cortex function reduces strength and muscle function. One thing
 that we know about muscle recruitment is that if you work to fail-
 ure/fatigue, you will recruit all possible motor units within a muscle
 group. This results in an increase in protein synthesis and muscle
 hypertrophy even when you don't lift heavy weights. Therefore I
 think that the way forward for these athletes is to push them to at
 least positive failure in each exercise. They don't have to lift a lot
 of weight, but they do have to try to lift until they physically can't
 anymore. This will cause a significant increase in muscle size, and
 strength will increase in proportion to the weight lifted. With this
 type of strategy, these athletes will not only improve performance,
 but they will also have a dramatic effect on other health outcomes.

---

energy demands for activity may differ from their able-bodied counterparts and
these issues must be considered in any nutritional strategies.

5.3 NUTRITION

5.3.1 Nutrition Issues in Cerebral Palsy

The characteristics relating to each class of CP are important indicators or sign-
posts when considering the nutritional requirements of athletes with CP. The wide
variation observed in these characteristics from class CP1 to CP8 is reflected in a
range of nutritional issues that need consideration. Classification therefore is a useful tool in beginning to understand the potential nutritional issues that may arise for
an individual. Ultimately, understanding the specific conditions and impairments
individuals possess is of most importance. The ambulation status, and presence or
absence of athetosis, spasticity and ataxia will impact upon the energy requirements.
In more extreme cases, some of these factors, as well as oral motor dysfunction, will
also impact on an individual's ability to eat and hence may limit their nutritional
intake. Finally there are social and psychological factors that may also need to be
considered. Consequently, calculating the nutritional requirements of an individual
with CP is a multifaceted task.

There is a lack of research regarding the nutritional requirements of athletes with
CP. It is possible that the broad spectrum of factors that need consideration when
conducting such research are partly responsible for the dearth of information in

this area. Where possible this chapter has drawn on the limited amount of research available in adult and, more commonly, childhood CP and used this to draw logical conclusions, helping provide practical advice for those working with athletes with CP. However, the chapter will emphasise that it is vital an individual case-to-case assessment is adopted.

5.3.2 ENERGY EXPENDITURE

The classification of an athlete may be a useful first indicator when considering energy expenditure, and could offer some guidance. For example, athletes in CP class 7 and 8 generally train and compete in sports such as football, cycling, swimming or athletics (see Table 5.1) and their energy expenditure is likely to be more aligned with the requirements of able-bodied athletes in those sports. In contrast, athletes in class 1 or 2 are likely to be electric wheelchair users and are likely to participate in sports such as boccia. In sporting terms their energy expenditure during sporting activity and mobilisation may be relatively low, but the ataxic or athetosis symptoms often associated with this level of impairment may mean that uncontrolled shakes and twitches lead to an unduly elevated basal metabolic rate (BMR). Early work by Johnson et al. (1997) examining non-sporting populations reported elevated BMR is non-ambulatory individuals. However some researchers have found lower resting energy expenditure even in those with severe spasticity (Stallings et al. 1996) and concluded that low energy intakes (i.e. low energy availability, as outlined in Chapter 3) may be the issue.

Research in this field is clearly limited, however the first work undertaken in free living non-athletic male and female, ambulatory and non-ambulatory adults with CP using the doubly labelled water method (Johnson et al. 1997) produced some interesting findings. On average, the total energy expenditure (TEE) of these individuals was lower than that of able-bodied individuals. However, it was noticeable that there was a wide variation in TEE ranging from 5844 to 16,284 kJ/d (1396–3890 kcal/d) and BMR ranged from 4060 to 8916 kJ/d (970–2130 kcal/d). After adjusting for fat free mass, a trend towards a higher resting metabolic rate in the non-ambulatory individuals was reported, possibly due to athetosis. While considering a number of factors that may affect energy requirements, the authors concluded that the only single measure to be a significant predictor of total energy requirements was ambulation status. Similarly, energy expenditure in children with CP has been related to ambulation status (Bandini et al. 1991) and in children with mild CP it has been observed that although energy expended during walking is higher than that expended by their able-bodied peers (Piccinini et al. 2007), physical activity levels (PAL) and TEE were observed to be lower, resulting in a lower overall energy requirement (Bell and Davies 2010). This could lend credence to the assumption that those with athetosis do indeed have higher energy requirements, and even in the absence of athetosis, walking gait can increase energy expenditure.

Producing guidelines for the estimating energy expenditure of individuals with CP has proved difficult (Johnson et al. 1997). The wide variation in results suggests that traditional methods of estimating energy requirements using equations for resting metabolic rate, and adding subjective factors for other components may not be applicable for many individuals in this population. The guidelines considered best

---

COMMENTARY BOX 5.2

COACH'S INSIGHT: What do you believe are the biggest differences in coaching athletes with a disability compared to able-bodied athletes?

> I have found using video feedback a key coaching method with many of the cerebral palsy athletes I work with. The athlete's body often provides limited or disrupted feedback, so it is very helpful to be able to see what positions look like, or what the skill looks like, so the athlete can learn to relate a certain sensation they experience to a position and whether it is technically good or bad.

—Emily Nolan, strength and conditioning coach

---

practice by Johnson et al. (1997) were to use RMR, percentage body fat (as measured by DXA), ambulation status, and gender as the best predictors of requirement. Since the early studies, DXA has become more commonly available and this framework, combined with dietary assessment, is perhaps a good starting point for the assessment of energy expenditure and hence energy requirements of athletes with CP.

5.3.3 BODY COMPOSITION ASSESSMENT

One tool available to help the practitioner determine the appropriateness of energy intake relative to expenditure in an athlete with CP is to track changes in body composition over time, in addition to the impact of genetic traits, training and the physical impact of their CP. As outlined in Chapter 12, assessment procedures in CP populations may require some modification or careful selection due to the variable influence of the impairment on bone mineral density (BMD) and muscular and postural asymmetry. Figure 5.1 summarises some unique problems in assessing body composition in athletes with CP and gives suggestions as to appropriate methods to utilise.

Reliability and validity of standard body composition procedures must be considered, and so adjustments for the individual may have to be made, and noted in the records, to ensure repeatability in sequential measures. For example, in an athlete with right sided hemiplegia, it may be more appropriate to undertake skinfold and girth measures on the left side of their body. Similarly, bilateral girth measures can be useful to track responses to training in instances where the training modality aims to preferentially improve strength on the more affected side of the body. As discussed in Chapter 12, anthropometric measures should be undertaken using standardised procedures and repeat measures undertaken by the same skilled practitioner wherever possible.

5.3.4 DIETARY INTAKES AND FEEDING DIFFICULTIES

Research into the nutritional intake, adequacy, and needs of athletes with CP is lacking. Some research is established in the nutritional issues of children with CP, and while we cannot presume that it is directly transferable, it gives us some indictors of

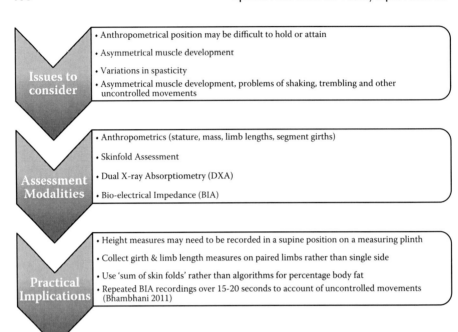

FIGURE 5.1 Assessment of body composition in cerebral palsy. (Section adapted from Bhambhani 2011.)

potential problems in some athletes. Athletes with CP in the lower level classes are likely to have some feeding difficulties that will have been part of the athlete's life since childhood. Kuperminc and Stevenson (2008) summarise that growth and nutritional problems are common in children with CP and that these problems are more common in those with greater motor impairment. An individual's inability to feed can restrict intake, and repeated bouts of illness could potentially make nutritional requirements higher, potentially resulting in malnutrition and consequently adverse effects on muscle strength, respiratory function, wound healing and immune function.

It is important that those with feeding problems have appropriate help from staff or carers to assist them at meal times. Meal times will take longer and the process of eating may be quite messy. Staff must handle this practically and sympathetically to help the athlete optimise their nutritional intake. In some instances it may be necessary to order food with a modified texture appropriate to the individual feeding difficulty.

Food choices and behaviour changes can go beyond texture modification requirements and normal fussy eating behaviour depending on the area of the brain affected by the individual's CP. For example:

- Difficulty eating new textures
- Increased sensory sensitivity
- Aversion to accepting new foods
- Poor tolerance of certain colours or packaging
- Dislike of certain temperatures (e.g. hot or cold food)
- Changes in eating time or surroundings

As a result, potential deficiencies of macro- and micronutrients may arise depending on the exact nature of the food aversion which may compromise nutritional adequacy during training phases and in particular the provision of food during residential training camps and competitions.

Assessing the actual intake of an athlete with CP who has a feeding difficulty can be difficult. Attempts have been made (Archer 1991; Lukens and Linscheid 2008) to validate assessment methods of eating and mealtime behaviour in individuals with autism and a range of other conditions that display selective eating habits. Some additional questions not normally included in dietary assessment by diet history have been suggested. Once assessment of intake has been made, behavioural change may be required to ensure an adequate intake for the individual's sporting requirements, and the support of a clinical dietitian and/or clinical psychologist may be useful alongside other team members to assist in this process.

Where feeding difficulties are significant and nutritional intake substantially restricted, food supplements may be warranted to include as part of the athlete's oral intake. A small number of those with CP may use enteral feeding, usually via a gastrostomy tube—an artificial tract created between the stomach and the abdominal surface. When working with an athlete using supplements or enteral feeding, it is vital that medical/clinical advice is sought. These individuals will normally have a support team including a doctor, clinical dietitian and nurse, who should be integrated into the overall support team for the athlete. The key message for the sports nutrition practitioner is the importance of individuality and the need to work carefully with other team members involved in the care and training of the athlete.

5.3.5 Micronutrient Intake

A review of vitamin and mineral status of children with CP was conducted by Schoendorfer et al. (2010) and concluded that the reduced food intake found in some individuals caused a reduction in all nutrients, increasing the possibility of nutrient deficiencies resulting in, for example, a compromised immune system. Henderson et al. (2004) reported that many young individuals with CP have a diminished bone density, which may be related to dietary deficiencies, the use of anticonvulsants, inability to undertake weight bearing exercise and possibly previous skeletal fractures. Therefore bone density, vitamin D status and dietary intake of calcium should all be assessed in athletes with CP. While the maintenance of an adequate dietary intake of calcium and maintaining adequate vitamin D status are important, supplementation and medical treatment using bone building drugs may be necessary in some cases.

Although much of the work cited here is taken from child populations, in the absence of any more specific research at this point it is pertinent to bear in mind that there will be a number of individuals with CP in sport who have these problems, which will most probably continue into adult life. Adequate micronutrient intake is important and the practitioner may have to be inventive in encouraging this to be achieved through dietary means. In some instances, oral nutritional supplements in the form of milk- or fruit-based drinks may be prescribed through the individual's medical team. Other individuals may use a vitamin and mineral supplement, which within Paralympic sport must then also comply with anti-doping regulations as outlined in Chapter 11.

5.3.6   Fibre Intake

If food intake is in any way compromised there is the possibility that fibre intake may be inadequate. Good bowel function requires:

- Adequate fibre intake
- Adequate fluid intake
- Physical activity

As with athletes with a spinal cord injury (outlined in Chapter 4), toilet access can be difficult for a wheelchair user, particularly those reliant on electric wheelchairs. As a consequence of this and more limited physical activity, care must be taken when altering dietary fibre intake for these athletes. The medical care team must be involved in any changes to fluid and fibre intake and the management of intake in situations which may impact on bowel function such as travel and eating in countries where the risk of food-related illness is greater.

5.3.7   Sweat Rates and Fluid Requirements during Exercise

As with all nutritional issues discussed in this chapter, there will be a wide variation in sweat rates and hence fluid requirements for athletes with CP. As with energy requirements, those in class 7 and 8 sports may be expected to show a range of sweat rates similar to able-bodied equivalent sports. Athletes displaying athetosis may have increased sweat rates due to the involuntary muscle action. Unnithan and Wilk (2005) reported some differences in sweat gland numbers between dominant and nondominant arms in children with hemiplegic CP but not sufficient to predict any difference in evaporative cooling effectiveness between sides. Korpelainen et al. (1993) found that there was an asymmetry to the sweat pattern, with increased sweating on the non-paretic side of adults with hemispheric brain infarction when they were exposed to a heat stimulus at rest. In contrast, Maltais et al. (2004a, 2004b) found that participants with CP demonstrate thermal strain responses that were similar to those without CP when tested using arm cranking exercise and a greater thermal strain when a treadmill was used. The sports nutrition practitioner must therefore understand the importance of considering each individual's needs carefully, and that fluid requirements, even within a team, may vary considerably. As outlined in Chapter 3, individual assessment of sweat loss and fluid intake is required in order to optimise hydration status before, during and after exercise in athletes with CP.

5.4   SUMMARY

Cerebral palsy involves a wide spectrum of physiological and medical issues which may be present to a greater or lesser extent in the athlete with CP. Within the sphere

---

COMMENTARY BOX 5.3

COACH'S INSIGHT: What sports nutrition practices have had the biggest impact on the training capability or performance of your athletes?

Recovery! Recovery is more specific to many athletes with an impairment. For example, in CP, the recovery of the nervous system is crucial to help them train effectively session after session and can take longer than in an AB athlete. If their nervous system does not recover quickly, they will tend to spasm more, which disrupts their sleep and further delays recovery.

—Iryna Dvoskina, athletics coach of multiple Paralympic medallists

---

of sporting competition, classification also encompasses impairments of a post-natal neurological origin such as stroke and acute head trauma.

From a muscle function perspective, the range of issues include imbalances through impairment of contractile function. Skeletal deformities are also often associated with CP and together they may lead to partial or total loss of ambulation and difficulties in maintaining a symmetrical posture. The sociopsychological challenges that often manifest themselves in childhood through feeding issues can be prevalent particularly in athletes who rely upon medical care support for daily needs.

The practitioner should consider the sporting classification of CP as a starting point in the evaluation of the needs of the individual. Classification encompasses a broad range of impairment within each class, and as such, individuals can vary even within a given classification. For appropriate and effective nutritional management, it is vital that as much information as possible is gathered about the physical demands for sport and daily living activities of the athlete as well as the typical nutritional intake of the individual. From this knowledge base an individual plan should be made for each athlete.

5.5 TAKE-HOME MESSAGES

1. CP results in a wide range of impairment, from a very low level of impairment to those who require daily care in all activities, all of whom have the opportunity to participate in sport and exercise. The limited research means that the nutritional assessment and support provided to each athlete must be individualised, with a full understanding of their specific capabilities in order to provide appropriate sports nutrition advice to optimise their training response and competition performance.

2. Estimating energy requirements of the individual requires an understanding of the physical capabilities of the athlete, and the following points are useful to integrate:
   - BMR in those with CP may be lower than in AB individuals
   - The presence of involuntary muscle spasm usually leads to elevated energy expenditure

---

COMMENTARY BOX 5.4

COACH'S INSIGHT: What are the biggest differences in coaching athletes with a disability compared to able-bodied athletes?

The general training concept and structure is the same, however with CP, the athlete will fatigue more quickly. Furthermore, the specific strength exercises you may prescribe will be different, as you have to balance their muscle structure and function and balance in an athlete with CP, and this will be very individual.

—Iryna Dvoskina, athletics coach of multiple Paralympic medallists

---

- Athetosis may restrict daily living activities and reduce total energy requirements
- Movement economy of the individual may elevate energy expenditure in ambulation
- Low energy availability may be present in wheelchair-reliant individuals where the focus has been the prevention of weight gain for the ease of carers.

3. Athletes with CP may exhibit food aversions and feeding difficulties which do not necessarily 'match' their physical impairment. The sports nutrition practitioner is encouraged to look beyond the possibility of 'fussy eating' to determine the true nature of these aversions and how they may impact on nutrient intake.

REFERENCES

Archer, L.A. 1991. The children's eating behavior inventory: reliability and validity results. *Journal of Pediatric Psychology* 16:629–642.

Bandini, L.G., Schoeller, D.A., Fukagawa, N.K., Wykes, L.J., and Dietz, W.H. 1991. Body composition and energy expenditure in adolescents with cerebral palsy or myelodysplasia. *Paediatric Research* 29:70–77.

Bax, M., Goldstein, M., Rosenbaum, P., et al. 2005. Proposed definition and classification of cerebral palsy. *Developmental Medicine and Child Neurology* 47:571–576.

Bell, K.L., and Davies, P.S. 2010. Energy expenditure and physical activity of ambulatory children with cerebral palsy and of typically developing children. *American Journal of Clinical Nutrition* 92:313–319.

Bhambhani, Y. 2011. Physiology. In *The Paralympic athlete*, ed. Y.C. Vanlandewijck and W.R. Thompson, 51–73. West Sussex: Wiley-Blackwell.

Bleck, E.E. 1994. The sense of balance. *Developmental Medicine and Child Neurology* 36:377–378.

Burtner, P.A., Qualls, C., and Woollacott, M.H. 1998. Muscle activation characteristics of stance balance control in children with spastic cerebral palsy. *Gait and Posture* 8:163–174.

CPISRA. 2011. http://www.cpisra.org/files/classification/Classification_CPISRA_Brochure_Classification_Profiles.pdf (accessed April 10, 2011).

Damiano, D.L., and Abel, M.F. 1998. Functional outcomes of strength training in spastic cerebral palsy. *Archive of Physical Medicine and Rehabilitation* 79:119–125.

Dobson, F., Morris, M.E., Baker, R., and Kerr, G.H. 2006. Gait classification in children with cerebral palsy: a systematic review. *Gait and Posture* 25:140–152.

Feltham, M.G., Ledebt, A., Deconnick, F.J.A., and Savelsbergh, G.J.P. 2010. Assessment of neuromuscular activation of the upper limbs in children with spastic hemiparetic cerebral palsy during a dynamical task. *Journal of Electromyography and Kinesiology* 20:448–456.

Henderson, R.C., Kairalla, B.S., Abbas, A., and Stevenson, R.D. 2004. Predicting low bone density in children and young adults with quadriplegic cerebral palsy. *Developmental Medicine and Child Neurology* 46:164–169.

Johnson, R.K., Hildreth, H.G., Contompasis, S.H., and Goran, M.L. 1997. Total energy expenditure in adults with cerebral palsy as assessed by doubly labelled water. *Journal of the American Dietetic Association* 97:966–970.

Korpelainen, J.T., Sotaniemi, K.A., and Myllyla, V.V. 1993. Asymmetric sweating in stroke: a prospective quantitative study of patients with hemispheral brain infarction. *Neurology* 43:1211–1214.

Kuperminc, M.N., and Stevenson, R.D. 2008. Growth and nutrition disorders in children with cerebral palsy. *Developmental Disabilities Research Reviews* 14:137–146.

Lukens, C.T., and Linscheid, T.R. 2008. Development and validation of an inventory to assess mealtime behaviour problems in children with autism. *Journal of Autism and Developmental Disorders* 38:342–352.

Maltais, D., Unnithan, V., Wilk, B., and Bar-Or, O. 2004a. Responses of children with cerebral palsy to arm-crank exercise in the heat. *Medicine and Science in Sports and Exercise* 36:191–197.

Maltais, D., Wilk, B., Unnithan, V., and Bar-Or, O. 2004b. Responses of children with cerebral palsy to treadmill walking exercise in the heat. *Medicine and Science in Sports and Exercise* 36:1674–1681.

Odding, E., Roebroeck, M.E., and Stam, H.J. 2006. The epidemiology of cerebral palsy: incidence, impairments and risk factors. *Disability and Rehabilitation* 28:183–191.

Piccinini, L., Cimolin, V., Galli, M., Berti, M., Crivellini, M., and Turconi, A.C. 2007. Quantification of energy expenditure during gait in children affected by cerebral palsy. *Europa Medicophysica* 43:7–12.

Rose, J., Wolff, D.R., Jones, V.K., Bloch, D.A., Oehlert, J.W., and Gamble, J.G. 2002. Postural balance in children with cerebral palsy. *Developmental Medicine and Child Neurology* 44:58–63.

Rosenbaum, P., Paneth, N., Leviton, A., Goldstein, M., and Bax, M. 2007. A report: the definition and classification of cerebral palsy. *Developmental Medicine and Child Neurology* 49:516–521.

Schoendorfer, N., Boyd, R., and Davies, P.S. 2010. Micronutrient adequacy and morbidity: paucity of information in children with cerebral palsy. *Nutrition Reviews* 68:739–748.

Sheean, G. 2002. The pathophysiology of spasticity. *European Journal of Neurology* 9:3–9.

Stallings, V.A., Zemel, B.S., Davies, J.C., Cronk, C.E., and Charney, E.B. 1996. Energy expenditure of children and adolescents with severe disabilities: a cerebral palsy model. *American Journal of Clinical Nutrition* 64:627–634.

Tweedy, S.M., and Vanlandewijck, Y.C. 2011. International Paralympic Committee position stand—background and scientific principles of classification in Paralympic sport. *British Journal of Sports Medicine* 45:259–269.

Unnithan, V.B., and Wilk, B. 2005. The effect of upper-limb dominance on forearm sweating patterns in children and adolescents with cerebral palsy. *Pediatric Exercise Science* 17:182–189.

6 Amputees

Nanna L. Meyer and Stephanie Edwards

CONTENTS

6.1 INTRODUCTION

Amputation of a limb generally means a permanent impairment with decreased mobility, at least in the short term but most likely also long term. In the United States about 82% of all amputations are due to vascular conditions, 16% of amputations are due to trauma, and 2% result from inflammatory causes, cancer, or birth defects (Dillingham et al. 2002). Athletes with an amputation are more commonly individuals who have suffered a congenital malformation or cancer leading to amputation, rather than vascular causes. Physical activity and sport participation are important to amputees' psychological and physiological wellbeing, being associated with favorable outcomes in a broad range of health parameters, including the cardio-pulmonary system, mental wellbeing, social integration, and general physical abilities (Bragaru et al. 2011). Data show that younger individuals with unilaterial transtibial amputations achieve greater physical performance with fewer issues when participating in sports compared with older individuals who may have bilateral transfemoral amputations (Bragaru et al. 2011). Based on the Paralympic classification system (International Paralympic Committee 2007), athletes with an amputation fit into the impairment type of loss of limb or limb deficiency. Full or partial absence of bones or joints, as a consequence of amputation due to illness, trauma, or congenital limb deficiency (e.g. dysmelia), is considered impairment. Athletes are classified not only relative to their impairment, but also based on sport (as outlined in Chapter 2).

Athletes with an upper extremity amputation or limb deficiency can easily participate in most sports, with or without the use of an adaptive device. Adaptive equipment for athletes with amputations has greatly improved and the variety of options are remarkable. Today, amputees can participate in virtually any sport, regardless of level of competition.

Skiing is very popular for amputees, partly due to the advanced technologies available for them to engage in winter sports. Due to the stiff ski boots, below-knee amputees can ski using a prosthesis with a multiaxial ankle or an ankle with a pre-fixed dorsiflexion. Those with above-knee amputation or hip disarticulation can use a three-track system, with skis attached to crutches and a third ski on the intact leg. Finally, skiers with bilateral above-knee amputations or hip disarticulation can choose a monoski, which is mounted under a sled (Bergeron 1999). A skier with an amputation can go as fast as an able-bodied skier and the feeling of speed and precision in a mountainous environment must provide a thrill to many amputees who may otherwise face barriers in their daily activities.

Cycling is also a popular sport for amputees. Pedaling devices such as toe clips facilitate the cycling amputee's up and down strokes. The more proximal the amputation, the more likely the athlete will choose to ride without their prosthesis.

While most Paralympic sports allow prostheses in competition, they are not permitted in swimming at international competitions. However, for recreational swimmers there are various prosthetic limbs, including fin attachments.

In running, prosthetics are commonly used if the amputation is, at a minimum, below-knee. In fact, these prostheses are so well designed that the athlete can develop a normal running cadence, contributing to the current debate of whether these devices put able-bodied athletes at a disadvantage. This topic will be discussed

---

COMMENTARY BOX 6.1

COACH'S INSIGHT: What are the biggest differences in coaching athletes with an impairment compared to able-bodied athletes?

Athletes with an amputation cannot undertake as much vertical loading as other track athletes due to the impact on their stump. Therefore you have to incorporate more water running/pool sessions.

—Iryna Dvoskina, athletics coach of multiple Paralympic medallists

later in the chapter. For athletes with above-knee amputations, running becomes more challenging; the running stride is more like a hop-skip type pattern, due to a prolonged swing phase of the prosthetic limb (Bragaru et al. 2011).

Interestingly, some athletes with an amputation choose not to use a prosthetic limb, preferring to use crutches instead. A famous American skiing amputee, Diana Golden-Brosnihan, who unfortunately passed away several years ago due to the return of the cancer that initially forced an above-knee amputation at age 12 years, completed both her dryland and her on-snow training and competitions without a prosthesis. A gold medalist at the Calgary 1988 Paralympics, she used one ski and two outriggers (forearm crutches with ski tips attached) in her initial years as a skier. In later years, she abandoned the outriggers in favor of regular ski poles so she could go faster. Diana never used an artificial leg and became well known for running with crutches. In fact, Diana Golden-Brosnihan ran up the mountains during a training camp in Austria alongside able-bodied athletes, including one of the authors of this chapter (unpublished observation, N. Meyer). Diana was not only an inspiration to European skiers at the time but changed the public's perspective and appreciation for athletes with an impairment in America. Diana was inducted into the Women's Sports Foundation International Hall of Fame and the National Ski Hall of Fame in 1997 (Litsky 2001).

The lack of limbs can present many challenges in active individuals, depending on the level of amputation. While athletes with amputations may not show compromised physiological responses to exercise, there are other issues related to the missing body part which athletes with an amputation manage daily. From a nutritional perspective, energy expenditure may be increased due to the inefficiency of movement, with or without fitted prostheses. It is common for athletes with an amputation to be naturally asymmetric. Swimmers, for example, have difficulty maintaining balance, thus oscillating more frequently with a less effective streamline position, which may increase energy expenditure and decrease performance capacity compared with able-bodied athletes (Bragaru et al. 2011). This higher energy demand also requires greater attention paid to macro- and micronutrients. Asymmetric movements may disrupt the kinetic chain and compensatory strategies may also overload other areas or links, increasing the risk of injury (Rice et al. 2011). In addition, athletes with an amputation can suffer from pressure sores and subsequent infection at the site where the prosthetic and stump of the amputation intersect, requiring immune-modulating nutritional strategies to be incorporated. Finally, depending on the sport, training environment, and physical discomfort, athletes with an amputation may be at risk of dehydration due to restrictions in being able to handle fluid (for example, an athlete using two crutches to "run" in a triathlon) or limited access to bathroom facilities (such as a sit-skier).

This chapter will focus on nutritional issues common to athletes with an amputation. First, common medical problems experienced by athletes with an amputation will be presented. Following, energy expenditure and body composition are discussed, underlining the difficulty of measuring each in amputees. Finally, specific nutritional issues in athletes with an amputation are highlighted. Due to the fact that almost no data exist on nutritional status in amputees, three elite athletes with an amputation were interviewed. Their unique challenges will be the entry point of the discussions related to nutrition issues of this population.

6.2 MEDICAL ISSUES IN ATHLETES WITH AN AMPUTATION

6.2.1 CHRONIC MEDICAL CONDITIONS

In general, athletes with an amputation are not at greater risk for injury compared to their able-bodied counterparts. However, some research shows that amputees have elevated risk for chronic complications to cardiovascular, metabolic, and musculoskeletal systems.

Modan et al. (1998) studied coronary risk factors of 201 traumatic unilateral lower-limb male amputees, each wounded during military service with a mean age of 58.6 years. Anthropometrics, heart rate, blood pressure, cholesterol and triglyceride levels were evaluated and a glucose tolerance test was administered. Anthropometric data, lipoprotein profiles, mean heart rate and blood pressure were similar between amputees and age-matched controls. Plasma glucose was also similar in the fasting state and after glucose load. Insulin levels, however, were significantly different, with higher insulin concentrations found in amputees both when fasted and after a glucose load. Although not significant, there was a trend toward an increased prevalence of hypertension, hyperlipidemia, and myocardial infarction in amputees. Coagulation measurements of blood samples showed increased coagulation in amputees compared to controls. All of these results may be attributed to chronic mental and physical stress endured by veteran amputees (Modan et al. 1998). Although many athletes with an amputation have endured a traumatic event that led to their amputation, many were also born with congenital defects that left them without a limb and are therefore at lower risk of this chronic mental and physical stress. In addition, daily exercise training as part of an active lifestyle most likely reduces health complications associated with the metabolic syndrome. Thus whether these medical findings can be generalized to all amputees is uncertain.

Athletes with an amputation are at greater risk for cardiovascular complications. The size of central and peripheral arteries and associated blood flow were compared between highly trained able-bodied athletes and those with an impairment. Diastolic inner vessel diameter of the thoracic and abdominal aorta and common femoral artery were measured by duplex sonography. The diameter of the femoral artery proximal to the lesion in athletes with a below-knee amputation was 21% smaller than that of able-bodied, untrained subjects. This may be attributed to the decreased metabolic and musculature needs of the amputated limb (Huonker et al. 2003).

6.2.2 INJURIES

Data on injuries in athletes with an impairment are difficult to collect due to differing definitions of an injury. Some of the research available describes the injury as upper or lower extremity but does not go into detail about what part of the limb was affected (i.e. shoulder, elbow, hip, knee, or ankle; Ferrara and Peterson 2000). The lack of uniformity in the definition of an injury makes it difficult to make generalizations about injuries endured by amputees. Ambulating athletes with an impairment (across all classes) are more likely to suffer injuries to the lower extremities than to the upper extremities and also more commonly than those who use a wheelchair for daily mobilization (Ferrara and Peterson 2000). Lower extremity injuries to the stump, spine, and intact limbs are most common in athletes with a lower-limb amputation. Stump injuries are frequent and include skin abrasions, pressure sores, blisters and rashes due to interaction with an improperly fitted prosthetic. Keeping the stump clean with appropriate skin care, particularly after sweating, can decrease the prevalence of abrasions and sores.

Back injuries are also common with upper-extremity amputations and occur predominantly at the cervical and thoracic spine. These injuries are attributed to imbalance, unequal movements and compensatory strategies of limbs during physical activity. On the other hand, lower-limb amputations are associated with low back pain due to excessive lumbar spine lateral flexion and extension as a compensatory mechanism. Particular attention should be focused on core and back strengthening and flexibility to alleviate these problems. Injuries to the intact limb result in overuse injuries like plantar fasciitis, Achilles tendonitis, and stress fractures. Repeated assessment of running and walking gaits may prevent these overuse injuries (Klenck and Gebke 2007).

Bone mass in unilateral below-knee amputees differs between impaired and intact limbs. Intact proximal tibia bone mineral density (BMD) has been reported to be 45% greater than in the impaired side (Royer and Koenig 2005). A possible explanation for this difference is the increased load on the knee compartment of the intact limb. Despite the increase in BMD, the intact limb of unilateral below-knee amputees is susceptible to irreversible degeneration and osteoarthritis due to repeated stress on the joint (Royer and Koenig 2005). Melzer et al. (2001) found some degree of knee osteoarthritis in 65.6% of unilateral, lower-extremity amputees, which was significantly higher than in able-bodied controls. Knee injuries consisted of patellar and medial osteophytosis. Osteoarthritis is not dependent on BMD but is a multifactorial disease impacted by age, body mass, joint injury and genetic factors (Royer and Koenig 2005).

Finally, sport-related muscle pain (SRMP) is also common in active individuals and athletes, whether able-bodied or with an impairment. Bernardi et al. (2003) conducted a survey on 227 members of the Italian Federation of Sports for Disabled (FISD). SRMP was defined as muscle pain experienced in the past 12 months, lasting at least 1 day, endured from physical activity in sport and not due to systemic disease. SRMP was recognized when it forced the athlete to stop, limit, or modify participation in sport. Although the study sample was predominantly athletes with a spinal cord injury, 12.3% of subjects were amputees. Demographics also included a majority of males (74.4%), participating in swimming (44.1%) and track and field events (29.5%). The most common SRMP reported was of the shoulder muscle (56%), followed by upper limbs (33%) and lumbar muscles (13.1%); this may be attributed to the high representation of athletes with spinal cord injuries. Increased training volume was a key determinant in the onset of SRMP. The authors acknowledged that athletes with an amputation may be at risk of injury due to the increased ambulatory activity compared to athletes with spinal cord injuries. This may result in increased overload of muscle use in these athletes. Finally, the improper fit of prostheses can result in lower coordination of muscle groups and increased susceptibility of SRMP due to overcompensation when unstable.

In summary, athletes with an amputation are not expected to suffer from greater injuries due to sport participation than their able-bodied counterparts. However, there may be long-term effects on bone, muscle, and connective tissue in amputees because of asymmetry, leading to acute SRMP as well as osteoarthritis. Prevention includes careful fitting of prosthetics, maintenance of body mass and composition, and a properly periodized training and competition plan supported by performance-based fueling strategies.

6.3 ENERGY EXPENDITURE IN ATHLETES WITH AN AMPUTATION

The assessment and analysis of components of energy expenditure used for able-bodied athletes may not be consistently applicable to athletes with an amputation (Van de Vliet et al. 2011). Resting metabolic rate (RMR) is often estimated using prediction equations; however, these cannot be applied to athletes with an amputation unless the amputation is of small magnitude or adjustments are made for the missing limb. In fact, estimating RMR using formulae in amputees will overestimate it by 5 to 32% (Buchholz and Pencharz 2004). In addition, prediction equations often require the determination of height and body mass. For a lower limb amputee, height assessment may be challenging due to the possible inability of the athlete to stand upright. Other methods of measuring height, such as supine or sitting height, may be applied in this population and considered within their own limitations. As outlined in Chapter 3, the Cunningham equation (1980) is often used to estimate RMR but it requires lean body mass from body composition assessment, however this relies on there being a validated method of measuring lean body mass (refer to Chapter 12).

Osterkamp (1995) reviewed body proportions for the determination of energy requirements of subjects with amputations. In a total of 21 subjects Dempster (1955) and Clauser et al. (1969) reported the following body proportional values: 8% head, 50% trunk, 5% total arm (1.6% forearm, 2.7% upper arm, 0.7% hand), and 16% total leg (10.1% thigh, 4.4% calf, 1.5% foot). These body proportions may be used for adjustments of RMR in amputees, however there are currently no data to validate this in an athlete population. Future research should compare measured RMR to proportionally adjusted RMR using prediction equations in athletes with an amputation.

Other components of total daily energy expenditure (TDEE) of relevance to athletes are non-exercise adaptive thermogenesis (NEAT) and energy expenditure of exercise (EEE), both having a great potential to increase TDEE. In able-bodied athletes, EEE is often assessed using the Compendium for Physical Activities (Ainsworth et al. 2011). Unfortunately, there are no published metabolic equivalents (METs) for amputees that could estimate energy expenditure during daily activities and, most importantly, during exercise. Further, there are currently no guidelines that could be used to adjust able-bodied MET values to an athlete with an amputation, particularly lower body amputees. The current literature, although limited, provides some insight into the differences in energy expenditure. Research investigating oxygen consumption (VO_2) during exercise in amputees shows greater VO_2

for proximal versus distal leg amputations. Schmalz et al. (2002) showed that the VO_2 for treadmill or free walking is about 25% higher in transtibial amputees using a prosthesis, while transfemoral amputees using a prosthesis exhibited a remarkable 55–65% increase in VO_2 during exercise compared with able-bodied counterparts. Thus the more proximal the amputation, the greater the tissue loss and the higher EEE during movement. Concurrently, RMR is expected to be lower the more proximal the amputation, and therefore TDEE may not be different to an able-bodied counterpart, depending on the volume of exercise undertaken. Interestingly, it is not only the location of the amputation that determines energy expenditure, but data suggest a direct link between the cause of the amputation (e.g. peripheral vascular disease and diabetes versus traumatic injury or congenital causes) and energy expenditure, with disease-related removal of limbs creating a 20–35% increase in energy expenditure (Schmalz et al. 2002) most likely due to pre-existing health, mobility and fitness status.

Applying this information, it appears that the best practice strategies to estimate EEE and TDEE in an athlete with an amputation may include measuring RMR or estimating RMR using proportionally adjusted prediction equations. For EEE, there is no doubt that measuring VO_2 during exercise would provide a more valid assessment. Portable devices are available and future research should attempt to measure VO_2 in athletes with various degrees of amputations participating in different sports in order to present a likely proportional difference. If indirect calorimetry is not available, portable devices such as heart rate monitors and accelerometers may be valid in ambulating athletes with an amputation, but cross-validation with VO_2 would still be required. Finally, the Compendium for Physical Activities (Ainsworth et al. 2011) could also be used for both ambulating activities and general and sport-specific training, particularly for arm amputees. Adjustments, as identified by Schmalz et al. (2002) for transtibial (25%) and transfemoral (~60%) amputations, are needed to account for inefficiency of movement in certain, but possibly not all, activities.

6.3.1 Do Prostheses Offer an Advantage to Athletes with an Amputation?

Advances in prosthetic technology have resulted in dramatic improvements of energy-storing properties of the prosthesis. This may alter the efficiency of a lower-limb amputee's gait, potentially diminishing the higher energy demands placed on the athlete. Significant metabolic differences appear nonexistent at normal walking speeds among transtibial amputees using prosthetics with various foot designs and carbon fibre springs. Increased energy efficiency is noted at speeds at or above 4.8 km/h, transitioning from walking to running (Schmalz et al. 2002). However, the placement and alignment of the prosthesis is critical. Schmalz et al. (2002) found that a small (i.e. 2 cm) anterior shift of the single axis knee joint significantly increased energy expenditure by 13%, probably attributed to the increased demand on the hip extensors to prevent prosthetic knee collapse. Thus, a prosthesis, if not aligned optimally, can be more energy inefficient and may also lead to compensatory strategies that may result in overload of other areas and potential injury.

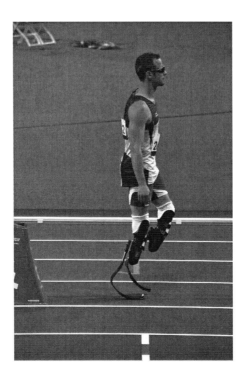

FIGURE 6.1   Oscar Pistorius. (Photograph courtesy of Scott Reardon.)

Lately, new research and development of prostheses have advanced while technology continues to aim at improving the options for amputees. Throughout 2011/2012, South African sprinter Oscar Pistorius brought international attention to the question of whether artificial legs can prove advantageous among athletes with amputations, and whether this puts able-bodied athletes at a disadvantage (Figure 6.1). An article published by the *New York Times* (Rohan 2012) highlighted an interview with Massachusetts Institute of Technology's (MIT) director of the Biomechatronics Group, H. Herr. According to Herr, artificial ankles have achieved biological-like functioning, as have legs for walking, but legs for running have not yet. Herr predicts, however, that the next-generation artificial legs will probably be developed, and the sporting community will have to re-evaluate athletes like Pistorius and amputees in general, identifying the point at which human meets "superhuman", and hopefully concluding the debate of whether an advantage exists for those using artificial legs or arms.

To date, running with prosthetics continues to offer no overall performance advantage to amputees over able-bodied athletes. Nolan (2008) investigated the metabolic cost of a carbon fibre prosthesis versus a prosthesis not specifically designed for running among bilateral and unilateral amputee and able-bodied counterparts. Use of a carbon fibre prosthetic made for running resulted in lower heart rates and VO_2 while running compared with the use of a prosthesis not designed for running. Interestingly, VO_2, heart rate, and VO_{2peak} between able-bodied individuals and amputees using the carbon fibre prosthesis were not different. The authors concluded that the use of carbon fibre prostheses would allow an amputee to reach equal but not greater running economy than able-bodied counterparts. Weyand et al. (2009) investigated the metabolic cost and mechanics during constant speed treadmill running in a bilateral, transtibial amputee sprinter versus competitive male runners with intact limbs. The amputee sprinter exhibited a metabolic cost 3.8% lower than able-bodied elite distance runners, 6.7% lower than sub-elite able-bodied distance runners and 17% lower than able-bodied 400 m sprinters. Physiologically, relative sprinting endurance during all-out speed trials was almost identical between amputee and able-bodied runners. However, at higher speeds, running mechanics differed between amputee and able-bodied athletes. The athletes with an amputation had longer foot-ground contact times and shorter aerial and swing times than intact-limb sprinters. The authors mentioned that these mechanical discrepancies between intact and amputee limbs are a good example of the functional trade-offs that may exist between biological and artificial limbs (Weyand et al. 2009). Thus, the debate of whether the use of prosthetics offers an advantage to amputees remains unsettled. Nevertheless, in running amputees, especially sprinters using advanced technology prosthetics, it can be assumed that EEE is similar to that of able-bodied athletes. This should, however, not be assumed in other athletes with an amputation, as it is likely that TDEE is higher due to increases in both NEAT and EEE. Sport nutritionists and physiologists working with athletes with an amputation are therefore required to carefully assess each individual athlete's degree and location of amputation and prosthetic devices used in both daily living and/or sport in order to accurately quantify energy needs. Measuring VO_2 under resting, ambulating, and various exercising conditions is likely the most accurate assessment of individual needs.

6.4 BODY COMPOSITION OF ATHLETES WITH AN AMPUTATION

As in able-bodied athletic populations, assessment of body composition can assist in evaluating the health and fitness status of the athlete with an amputation. However, it is imperative to recognize that body composition methods have inherent problems of validity and reliability, even in the able-bodied population (Ackland et al. 2012). Body composition assessment in amputees is further complicated by the location and degree of amputation and the lack of standardized methods and normative data established in this population.

There are several methods to assess body composition. While Chapter 12 will focus in more detail on body composition assessment in athletes with impairments, we will summarize the key issues regarding the most common laboratory and field methods in the amputee population. For an excellent resource for body composition in chronic disease and impairments see also Goosey-Tolfrey and Sutton (2012).

Densitometry such as hydro-densitometry or air displacement plethysmography (ADP) are common laboratory method using a two-component model. While these methods already use invalid assumptions for the estimation of fat free tissue densities in able-bodied populations (Ackland et al. 2012), an additional concern in amputees is the reduced body volume as a result of missing a limb. In addition, amputees will also present lower whole-body BMD, which is a part of the fat free mass (FFM) component, and would therefore underestimate FFM in amputees versus able-bodied counterparts (Van de Vliet et al. 2011).

Dual energy x-ray absorptiometry (DXA) measures fat, bone mineral and other fat free soft tissues (Ackland et al. 2012) and shows the greatest potential to accurately measure body composition in the amputee population. The ability of DXA to measure specific body segments makes it an optimal choice where regional differences are of interest. It is also useful for monitoring body composition changes over time when used in a standardized fashion (Van de Vliet et al. 2011) and for assessing the centre of mass for the purpose of optimizing prosthetic fittings because DXA allows for segmentalisation.

Body composition field methods include surface anthropometry, bioelectrical impedance analysis (BIA), body mass index (BMI) and various others, some of which propose a combination of measures and are briefly discussed below. Surface anthropometry, if conducted by a International Society for the Advancement of Kinanthropometry (ISAK) certified anthropometrist, is reliable (Ackland et al. 2012). Additional limb girths, bone lengths and bone breadths can be utilized to attain a more accurate representation of an individual's anthropometry. While ISAK does not preclude the use of raw skinfold data in estimating body density and percent body fat (% BF), it emphasizes the sum of skinfolds and skinfold ratios over % BF, as these additional steps introduce error (Ackland et al. 2012). Since there are currently no equations developed for amputees that convert the sum of skinfolds to body density and % BF, the sum of skinfolds should be reported in amputees. Another issue relates to the location of skinfold sites; standardization requires skinfold measures to be taken on the right side of the body. If an athlete is missing a right limb the measurement should be taken on the left side. This needs to be noted by the anthropometrist for future reference and/or comparison (Van de Vliet et al. 2011). For further guidelines and tools specifically using ISAK methodology in populations with impairments, including amputees, see Sutton and Stewart (2012) and Chapter 12.

In addition to skinfold measurements, body mass plays a key role in surface anthropometry assessment. However, issues exist regarding data interpretation. Body mass of an athlete with an amputation will be lower than that of an able-bodied counterpart. This factor alone makes it impossible to compare able-bodied athletes to those with amputations. Thus, monitoring the sum of skinfolds and body mass is only useful if performed over time and an athlete-specific range is established.

Determining stretch stature also poses multiple problems in athletes with lower limb amputations. Whether an athlete with an amputation has a unilateral or bilateral below-knee amputation, stretch stature may be difficult to measure. An athlete with a unilateral below-knee amputation will be standing on one leg for this measurement; this can alter the athlete's standing position and curvature of the spine, hence care must be taken to ensure the stretch stature is appropriate and the athlete is able to remain stable standing on one leg. An athlete with a bilateral amputation will be missing a whole segment of body length compared to an able-bodied counterpart. Therefore, stretch stature may not be appropriate for this population. Instead, sitting height may be utilized. This method allows the individual to sit on a surface and have their torso measured for height evaluation. If sitting height is used, it is crucial to note that it cannot be correlated with a stretch stature; it must be used as a stand-alone measure. The severity of amputation and impairment will determine the appropriate method of assessment (Van de Vliet et al. 2011).

Finally, BIA estimates total body water, % BF and % FFM and assumes geometric similarity between subjects (Ackland et al. 2012), which is not met in amputee populations. BIA also underrepresents the trunk over the extremities, which poses problems in amputees, as the trunk most likely represents the largest body part in an amputee. If an athlete is able to successfully complete this assessment with either lower or upper limbs intact, values should still not be compared to normative data but to individual changes over time (Van de Vliet et al. 2011).

Anthropometry, including body mass and body mass index (BMI), has been used to acquire a general idea of an individual's nutritional status. In the general population, BMI has been particularly common for classification of overweight and obesity. It is well known that BMI can be misleading in athletes as it tends to overestimate body fatness due to the higher body mass from lean as opposed to fat mass. BMI also assumes constant body segment proportions (Ackland et al. 2012), which is an issue in amputees. Interestingly, BMI underestimates body fatness in those with unilateral amputations, while it overestimates fatness in individuals with bilateral amputations due to the lower stature. A study by Tzamaloukas et al. (1994) suggests there is premise for a corrected BMI formula to accurately reflect the amputee population. Through the use of pre- and post-amputation body weight a new formula for BMI was derived. Of the 23 subjects, two who were obese unilateral amputees were classified correctly as obese using the corrected BMI but classified nonobese by the uncorrected BMI equation. Similarly, four lean or wasting amputees were classified as obese using the uncorrected BMI equation, while the corrected BMI formula correctly identified them as nonobese. While the corrected BMI formula is useful in nonathletes, it is questionable if its application would have any merit in the athletic population. It remains unclear whether the BMI is a reliable indicator of nutritional state in athletes with an amputation.

Rather than the BMI, the corrected-arm-muscle area (CAMA) has been suggested to be useful. CAMA and other upper-arm anthropometry measurements may be a more accurate assessment of general body fatness and nutritional state compared with BMI. CAMA, mid-upper-arm circumference (MUAC) and triceps skinfold thickness (TST) were compared to corrected BMI (cBMI) and uncorrected BMI (uBMI). cBMI was calculated with a weight corrected by multiplying actual weight by 5.9% for transtibial subjects and 16% for transfemoral subjects. Height was estimated from knee height. The findings showed that CAMA, MUAC, and TST were all associated with both uBMI and cBMI; however, MUAC showed the strongest relationship to uBMI and cBMI compared with the other methods (Miller et al. 2008). This particular study was conducted in nonathletes with amputations. There are currently no studies that have examined this method with athletes with an amputation. More research is needed to determine whether CAMA, MUAC or TST are of any value in the athletic population. Previous work suggested MUAC is the gold standard (Mozumdar and Roy 2004) while other researchers state that MUAC and TST are not reliable predictive measurements (Burden et al. 2005).

In summary, as outlined in Chapter 12, DXA and anthropometry using ISAK standards probably offer the most valid and reliable body composition assessment in athletes with an amputation. To further examine whether other parameters such as CAMA may prove useful in athletes with an amputation, ISAK certified examiners could carefully monitor variables such as mid-arm circumference, in addition to skinfolds.

6.5 SPECIFIC NUTRITION ISSUES IN ATHLETES WITH AN AMPUTATION

The Paralympic movement is growing, with more athletes, including amputees, competing at international Games, yet very little is known about these athletes' specific nutritional needs. Silva Gomes et al. (2006) assessed anthropometrics and nutritional intake of the Brazilian amputee men's soccer team. Data presented in this article are one of a kind and essential for the advancement in understanding nutritional intake and needs of this population. The authors of this study reported data from 15 male amputees: two goalkeepers with upper limb amputation, four fullbacks, three midfielders, and six forwards. Twelve of 13 field players had a transfemoral amputation while the thirteenth had a transtibial amputation. Thirteen amputations were caused by trauma, one was congenital, and the last was attributed to complications of cancer. Using a 6-day dietary record, mean daily energy intake was 16 ± 4.4 MJ (241 ± 66.5 kJ/kg/d, 3830 ± 1040 kcal/d, 57.6 ± 15.9 kcal/kg/d), protein intake was 3.1 ± 0.8 g/kg/d and carbohydrate intake was 7.3 ± 2.1 g/kg/d. Fat intake was 29% of total energy intake. From these data, it appears that the average carbohydrate intake in Brazilian amputee soccer athletes was sufficient. Goalkeepers showed the highest intake of fat and lowest of carbohydrate, while midfielders and forwards had higher carbohydrate intake. Considering the high carbohydrate needs of team sport athletes (Holway and Spriet 2011), sport dietitians need to individualize carbohydrate recommendations, especially in athletes with an amputation playing in various positions. Unfortunately, this study did not report any data on training volume and/or intensity; thus these data are difficult to put into context of energy balance or availability. Future research should focus on assessing TDEE in athletes with an amputation, especially because the inefficiency of movement may increase energy expenditure, and thus energy and nutrient requirements.

In the study by Silva Gomes et al. (2006), percent body fat was also measured using three skinfold sites and the equation by Jackson and Pollock (1978). Goalkeepers had the lowest percent body fat of all positions ($13.5 \pm 10\%$) with mean % body fat of $14.4 \pm 4.4\%$ for all players. Jackson and Pollock (1978), however, did not develop this particular formula based on a sample of athletes with an amputation; thus, whether this equation is suitable for this population is questionable.

Considering the limited research related to nutrition in athletes with an amputation, it is not surprising that nutrition recommendations for this population are almost non-existent. Common nutritional issues in non-wheelchair-bound athletes such as amputees (if ambulating) include increased energy needs due to inefficiency of movement, heightened risk for discomfort, pressure sores and infection at contact site between prosthetics and amputation, and possible problems with digestion and associated bowel movements as well as hydration and urination (Broad 2001). When working with athletes with an amputation, it is imperative to assess each athlete thoroughly in order to develop an individual plan targeting the unique issues of each athlete based on their background and level of impairment.

6.5.1 NUTRITIONAL INTERVIEWS WITH AMPUTEE PARALYMPIANS

Due to the scarcity of data on nutrition in athletes with an amputation, nutrition issues for this chapter are based on interviews with three successful Paralympic athletes, which were conducted in 2011 prior to the 2012 London Paralympic Games. The interviews included one athlete with a unilateral above-knee amputation, one athlete with a bilateral below-knee amputation and another athlete with a bilateral above-knee amputation. Two of the three athletes were swimmers and currently ambulating; the third was a skier utilizing a wheelchair for transportation. Each of these individuals reported differing views of sport nutrition and managing their impairment. Challenges facing these athletes include demanding nutritional issues, maintaining body weight, combating overall health concerns, and managing activities of daily living.

Nutritional issues addressing body mass/composition management included portion control, hydration, and sodium intake. The wheelchair-bound, bilateral above-knee athletes with an amputation reported portion size and weight management along with hydration as daily challenges. This male skier was born with lumbar sacral agenesis, a genetic disorder where he was born with no lumbar vertebrae or sacrum. The muscles in his legs did not develop and were amputated at age four. It is crucial for this athlete to control portion size to maintain weight; while operating his wheelchair, almost 100% of his body weight is resting on his stomach creating a constant feeling of fullness. To relieve this 'full' sensation, the athlete must hold himself up on the armrests of his chair. Further, maintaining adequate hydration is a challenge for this skier. His body weight rests not only on his stomach but also on his bladder. When strapped into his ski while training and racing on the mountain, it is extremely inconvenient for him to use the bathroom. Unlike other skiers with an impairment, he cannot utilize a leg bag for urine collection due to limited space in his sit-ski. Although he knows it may be detrimental to his performance, he will purposely dehydrate the day of practice or on race day. He reports that the alternative to competing dehydrated is not worth the consequences or discomfort of an accident. Whereas the typical approach would be to find a strategy for this athlete to maintain euhydration during skiing, it is critical to individualize sport nutrition approaches, even if they may not align with current recommendations. Guiding this athlete to consume cranberry juice pre- and post-exercise to decrease the risk of urinary tract infection (UTI) and/or some electrolytes to promote the uptake and absorption of the fluid he consumes is probably a better strategy than forcing him to change his hydration routine on the mountain.

Both the athlete with the unilateral above-knee amputation and the athlete with the bilateral below-knee amputation reported weight maintenance through energy balance, and monitoring sodium intake as nutritional challenges. Both of these athletes were swimmers. The athlete with the unilateral above-knee amputation was born with proximal femoral focal deficiency, a condition where she was born without a femur in her right leg. The other athlete with the bilateral below-knee amputation was born with fibular hemimelia, or without a fibula in either leg. Both of these athletes were ambulating. One key component to their ambulation is the proper fit of their prostheses.

Prosthetic fittings take place once a year, at the most. It is important to maintain weight to adequately fit into the socket of the prosthetics. In addition, increased sodium intake, heat, or travel can cause these athletes' limbs and/or thighs to swell, making their prosthetic fit extremely uncomfortable. The swimmer with the unilateral above-knee amputation reported she will resort to crutches or her wheelchair if her prosthesis is not fitting properly. A frequent outcome of a misaligned prosthesis fit is the development of pressure sores, wounds, and infection, which may take weeks to heal and require time out of the water (i.e. not training).

The current training/competition routines in which these athletes engage can put them at risk for greater health complications later in life such as hip and knee replacements. The amount of force placed on their joints without adequate support, from either another leg or joint, can be overwhelming. One of the athletes expressed concern of being confined to a wheelchair; this would be a devastating progression to any ambulating athlete, able-bodied or amputee.

Daily barriers faced by athletes with amputations are unique to each individual athlete. The skier confined to a wheelchair expressed quite different challenges than did the ambulating bilateral below-knee swimmer. The wheelchair-bound athlete described challenges related to housing layout and accessibility to public places as daily barriers. The heights of countertops in most apartments are not conducive to access by an individual in a wheelchair. If this athlete wants to unload the dishwasher, he must first unload the dishes to the countertop, then climb on the counter and put them away into the cupboards. He also expressed difficulties with narrow kitchens; if the refrigerator door opens the wrong way it is impossible to get his wheelchair around to get into it. This athlete will ambulate on his hands while at home to overcome these obstacles. Difficulty accessing food may hinder this athlete from fueling properly on training days. Traveling to competitions has exposed this skier to many cultures. Some social groups tend to give him a sense of disapproval toward his impairment but are amazed by his resourcefulness. He says people often just stare however those who do attempt to help are often overzealous. This athlete says, "You can't be anonymous. You can't just go to the grocery store. I'm either going to be stared at, or be such an *amazing inspiration* to a group of people". He shows his frustration toward the stigmatism associated with his impairment.

The swimmer with the bilateral below-knee amputation described ambulating to be a daily challenge. The amount of energy required to walk is physically draining. During the 2012 Summer Paralympic Games in London, both swimmers used wheelchairs while traveling from the Olympic Village to the Aquatics Center, to conserve energy for competition. Daily challenges faced by the athlete with a bilateral below-knee amputation include walking on different textured floors. For example, she described hardwood and tile floors easier to navigate than floors covered in rug. Transitioning from one surface to another also poses a challenge. Besides the physical act of walking, stopping presents another difficulty; it is almost impossible for this athlete to stop short if someone ahead of her stops quickly or intersects her path. Despite the challenges faced, this athlete does not consider herself impaired. She says, "This is part of me. You don't leave the house without your keys or cell phone. I don't leave the house without my legs. I don't think of myself as disabled. I do have legs. I just put them on. There's not anything I can't do".

6.5.2 NUTRITIONAL PRIORITIES WHEN WORKING WITH ATHLETES WITH AN AMPUTATION

Integrating the interviews, our knowledge of sport nutrition for able-bodied athletes, and the unique challenges of athletes with an amputation, we summarize below the nutritional priorities when working with these athletes.

6.5.2.1 Energy Balance

Athletes with an amputation may have increased energy requirements; however, these athletes also need to be supported in using healthy approaches to maintaining an appropriate body mass and body composition. Their energy requirements must be evaluated based on individual circumstances.

6.5.2.2 Macronutrients

Athletes with an amputation may be at risk of poor nutritional habits, be it due to difficulties accessing, purchasing, and preparing food or simply due to poor nutrition knowledge (Rastmanesh et al. 2007). Educating the athletes relative to their nutrient needs, particularly carbohydrate, is imperative especially if inefficiency of movement may increase glycogen utilization. Further, ingesting adequate protein and integrating fats from fish, nuts, avocado and plant oils (e.g. olive) will further promote healthy eating patterns. If athletes prepare their own meals, it is crucial to develop simple strategies to adopt at home, and some may need help in learning how to cook. Depending on caretakers and/or the athlete's ability, cooking larger quantities and freezing them appropriately portioned may be useful. Athletes with an amputation must also learn that eating at least three meals and several snacks throughout the day is necessary to meet energy and nutrient needs.

6.5.2.3 Fueling and Recovery

Most athletes with an amputation can follow general fueling guidelines for before, during and after exercise as outlined in Chapter 3. Athletes in wheelchairs may need special attention and customizing, particularly targeting fluid replacement strategies before and after exercise. Sodium aids in fluid retention (Shirreffs and Sawka 2011) and may be used before and after exercise. Adding salt to both fluids (e.g. broths, sport drinks) and meals can be a useful strategy, especially for athletes training and competing seated in a sit ski or wheelchair (or similar) in environments where restroom access is both limited and burdensome. Athletes with an amputation should adopt similar recovery nutrition strategies as able-bodied athletes, as has been outlined in Chapter 3. Convenient, readily available sources such as non-perishable dairy or soy beverages, breads with nut butters, yogurt with fruit, or sport bars are all good options.

COMMENTARY BOX 6.2

EXPERT COMMENTARY: Protein requirements in amputee athletes
  Dr. Luc van Loon, Maastricht University, and Professor Kevin Tipton, Stirling University

Question: Do you believe the protein requirements for optimizing muscle protein synthesis (i.e. 20–25 g post-exercise) are the same in amputee athletes (especially bilateral leg amputees) as in able-bodied individuals?

Answer: Quite possibly the protein requirements are very similar, despite their reduced absolute amount of active muscle tissue. A lot of the protein ingested is utilized in the gut, and this component is unlikely to change. Unlike carbohydrate requirements, it doesn't appear as though (minimal) protein requirements can be advised on "a per kg body mass" basis directly. Therefore, if requirements are different, it's likely that differences are small (i.e. 5 g lower).

6.5.2.4 Thermoregulation and Hydration

Thermoregulation may be impaired in some athletes with an amputation. An amputee lacks part or all of a limb, resulting in comparable decreases in functional surface area, which reduces the athlete's ability to dissipate heat. Impaired thermoregulation may slow acclimatization in hot and humid environments (Van de Vliet et al. 2011). Assessing athletes' individual hydration status, using urine specific gravity and urine color charts prior to exercise, and estimating sweat rates during exercise are necessary to implement individualized fluid replacement and hydration guidelines.

If athletes purposefully refrain from drinking to avoid discomfort and lengthy bathroom breaks, they may risk dehydration and UTI. Prehydration and vigorous fluid replacement post-exercise are key to ensuring timely recovery. In addition, cranberry-containing preparations (e.g. juice, concentrate, tablets) may assist through their antimicrobial and antibacterial properties, although a recent review does not suggest cranberry preparations to be effective in preventing UTIs (Jepson et al. 2012).

6.5.2.5 Nutrition Issues Related to Prostheses

Prosthetic fit can be influenced by nutritional factors such as hydration. Gailey and Harsch (2009) suggested that the body fluids lost during long-distance cycling and running can reduce residual limb volume of amputees, resulting in excessive movement of the limb in the prosthetic socket. Attenuating fluid loss during exercise and adopting effective fluid replacement post-exercise strategies may be extremely important in this population of athletes. Likewise, body mass changes, both gain and loss, can negatively affect prosthetic fit, and thus require individual attention.

Pressure sores and infection risk are high in athletes with an amputation who are ambulating using prosthetics or for those using wheelchairs. If problems arise, nutritional approaches that increase wound healing may be helpful. These include increasing consumption of calories from carbohydrate, protein, and fat. In addition, foods rich in vitamin C (e.g. citrus fruit, kiwi), fish oils (e.g. wild salmon), and zinc supplements to speed wound healing may be helpful. Refer to Chapters 4 and 10 for further information concerning wound healing.

6.5.2.6   Ergonomic Issues with Nutritional Relevance

Unless athletes are thoroughly assessed in training, home and competition environments, it is difficult to evaluate what specific needs they may have and what strategies can help to overcome their barriers to good nutrition. While observation works best, a detailed query can also suffice to help understand what hurdles must be overcome daily and which part, from food purchasing to preparation and transport to training/competition venues, may be difficult to accomplish. In addition, when athletes are traveling, it is critical to incorporate necessities such as access to grocery stores and accessible kitchenettes in hotel rooms in addition to scoping out restaurants in close proximity to hotel or competition venue. Athletes may need special equipment in order to transfer nutritional practices from home to training and competition environments, and if not planned for, may develop into a major issue.

In summary, athletes with an amputation probably have similar or greater energy and macro- and micronutrient needs compared with able-bodied athletes, especially in training and competition. Greater energy and nutrient needs most likely occur due to the inefficiency of movement and over-compensation of intact limbs and possibly from poorly fitting prosthetics and associated inflammatory issues. Athletes with an amputation may deliberately dehydrate, depending on their level of injury and associated discomfort during exercise. Most importantly, athletes with an amputation need to be individually assessed in order to optimize nutritional strategies by removing daily obstacles that may occur inherent to their physical state. Practitioners working with athletes with an amputation, however, should also realize that these athletes are relatively self-sufficient and are just as able to adopt healthy, performance-based strategies as able-bodied athletes.

COMMENTARY BOX 6.3

COACH'S INSIGHT: What do you think is the most important thing a sports nutrition practitioner can do to assist your athletes?

Teach them how to eat right, including how to cook well. It's important for the sports nutrition practitioner to watch what the athlete actually does in training so that they understand how much food they need to eat. For example, my athletes don't need to eat as much as able-bodied track athletes do because they don't undertake the same volume of training since they fatigue more quickly.

—Iryna Dvoskina, athletics coach of multiple Paralympic medallists

6.6 FUTURE RESEARCH

There is a great need for research in athletes with an amputation. Studies are needed to describe energy expenditure in athletes with an amputation at rest, during daily activities, and during various types of exercise using methods such as doubly labeled water and indirect calorimetry. Studies should also compare RMR using prediction equations, incorporating body proportions as suggested by Dempster (1955) and Clauser et al. (1969), to indirect calorimetry in amputees. Future research should also include amputees for the study of body composition and sport scientists should establish norms for athletes with impairments. Due to the lack of nutrition data on athletes with an impairment, including amputees, research is needed that characterizes not only the diets of athletes with an amputation, but also their nutritional and hydration status. While it is assumed that fueling needs are similar among athletes regardless of an impairment, there is a need for research in athletes with impairments related to carbohydrate oxidation rates during exercise and post-exercise protein balance. Finally, research in this population should also focus on wound healing using nutritional interventions.

REFERENCES

Ackland, T.R., Lohman, T.G., Sundgot-Borgen, J., et al. 2012. Current status of body composition assessment in sport: review and position statement on behalf of the ad hoc research working group on body composition health and performance, under the auspices of the I.O.C. Medical Commission. *Sports Medicine* 42:227–249.

Ainsworth, B.E., Haskell, W.L., Herrmann, S.D., et al. 2011. Compendium of Physical Activities: a second update of codes and MET values. *Medicine and Science in Sports and Exercise* 43:1575–1581.

Bergeron, J.W. 1999. Athletes with disabilities. *Physical Medicine & Rehabilitation Clinics of North America* 10:213–228.

Bernardi, M., Castellano, V., Ferrara, M.S., Sbriccoli, P., Sera, F., and Marchetti, M. 2003. Muscle pain in athletes with locomotor disability. *Medicine and Science in Sports and Exercise* 35:199–206.

Buchholz, A.C., and Pencharz, P.B. 2004. Energy expenditure in chronic spinal cord injury. *Current Opinion in Clinical Nutrition and Metabolic Care* 7:635–639.

Burden, S.T., Stoppard, E., Shaffer, J., Makin, A., and Todd, C. 2005. Can we use mid upper arm anthropometry to detect malnutrition in medical inpatients? A validation study. *Journal of Human Nutrition and Dietetics* 18:287–294.

Bragaru, M., Dekker, R., Geertzen, J.H., and Dijkstra, P.U. 2011. Amputees and sports: a systematic review. *Sports Medicine* 41:721–740.

Broad, E. 2001. Sports nutrition for athletes with disabilities. *International Sports Medicine Journal* 1:1–4.

Clauser, C.E., McConville, J.T., and Young, J.W. 1969. Weight, volume, and center of mass of segments of the human body. In *AMRL technical report*, 69–70. Wright-Patterson Air Force Base, OH: U.S. Air Force.

Cunningham, J.J. 1980. A reanalysis of the factors influencing basal metabolic rate in normal adults. *American Journal of Clinical Nutrition* 33:2372–2374.

Dempster, W.T. 1955. Space requirements of the seated operator. In *WADC technical report*, 55–159. Wright-Patterson Air Force Base, OH: U.S. Air Force.

Dillingham, T.R., Pezzin, L.E., and MacKenzie, E.J. 2002. Limb amputation and limb deficiency: epidemiology and recent trends in the United States. *Southern Medical Journal* 95:875–883.

Ferrara, M.S., and Peterson, C.L. 2000. Injuries to athletes with disabilities: identifying injury patterns. *Sports Medicine* 30:137–143.

Gailey, R., and Harsch, P. 2009. Introduction to triathlon for the lower limb amputee triathlete. *Prosthetics and Orthotics International* 33:242–255.

Goosey-Tolfrey, V., and Sutton, L. 2012. Body composition in disease and disability. In *Body composition in sport, exercise and health*, ed. A.D. Stewart and L. Sutton, 166–186. Abingdon, UK: Routledge.

Holway, F.E., and Spriet, L.L. 2011. Sport-specific nutrition: practical strategies for team sports. *Journal of Sports Sciences* 29(Suppl 1):S115–S125.

Huonker, M., Schmid, A., Schmidt-Trucksass, A., Grathwohl, D., and Keul, J. 2003. Size and blood flow of central and peripheral arteries in highly trained able-bodied and disabled athletes. *Journal of Applied Physiology* 95:685–691.

International Paralympic Committee. 2007. IPC classification code and standards. http://www.paralympic.org – The IPC – IPC Handbook (accessed November 1, 2012).

Jackson, A.S., and Pollock, M.L. 1978. Generalized equations for predicting body density of men. *British Journal of Nutrition* 40:497–504.

Jepson, R.G., Williams, G., and Craig, J.C. 2012. Cranberries for preventing urinary tract infections. *Cochrane Database Systematic Reviews* Oct 17;10:CD001321 (retrieved November 1, 2012).

Klenck, C., and Gebke, K. 2007. Practical management: common medical problems in disabled athletes. *Clinical Journal of Sports Medicine* 17:55–60.

Litsky, F. 2001. Diana Goldon-Brosnihan dies at 38. *New York Times*. http://www.nytimes.com/2001/08/28/sports/diana-golden-brosnihan-skier-dies-at-38.html?src=pm; (accessed November 1, 2012).

Melzer, I., Yekutiel, M., and Sukenik, S. 2001. Comparative study of osteoarthritis of the contralateral knee joint of male amputees who do and do not play volleyball. *Journal of Rheumatology* 28:169–172.

Miller, M., Wong, W.K., Wu, J., Cavenett, S., Daniels, L., and Crotty, M. 2008. Upper-arm anthropometry: an alternative indicator of nutritional health to body mass index in unilateral lower-extremity amputees? *Archives of Physical Medicine and Rehabilitation* 89:2031–2033.

Modan, M., Peles, E., Halkin, H., et al. 1998. Increased cardiovascular disease mortality rates in traumatic lower limb amputees. *American Journal of Cardiology* 82:1242–1247.

Mozumdar, A., and Roy, S.K. 2004. Method for estimating body weight in persons with lower-limb amputation and its implication for their nutritional assessment. *American Journal of Clinical Nutrition* 80:868–875.

Nolan, L. 2008. Carbon fibre prostheses and running in amputees: a review. *Journal of Foot and Ankle Surgery* 14:125–129.

Osterkamp, L. 1995. Current perspective on assessment of human body proportions of relevance to amputees. *Journal of the American Dietetic Association* 95:215–218.

Rastmanesh, R., Taleban, F.A., Kimiagar, M., Mehrabi, Y., and Salehi, M. 2007. Nutritional knowledge and attitudes in athletes with physical disabilities. *Journal of Athletic Training* 42:99–105.

Rice, I., Hettinga, F.J., Lafferrier, J., et al. 2011. Biomechanics. In *The Paralympic athlete*, ed. Y.C. Vandlandewijck and W.R. Thompson, 33–50. 1st ed. West Sussex, UK: Wiley-Blackwell.

Rohan, T. 2012. *New York Times*. http://london2012.blogs.nytimes.com/2012/07/05/will-technology-solve-tracks-debate-over-amputees (retrieved October 26, 2012).

Royer, T., and Koenig, M. 2005. Joint loading and bone mineral density in persons with unilateral, trans-tibial amputation. *Clinical Biomechanics* 20:1119–1125.

Schmalz, T., Blumentritt, S., and Jarasch, R. 2002. Energy expenditure and biochemical characteristics of lower limb amputee gait: the influence of prosthetic alignment and different prosthetic components. *Gait and Posture* 16:255–263.

Shirreffs, S.M., and Sawka, M.N. 2011. Fluid and electrolyte needs for training, competition, and recovery. *Journal of Sports Sciences* 29(Suppl 1):S39–S46.

Silva Gomes, A.I., Goncalves Ribeiro, B., and Abreu Soares, E. 2006. Nutritional profile of the Brazilian amputee soccer team during the precompetition period for the world championship. *Nutrition* 22:989–995.

Sutton, L., and Stewart, A. 2012. Body composition: a professional discipline and inter-disciplinary toolkit. In *Body composition in sport, exercise and health*, ed. A.D. Stewart and L. Sutton, 187–208. Abingdon, UK: Routledge.

Tzamaloukas, A.H., Patron, A., and Malhotra, D. 1994. Body mass index in amputees. *Journal of Parenteral and Enteral Nutrition* 18:355–358.

Van de Vliet, P., Broad, E., and Strupler, M. 2011. In *The Paralympic athlete*, ed. Y.C. Vandlandewijck and W.R. Thompson, 172–197. West Sussex, UK: Wiley-Blackwell.

Weyand, P.G., Bundle, M.W., McGowan, C.P., et al. 2009. The fastest runner on artificial legs: different limbs, similar function? *Journal of Applied Physiology* 107:903–911.

7 Les Autres

Elizabeth Broad

CONTENTS

7.1 INTRODUCTION

The classification of 'les autres' (French for 'the others') encompasses a range of impairment types which do not fall into the other primary classes and are not covered by specific sporting organisations. Les autres includes dwarfism, Friedreich's ataxia, multiple sclerosis, severe burns, polio, severe forms of arthritis, arthrogryposis, osteogenesis imperfecta, congenital limb deformities (such as club foot) and muscular dystrophies. Due to their relatively small numbers, very little is known about the impact of these impairments within an exercise environment, however some valuable information can be gained from the clinical literature. This chapter describes the major impairments that comprise les autres and provides some insight into potential nutrition issues the athlete may face.

7.2 DWARFISM

Dwarfism generally refers to a group of genetic disorders characterised by shorter than normal skeletal growth and caused by one of over 300 conditions. Achondroplasia is the most common type of dwarfism, the majority of these children having average-sized parents. In achondroplasia, the head is relatively large, the trunk is a relatively normal length, however the arms and legs are disproportionately short. Such disproportionate dwarfism is characterised by one or more body parts being relatively large or small in comparison to those of an average sized adult, whereas an alternate type is proportionate dwarfism whereby the body is normally proportioned but unusually small.

While the majority of causes for dwarfism do not coincide with other medical conditions, it is important to know the primary diagnosis and cause of the athlete's short stature. Bloom's syndrome is one rare genetic disorder where the primary feature is proportional dwarfism but also results in other clinical manifestations such as chronic lung disease, diabetes and cancer (Diaz et al. 2006). Impaired glucose tolerance and insulin resistance are also present even at very young ages, along with low immunoglobulin concentrations (Diaz et al. 2006). Similarly, individuals with lifetime congenital growth hormone deficiency who remain untreated display reduced β-cell function and a higher frequency of impaired glucose tolerance (Oliveira et al. 2012). While regular exercise is known to reduce insulin resistance and be protective against diabetes, it may be prudent to consider the use of lower glycemic index and glycemic load of carbohydrate when managing an athlete who has Bloom's syndrome or congenital growth hormone deficiency (see Chapter 8 with regard to diabetes).

Some information sources state that dwarfs experience difficulties in maintaining a healthy weight for height in adulthood (Hunter et al. 1996), although it may be particularly noticeable due to their short stature (Owen et al. 1990). There is limited research regarding the energy requirements of dwarfs, with only one study in achondroplastic dwarfs indicating their resting metabolic rate (RMR) relative to fat free mass was higher than the reference, normal height population (Owen et al. 1990). Interestingly, the researchers noted that the RMR calculated using the Cunningham equation (see Chapter 3) overestimated the energy requirements of these individuals, however there was no description of activity provided for these subjects. Specific RMR prediction equations were developed by Owen and colleagues (1990), however the population was small ($n = 32$), the data have not been validated, and the authors themselves note the variability between individuals and recommended assessment on a case by case basis in future. While it is likely that athletes who are dwarfs have similar energy requirements per kg body mass to normal height athletes in similar sports, in absolute terms their energy requirements are reduced which means that the nutrient density of their diets must be greater to ensure all nutrient requirements are adequately met. It may be necessary to specifically educate dwarf athletes with short stature to understand their own individual nutritional needs rather than being influenced by what other athletes eat, especially where body composition management is required.

Undertaking anthropometrical assessments in a dwarf is effectively the same as for a standard height individual although it must be acknowledged that reference data may not be relevant for comparison and many assumptions may be violated (see Chapter 12), especially where the body is disproportionately short. Standard weight for height curves have been developed for individuals with achondroplasia ranging from birth to adulthood (Hunter et al. 1996), which can be useful when assessing growth and development of younger athletes or estimating appropriate weight for height in adults. While this dataset is unique, it also has some limitations (particularly for adults) in that it is based on 1147 observations undertaken on 409 Caucasian subjects, mostly during childhood. Waist to hip ratio and body mass index do not appear to be useful indicators of body fatness in this population (Hunter et al. 1996; Owen et al. 1990). Skinfold thicknesses were found to correlate with weight and body density in adult dwarfs with achondroplasia, so are believed to be a useful indicator of body fatness in this population (Hunter et al. 1996; Owen et al. 1990). Owen and colleagues (1990) developed equations to estimate body density from anthropometrical measures in achondroplastic dwarfs, however it must be recognised that the population used was small and has not been validated by other researchers. Therefore, in the hands of an appropriately trained practitioner, skinfold measures most likely remain a relevant tool to use for athletes who are dwarfs to assess body composition changes over time.

From a practical perspective, consideration must be taken in regards to catering facilities (for example, height of serveries) and self-catering kitchen facilities (for example, when undertaking cooking classes or where athletes must self-cater) in regards to safe access to stovetops, ovens and benchtops.

7.3 SEVERE BURNS

Individuals with severe burns can be classed within les autres, but there may also be individuals in other classes where burns coexist with another form of impairment, such as amputees. In the acute phase of healing from severe burns, energy and protein requirements are substantially higher than normal. Evidence suggests that an increased energy expenditure and negative nitrogen balance may persist for up to 18 months post-burn injury, but insulin resistance induced by this hypermetabolic response to burns can persist for up to 3 years (Gauglitz et al. 2009; Klein 2008). By the time a burn victim has healed sufficiently to become actively involved in exercise this hypermetabolic response will most likely have resolved and their energy and protein requirements returned to normal, however it is worthwhile checking the period since initial burn injury. Bone loss also occurs as a consequence of burns (Klein 2008), therefore it is important to consider nutrition support which optimises bone mineralisation and limits any further loss of bone density for athletes who have burns.

One key nutrient which may be at risk of deficiency in burn victims is vitamin D. It has been reported that acute burn injury that covers 40% or more of the total body surface area is associated with reduction in bone formation and resorption, hypocalcaemia, hypercalciuria, and hypoparathyroidism (Klein et al. 2004), the long term outcome being reduced bone mineral density. Disruption to the skin integrity from burns has been shown to reduce both the levels of 7-dehydrocholesterol and also the percentage conversion to vitamin D_3, not only where the burn scar is but also in adjacent normal skin (Klein et al. 2004). Since the majority of vitamin D is obtained through skin exposure to ultraviolet B rays, serum 25-hydroxyvitamin D concentrations are consequently low (Klein 2008). This is exacerbated by a reluctance of individuals to expose their skin (particularly outdoors) and spend time outside since sweat glands are destroyed by the injury (Klein 2008), thereby limiting the exposure to sunlight. As outlined in Chapter 4, vitamin D deficiency has been associated with reduced bone mineral density, abnormalities in calcium homeostasis, reduced muscle strength and a disrupted immune response (Solomon and Whithard 2010), all factors which are important to prevent in order to optimise training capacity and the health and well-being of an athlete. Hence it is recommended that athletes with severe burns are assessed at least annually for vitamin D status and supplemented appropriately (as outlined in Chapter 10).

Where a burn victim has substantial skin grafts, their response to heat from the perspective of both cutaneous vasodilation and sweat response is limited at the graft site (particularly in split-thickness grafts as opposed to full-thickness grafts) and unlikely to recover over time (Crandall and Davis 2010). Donor sites appear to be unaffected, and while total sweat rates per area of normal skin may be higher in burn victims (Ben-Simchon et al. 1981) there is little clarity as to whether this compensatory sweating is effective in managing thermoregulatory capacity. Indeed, individuals who have skin grafts covering more than 40% surface area of their body are at higher risk for hyperthermia if exercising in the heat or exposed to hot conditions over an extended period of time (Ben-Simchon et al. 1981; Shapiro et al. 1982). One study reported no difference in rectal temperature or heart rate response to cycling at low intensity for 14–60 min in hot conditions in subjects with over 60% surface area burns compared to 30–40% surface area burns and unburned controls. However, study limitations included small subject numbers ($n = 3$ in both burned groups, $n = 2$ controls), groups included both males and females, with a wide variance in activity levels, age, body mass and exercise duration, plus statistical analysis was not undertaken by the authors (Austin et al. 2003). Furthermore, three of the six burned subjects were unable to complete 60 min of exercise (in fact, one only completed 14 min), making the results very difficult to interpret, and after close scrutiny of the data it is noted that core temperature rise in those with burns who completed the full 60 min was twice that of the control group despite similar reported sweat rates. Currently there is no published literature describing the sweat rates or fluid intake practices of athletes with severe burns or skin grafts. It is therefore important for the practitioner to investigate individual sweat rates in these athletes, and where possible changes in core temperature, and work with them to determine an individualised fluid intake plan and consider the need for alternative cooling devices when exercising in the heat.

The choice of anthropometrical assessment for athletes with severe burns may require modification depending on the location of those burns. Skin grafts, and sites where skin grafts have been taken from, have different compressibility of the skin, which may lead to difficulty in taking consistent skinfold measurements. An anthropometrist may choose to alter the location of a skinfold site (provided this is well documented and used consistently in repeat measurements), omit one site, or elect not to take skinfolds in situations where skin grafts are widespread. In this case, alternative methods of body composition assessment may be considered, such as the use of dual energy x-ray absorptiometry (DXA) or air displacement plethsmography, as discussed in Chapter 12.

7.4   FRIEDREICH'S ATAXIA AND MUSCULAR DYSTROPHIES

Muscular dystrophy is a range of neuromuscular disorders which involve the progressive and irreversible wasting of voluntary muscle tissue. There are approximately 60 muscular dystrophy diseases, each with a separate cause, and symptoms of the disorder and the muscles it impacts upon will vary across causes. Since the disease impacts directly on muscle, the likely sports nutrition issues include a reduced energy expenditure and fuel utilisation during exercise, particularly the more immobile an athlete becomes. Athletes will need to be assessed on a case by case basis according to their functional capabilities, body size and the sport they are involved in.

Friedreich's ataxia is one form of muscular dystrophy and is a genetic disease causing progressive degeneration in the central and peripheral nervous systems, cardiomyopathy, skeletal abnormalities and an increased risk of diabetes (Pandolfo 2002; Santos et al. 2010). The neurological deficits result in a range of symptoms from muscle weakness to speech problems, with symptoms usually beginning between the ages of 5 and 15, and within 8 to 10 years the majority of sufferers are unable to walk. Friedreich's ataxia is caused by the decreased function of frataxin, a protein that binds iron in the mitochondrial matrix (Santos et al. 2010). Decreased frataxin function results in iron accumulation in the mitochondria, resulting in dysfunction of mitochondria, iron-mediated oxidative stress and iron depletion in the cytosol (Wilson 2012). This localised iron accumulation does not appear to be associated with systemic iron deficiency (Santos et al. 2010). A number of therapies are being trialled to manage this disease, each of which has a tendency for adverse outcomes related to iron (including low serum ferritin or elevated haematocrit; Nachbauer and Boesch 2011; Wilson 2012), therefore it should be determined whether the athlete is on any treatment (and if so, which) since this may impact on dietary iron requirements. The recommendation to increase antioxidant nutrient consumption in athletes remains valid in this population to help counterbalance the increased oxidative stress within the mitochondria.

7.5   MULTIPLE SCLEROSIS

Multiple sclerosis (MS) is the most common degenerative auto-immune disorder of the central nervous system resulting in a range of neurological symptoms depending on the site of inflammation and scarring of the myelin sheath around nerve fibres (Payne 2001). Common symptoms of MS include fatigue, depression, cognitive impairment, spasticity, pain and imbalance. There are several forms of MS depending on the nature of progression (e.g. relapsing-remitting, primary progressive, or secondary/chronic progressive) and while the neurological dysfunction may be minimal in the early stages, it will progressively worsen. It is therefore more likely that individuals whose MS results in limitations that would enable them to be classified as an athlete with an impairment will have had the disease for some time and their neurological symptoms will most likely change and/or worsen in due course.

Athletes with MS need nutrition advice to account for the primary symptoms and the impact they have on motor function (and hence energy requirements). A diet rich in essential fatty acids (omega-3 and omega-6 fatty acids) and low in saturated fatty acids via increased intake of fish and vegetable oils, and reduced animal fat intake, has been recommended due to their essential role in membrane phospholipids (Harbige and Sharief 2007; Payne 2001). Similarly, increased intakes of antioxidant nutrients have been advised (particularly vitamin E) as there are indications of increased oxidative stress in MS sufferers. Where neurological changes impact on gut motility or swallowing, increased fibre and fluid intake or alterations in the consistency of food (respectively) are also advised (Payne 2001). There has also been interest in the association between vitamin D and MS, in terms of both the risk of developing the

---

COMMENTARY BOX 7.1

ATHLETE INSIGHT: Training and multiple sclerosis.

The biggest challenge to me being able to train consistently and optimise my sporting performance is being extremely careful about managing my training so that my MS doesn't flare up, knowing where that fine line is.

—**Carol Cooke, cyclist, Paralympic medallist;
ex-rower and able-bodied swimmer**

---

disease and its management, the evidence for which has been reviewed by Solomon and Whitham (2010). They recommend screening MS sufferers for vitamin D status and supplementing where blood levels are deficient or insufficient.

7.6 POLIOMYELITIS

Poliomyelitis is an acute viral infection which results in inflammation of the spinal cord grey matter and destruction of motor neurons. This leads to muscle weakness and flaccid paralysis and in a relatively small number of individuals (<0.5% of those infected) it will be permanent. For these individuals sports nutrition requirements will be based on the severity of the paralysis—often it only affects one limb or one component of a limb (such as the foot).

7.7 SEVERE ARTHRITIS

Arthritis is a disorder which involves inflammation of one or more bone joints. There are over 100 forms of arthritis and associated autoimmune diseases, of which some forms can onset in young individuals. Over time joints can become further damaged and mobility more limited due to stiffness and chronic pain. In rheumatoid arthritis, the immune system attacks tissues including joint lining and cartilage and can lead to severe deformity in only a few years if not treated.

There is some documentation that rheumatoid arthritis can result in increased metabolic rate and catabolism due to the inflammatory processes (Martin 1998). There may also be influences of regular medications on either gastrointestinal function, hormone balance or micronutrient interactions, so use of medication should be checked. Finally, there has been interest in the use of omega-3 fatty acids (e.g. fish oils) and vitamin E supplementation for their anti-inflammatory and anti-oxidant roles as part of the management of pain and inflammation in arthritis (particularly rheumatoid forms; Tidow-Kebritchi and Mobarhan 2001). Practitioners are encouraged to assess athlete usage of these adjunct therapies and consider recent literature prior to giving advice. As with polio, the impact of arthritis varies enormously between individuals, hence the practitioner must assess sports nutrition needs and modifications to recommendations on a case by case basis.

COMMENTARY BOX 7.2

ATHLETE INSIGHT: The value of a sports nutrition practitioner.

I think the most important thing my sports nutrition practitioner did to assist me was recommend what I could do or what I could eat when I found that I was lacking in energy during a specific training block. We also talked about and tried different ways of getting ready on race day, well before the race day, to make sure that my energy levels were at their best in order to make my racing the best it could be. She also was there to listen when I wanted a whinge! She praised me when things were going well (with weight loss) but didn't come down on me when things had stalled. She was extremely supportive.

—Carol Cooke, cyclist, Paralympic medallist;
ex-rower and able-bodied swimmer

7.8   ARTHROGRYPOSIS AND OSTEOGENESIS IMPERFECTA

Arthrogryposis is a non-progressive disease characterised by multiple joint contractures usually in all four limbs. Muscle weakness can result from the contractures, which further limits movement. Osteogenesis imperfecta is a genetic mutation whereby collagen production is reduced or of poorer quality than normal. The primary outcome is weak bones which fracture easily. Neither of these disorders has specific nutrition management nor are the nutritional requirements during exercise documented. However, considering both are likely to require the athlete to be involved in minimal impact, low intensity forms of exercise, it is most likely that sports nutrition education would focus on optimising neurological function and general health and wellbeing.

REFERENCES

Austin, K.G., Hansbrough, J.F., Dore, C., Noordenbos, J., and Buono, M.J. 2003. Thermoregulation in burn patients during exercise. *Journal of Burn Care and Rehabilitation* 24:9–14.

Ben-Simchon, C., Tsur, H., Keren, G., Epstain, Y., and Shapiro, Y. 1981. Heat tolerance in patients with extensive healed burns. *Plastic and Reconstructive Surgery* 67:499–504.

Crandall, C.G., and Davis, S.L. 2010. Cutaneous vascular and sudomotor responses in human skin grafts. *Journal of Applied Physiology* 109:1524–1530.

Diaz, A., Vogiatzi, M.G., Sanz, M.M., and German, J. 2006. Evaluation of short stature, carbohydrate metabolism and other endocrinopathies in Bloom's syndrome. *Hormone Research* 66:111–117.

Gauglitz, G.G., Herndon, D.N., Kulp, G.A., Meyer, W.J., and Jeschte, M.G. 2009. Abnormal insulin sensitivity persists up to three years in pediatric patients post-burn. *Journal of Clinical Endocrinology and Metabolism* 94:1656–1664.

Harbige, L.S., and Sharief, M.K. 2007. Polyunsaturated fatty acids in the pathogenesis and treatment of multiple sclerosis. *British Journal of Nutrition* 98(Suppl 1):S46–S53.

Hunter, A.G.W., Hecht, J.T., and Scott, C.I., Jr. 1996. Standard weight for height curves in achondroplasia. *American Journal of Medical Genetics* 62:255–261.

Klein, G.L. 2008. The interaction between burn injury and vitamin D metabolism and consequences for the patient. *Current Clinical Pharmacology* 3:204–210.

Klein, G.L., Chen, T.C., Holick, M.F., et al. 2004. Synthesis of vitamin D in skin after burns. *Lancet* 363:291–292.

Martin, R.H. 1998. The role of nutrition and diet in rheumatoid arthritis. *Proceedings of the Nutrition Society* 57:231–234.

Nachbauer, W., and Boesch, S. 2011. New advances in the treatment of Friedreich ataxia: promises and pitfalls. *Clinical Investigation* 1:1095–1106.

Oliveira, C.R.P., Salvatori, R., Barreto-Filho, J.A.S., et al. 2012. Insulin sensitivity and β-cell function in adults with lifetime, untreated isolated growth hormone deficiency. *Journal of Clinical Endocrinology and Metabolism* 97:1013–1019.

Owen, O.E., Smalley, K.J., D'Alessio, D.A., et al. 1990. Resting metabolic rate and body composition of achondroplastic dwarfs. *Medicine* 69:56–67.

Pandolfo, M. 2002. Iron metabolism and mitochondrial abnormalities in Friedreich ataxia. *Blood Cells, Molecules and Diseases* 29:536–547.

Payne, A. 2001. Nutrition and diet in the clinical management of multiple sclerosis. *Journal of Human Nutrition and Dietetics* 14:349–357.

Santos, R., Lefevre, S., Sliwa, D., Seguin, A., Camadro, J., and Lesuisse, E. 2010. Friedreich ataxia: molecular mechanisms, redox considerations, and therapeutic opportunities. *Antioxidants and Redox Signaling* 13:651–690.

Shapiro, Y., Epstein, Y., Ben-Simchon, C., and Tsur, H. 1982. Thermoregulatory response of patients with extensive healed burns. *Journal of Applied Physiology* 53:1019–1022.

Solomon, A.J., and Whitham, R.H. 2010. Multiple sclerosis and vitamin D: a review and recommendations. *Current Neurology and Neuroscience Reports* 10:389–396.

Tidow-Kebritchi, S., and Mobarhan, S. 2001. Effects of diets containing fish oil and vitamin E on rheumatoid arthritis. *Nutrition Reviews* 59:335–338.

Wilson, R.B. 2012. Therapeutic developments in Friedreich ataxia. *Journal of Child Neurology* 27:1212–1216.

8 Vision and Hearing Impairment

Elizabeth Broad

CONTENTS

8.1 INTRODUCTION

Individuals with vision impairment compete in a range of sports, have several subcategories and the terminology used to differentiate them is sport-specific. Those with the most visual acuity often compete without a support person, whereas those with the least vision will require a seeing guide, such as the lead rider on a tandem bike, or a guide calling instructions in alpine skiing. Consequently, the practitioner could be advising both the visually impaired athlete and their guide when providing sports nutrition advice. Many sports can be modified to enable participation by visually impaired individuals, especially in ways that take advantage of other senses such as hearing. In contrast, some sports such as goalball and 5-a-side football are specifically for this class of athletes. Team sports involve balls containing bells so that athletes are able to hear their location. To enable all categories of vision impairment to compete in these specialised sports at an equal level, blindfolds are used (other than the goalkeeper in football) and interestingly the audience is requested not to make any noise during play so that the competitors can hear the sound of the ball and be able to judge its location and direction of movement.

Deafness is defined (for the purposes of international sporting competitions) as having lost at least 55 decibels from normal values in the better hearing ear, although some countries may have different criteria for domestic competitions. Hearing impairment is not a category for competing in the Paralympic Games, however there are other major competitions including the Deaf Summer and Winter Games (Deaflympics) run every 4 years, and others such as regional competitions, plus hearing impaired individuals are often invited to compete in domestic competitions which include other athletes with an impairment.

8.2   VISION IMPAIRMENT

The most prevalent causes of vision loss in most developed countries are age-related degenerative eye diseases such as macular degeneration, diabetic retinopathy, glaucoma and cataract. Retinitis pigmentosa, hereditary retinal disorders (such as congenital nystagmus and albinism), optic nerve hypoplasia and eye trauma are more common causes of vision impairment (VI) in younger individuals. In developing countries, visual impairments in children are also due to infectious diseases such as toxoplasmic macular retinochoroiditis, retinal dystrophies and ocular malformation (Haddad et al. 2007).

Physiologically, there is no reason to believe there are any differences between VI athletes and seeing counterparts. The circadian rhythm of individuals with complete VI is longer than 24 h which may influence their strength and reaction times, and hence the optimal time for competition and performance may vary over time and repeatability of performance tests may be reduced compared to a non-VI population (Squarcini et al. 2013). VI athletes may also suffer sleep disturbances due to the disruption to their circadian rhythm, which can impact on recovery, dietary intake and timing of meals. VI athletes are most likely going to train and compete at a slower speed than their seeing counterparts, and rely more heavily on other senses (such as hearing). For example, the winning 400 m run times at the London Paralympic Games were 50.75 s for the men's T11 (most visually impaired) and 48.59 s for T13 (least visually impaired) compared to 43.94 s for the men's London Olympic Games results. It is not known to what degree this difference in speed impacts on sports nutrition requirements.

COMMENTARY BOX 8.1

COACH'S INSIGHT: Coaching VI athletes.

Visually impaired athletes are slower partly due to the longer processing time required to determine their body position in relationship to their environment— for example, where they are located in their lane, when the bend starts and finishes when running the bend on a track. In addition, some forms of VI are impacted by training load, so you cannot train them for as long and/or hard within an individual training session.

—Iryna Dvoskina, athletics coach (multiple Paralympic medallists)

8.2.1 RETINITIS PIGMENTOSA

Retinitis pigmentosa is a group of genetic eye diseases that cause the progressive degeneration of photoreceptor cells in the retina resulting in a loss of vision. Initially the individual may have difficulty seeing at night, but eventually their 'field of vision' reduces progressing from the periphery towards central vision.

Several nutrition interventions have been investigated for individuals with retinitis pigmentosa, primarily in the form of fat soluble vitamin supplementation. Berson (1999) suggests that consumption of 15,000 IU of vitamin A daily in supplemental form, under medical supervision, slows the rate of progression of the disease and has a low risk of toxicity in those over 18 years of age. Vitamin E supplementation, however, should be avoided. There has also been a small number of studies investigating supplemental omega-3 fatty acids in slowing the progression of retinitis pigmentosa since individuals with the disease have significantly reduced plasma docosahexanoic acid (DHA) which appears to have an important function in the retina (Hodge et al. 2006). The outcomes of these studies show possible small benefits, but importantly no detrimental effects, on progression of the disease (Hodge et al. 2006). Consequently it would appear prudent to advise athletes with retinitis pigmentosa to maintain an adequate intake of omega-3 containing foods such as oily fish, walnuts, flaxseed and canola oil.

8.2.2 DIABETIC RETINOPATHY

Diabetic retinopathy occurs when the blood vessels in the retina burst or are damaged and the blood leakage causes swelling or oedema in the retina. It is one of the known long term complications of poorly controlled diabetes (Deakin et al. 2010), and due to the age of most athletes who will seek sports nutrition advice, it is most likely that they will have Type 1 diabetes rather than Type 2. The management of Type 1 diabetes relies on insulin injections, whereas Type 2 can usually be managed through diet, exercise and oral medications. The inability to self-regulate insulin, and consequently other counter-regulatory hormones such as glucagon, in Type 1 diabetes increases the risk of hypoglycaemia which can be further potentiated by exercise if insulin and carbohydrate intakes are not managed carefully.

A complete overview of the dietary management of athletes with diabetes is a topic that is beyond the scope of this chapter and readers are referred to more specialised resources (for example, Deakin et al. 2010, www.runsweet.com, www.diabetes-exercise.org/index.asp and www.glycemicindex.com). In addition, an athlete's management should always be undertaken in conjunction with their endocrinologist and diabetes educator and involves regular monitoring of blood glucose response to exercise on an individual basis since everyone can respond differently. The use of real-time continuous glucose monitoring can be beneficial for athletes with Type 1 diabetes to help understand their blood glucose response to exercise, especially when exercise levels vary from day to day or increase as happens in a sports camp situation or in an athlete who trains two or three times daily. Carbohydrate intake algorithms have been developed to guide carbohydrate intake in response to blood glucose levels during exercise (Riddell and Milliken 2011; Robertson et al. 2009);

however it is important to remember that blood glucose response to exercise can be variable even under standardised conditions and will also vary according to pre-exercise blood glucose concentration, fitness levels, age, body mass, intensity and duration of exercise (Robertson et al. 2009). Therefore a standardised recommendation will be difficult to develop.

There are some key factors which are worth noting when working with an athlete who has diabetes. The current recommendations are to manage insulin doses around the carbohydrate requirements for exercise, as opposed to managing carbohydrate intake according to insulin. Since exercise itself results in the insulin-independent uptake of glucose into muscles, in most instances less insulin is required around an exercise bout (particularly afterwards) than in a sedentary situation. While carbohydrate requirements during exercise do not differ from those of other athletes, the diabetic may need to be more strategic with consuming carbohydrate during and immediately after exercise in order to prevent declines in blood glucose concentrations. Patterns of carbohydrate intake across the day will also need to be more regimented in athletes with diabetes and meal plans will require specificity especially where the vision impairment limits the athlete's ability to read food labels and readily monitor portion sizes. Finally, there may be other nutritional requirements which require attention if there are other diabetes complications present (such as high blood pressure or renal failure).

8.2.3 ALBINISM

Albinism is a congenital disorder where there is partial or complete absence of pigment in the skin, hair and eyes due to a defect in the production of melanin. Albinism is associated with a number of vision defects, such as photophobia, nystagmus and astigmatism. An additional complication of albinism is an increased tendency to sunburn and develop skin cancers, which generally results in limiting exposure to sunlight, thereby increasing the risk of low vitamin D status. As discussed in Chapters 4 and 7, vitamin D deficiency can impact on exercise performance and health, therefore all athletes with albinism should be screened for vitamin D status on an annual basis and supplemented as necessary (see Chapter 10).

8.2.4 STAGARDT DISEASE

Stagardt disease (or fundus flavimaculatus) is an inherited juvenile form of macular degeneration (MD) which begins before 20 years of age and progressively deteriorates with central vision affected more than peripheral.

The majority of nutrition interventions into reducing the incidence and progression of macular degeneration have been investigated in older-age-related MD. Research has highlighted the potential roles of linoleic acid (being implicated in the progression of the disease), while omega-3 fatty acids and antioxidant nutrients including vitamins C and E, beta carotene, lutein, zeaxanthin and zinc are all being investigated regarding potential protective effects against disease progression. There is consistent support for increased consumption of fish rich in omega-3 fatty acids in reducing the incidence of age-related MD (Chua et al. 2006). Whether this is also relevant at younger ages has not been determined, however there remains strong interest in the role of omega-3 oils, and a reduced ratio of omega-6:omega-3 fatty acid intake, in slowing the progression of a number of eye diseases (Fang et al. 2009). The research regarding the role of antioxidant nutrients and zinc remains limited (Berson 1999; Stone 2007), and the practitioner must be mindful of the evidence suggesting antioxidant supplementation has the potential to reduce adaptations to exercise (as discussed in Chapter 3) and high doses of some vitamins and zinc can have adverse effects (such as increased incidence of cancer, and Alzheimer's disease; Stone 2007). Consuming a diet rich in lutein- and zeaxanthin-rich foods such as carrots and green leafy vegetables (such as spinach) may improve macular pigment levels in individuals who initially have low levels of macular pigment (Graydon et al. 2012) and lutein has been shown to inhibit the expression of the proinflammatory gene cyclooxygenase-2 which has been linked to the pathogenesis of age-related MD (Fang et al. 2009). Therefore, together with the proposed anti-inflammatory properties of fish oils, there is efficacy in encouraging athletes with visual impairment to consume at least two or three servings of oily fish/week and maintain a diet rich in antioxidant nutrients, carotenoids and zinc sourced from foods (such as fruit, brightly coloured vegetables, whole grain cereals and animal products). Finally, recent research indicates the potential for saffron to be effective in improving vision in the early stages of MD (Falsini et al. 2010) so research trends in this area are worth following. Whether this is related to the antioxidant properties of saffron or other mechanisms remains unknown.

8.2.5 PRACTICAL ISSUES WITH VISUAL IMPAIRMENT

To optimally support athletes with visual impairments, it is important for the sports nutrition practitioner to discuss openly how best to provide information (for example, written or verbal) and to understand the athlete's range and accuracy of vision.

Much of the sports nutrition advice for athletes with visual impairment will be centred around practical modifications/applications. For example, vision impairments prevent athletes from being able to drive, so they are usually dependent upon public transport or transport by other individuals. Taking public transport to and from training and sporting venues usually extends the time frame of travel, however can also present an opportunity to eat and drink. Therefore pre-training and recovery nutrition suggestions need to be portable and the time spent in travel needs to be incorporated into meal plans. Similarly, vision impaired athletes are less able to recognise dehydration status through visual clues so may require additional external support (for example, a support person to undertake urine specific gravity (USG) measurements) when educating them about hydration and the impact of training and environment on this. Chapter 13 provides additional practical advice for these athletes.

It is important to ensure sports nutrition advice promotes optimal nervous system function and attention in order for the athlete to optimise their sensory receptors. As discussed in Chapter 3, maintaining adequate blood glucose concentrations and optimising hydration status are useful for ensuring optimal nervous system functioning.

COMMENTARY BOX 8.2

COACH'S INSIGHT: What do you believe are the biggest differences in coaching athletes with an impairment compared to able-bodied athletes?

With the visually impaired athletes your verbal communication is of paramount importance to achieving a result. You need an intimate understanding of the skill you are trying to teach, and must be able to relate the way it feels to these athletes, be confident in this and in guiding them into correct positions so they can develop the feeling you are after.

—Emily Nolan, strength and conditioning coach

8.3 HEARING IMPAIRMENT

There are several causes of hearing impairment, including injury, disease and genetic defects. The most common adjustment required for athletes with a hearing impairment is a visual form of the starter's gun, such as a starting light, to replace the auditory one. Coaches may also have to modify their communication process, for example in swimming, when hearing aids are unable to be used during aquatic training sessions. When educating an individual with a hearing impairment, it is important to speak directly to their face and provide written support wherever possible. It is also useful to check their understanding of what you have said to ensure the correct message has been received.

REFERENCES

Berson, E.L. 1999. Nutrition and retinal degenerations. In *Modern nutrition in health and disease*, ed. M.E. Shils, J.A. Olson, M. Shike, and A.C. Ross, 1491–1501. Baltimore: Williams & Wilkins.

Chua, B., Flood, V., Roohtchina, E., Wang, J.J., Smith, W., and Mitchell, P. 2006. Omega 3 fatty acids and age-related macular degeneration. *Archives of Opthalmology* 124:981–986.

Deakin, V., Wilson, D., and Cooper, G. 2010. Special needs: the athlete with diabetes. In *Clinical sports nutrition*, ed. L. Burke and V. Deakin, 578–601. 4th ed. Sydney: McGraw-Hill.

Falsini, B., Piccardi, M., Minnella, A., et al. 2010. Influence of saffron supplementation on retinal flicker sensitivity in early age-related macular degeneration. *Investigative Ophthalmology and Visual Science* 51:6118–6124.

Fang, I., Yang, C., Yang, C., and Chen, M. 2009. Comparative effects of fatty acids on proinflammatory gene cyclooxygenase 2 and inducible nitric oxide synthase expression in retinal pigment epithelial cells. *Molecular Nutrition and Food Research* 53:739–750.

Graydon, R., Hogg, R.E., Chakravarthy, U., Young, I.S., and Woodside, J.V. 2012. The effect of lutein- and zeathanin-rich foods v. supplements on macular pigment level and serological markers of endothelial activation, inflammation and oxidation: pilot studies in healthy volunteers. *British Journal of Nutrition* 108:334–342.

Haddad, M.A.O., Sei, M., Sampaio, M.W., and Kara-Jose, N. 2007. Causes of visual impairment in children: a study of 3210 cases. *Journal of Pediatric Ophthalmology and Strabismus* 44:232–240.

Hodge, W.G., Barnes, D., Schachter, H.M., et al. 2006. The evidence for efficacy of omega-3 fatty acids in preventing or slowing the progression of retinitis pigmentosa: a systematic review. *Canadian Journal of Opthalmology* 41:481–490.

Riddell, M.C., and Milliken, J. 2011. Preventing exercise-induced hypoglycaemia in type 1 diabetes using real-time continuous glucose monitoring and a new carbohydrate intake algorithm: an observational field study. *Diabetes Technology and Therapeutics* 13:1–7.

Robertson, K., Adolfsson, P., Scheiner, G., Hanas, R., and Riddell, M.C. 2009. Exercise in children and adolescents with diabetes. *Pediatric Diabetes* 10(Suppl 12):154–168.

Squarcini, C.F.R., Pires, M.L.N., Lopes, C., et al. 2013. Free-running circadian rhythms of muscle strength, reaction time, and body temperature in totally blind people. *European Journal of Applied Physiology* 113:157–165.

Stone, E.M. 2007. Macular degeneration. *Annual Reviews of Medicine* 58:477–490.

9 Intellectual Impairments

Elizabeth Broad

CONTENTS

9.1   INTRODUCTION

Intellectual impairments, as outlined in Chapter 2, are currently included in a limited range of sports such as table tennis, swimming and athletics at the Paralympic Games. Additionally they are included in a range of other major sporting events, including the Summer and Winter Special Olympics which are also run every 4 years. The most recent Summer Special Olympics held in 2011 attracted nearly 7000 athletes from 170 countries. Intellectual impairments cover a broad spectrum of disorders, with the overriding requirement being an IQ less than 75, age of onset under 18 years, and limitations in adaptive behaviour (such as self-care, communication, social interaction and learning). There are a large range of diagnoses, which include Down syndrome, autism, and Asperger syndrome. Some intellectual impairments also coincide with other clinical issues, including epilepsy, visual and auditory defects, and congenital heart disease.

Limited research is available on athletes with intellectual impairments, however there has been interest in non-athletes from the perspective of health since a lack of mobility and physical activity contributes to early mortality in this population (Fernhall and Pitetti 2001). In a review of studies investigating physical work capacity in individuals with intellectual impairments where care was taken to adequately familiarise participants with testing procedures, Fernhall and Pitetti (2001) reported lower than average maximal aerobic capacity (VO_{2max}) other than in one group of runners. Alarmingly, those with Down syndrome have even lower values than other individuals. The primary explanation for this has in the past been a sedentary lifestyle, however more recent research indicates autonomic dysfunction leading to a low maximal heart rate and poor leg strength in this population. Whether these data are skewed since many studies have been undertaken using subjects in institutions

---

COMMENTARY BOX 9.1

COACH'S INSIGHT: What do you believe are the biggest differences in coaching athletes with an impairment compared to able-bodied athletes?

I have found with more individualised and hands-on coaching of the athlete you can get some very significant results and performances, small group or one-on-one sessions is best, and allows you, as the coach, to observe and learn how their impairment impacts on their learning, movement, and performance.

—Emily Nolan, strength and conditioning coach

---

or specific care facilities is unknown. Fortunately, the adaptive response to exercise training appears to be in line with the general population (Frey et al. 1999; Pitetti and Tan 1991; Tsimaras et al. 2001). It is important to note that athletes with intellectual impairments appear to require more opportunities to familiarise themselves with testing equipment and procedures in order to be able to provide reproducible, meaningful results for physiological testing and this should be a requirement of any research studies in this population (Fernhall and Pitteti 2001).

Lante et al. (2010) investigated 31 intellectually impaired individuals (with and without Down syndrome) and found their energy expenditure at various walking speeds to be higher than both a non-intellectually impaired comparison group and also the typical range of values reported in the 'Compendium of Physical Activities' for all but the fastest walking speed (Ainsworth et al. 2011). Lante et al. (2010) believed the differences were due to uncoordinated and exaggerated gross motor movements, or biomechanical inefficiency, in the intellectually impaired group and this thesis has been supported by other investigations (Ohwada et al. 2005). Observing athletes with intellectual impairments in their activities of daily living and general patterns of movement outside of their sport is likely to be important when a practitioner is assessing energy intake guidelines to match estimated energy expenditure.

9.2 DOWN SYNDROME

Down syndrome (DS) (also known as trisomy 21) is a genetic condition which leads to physical and development delays and is responsible for about one third of all cases of moderate to severe intellectual impairment (Hayes and Batshaw 1993). Individuals with DS display joint laxity, muscle hypotonia, reduced strength and a more unstable gait in walking (Agiovlasitis et al. 2011). Additionally, they have higher rates of autoimmune diseases, hearing loss, morbidity and mortality than the general population (Hayes and Batshaw 1993; McKelvey et al. 2012), resulting in a reduced life expectancy which may be improved by involvement in regular physical exercise. Aerobic capacity has been reported to be lower in DS than both the general population (Fernhall and Pitetti 2001) and compared to other intellectually impaired individuals, which Fernhall et al. (2013) have recently proposed is due to autonomic dysfunction resulting in reduced maximal heart rate and muscle hypotonia. Balic et al. (2000) found higher aerobic capacity, maximal heart rate, endurance times and muscle strength in a DS group who had trained an average of 4.9 h per week for at least 1 year in order to compete in the Special Olympics compared to sedentary DS adults, indicating that there can be positive responses in these variables as a result of structured training. However, the values remained low compared to results frequently reported in the general population, and exercise training programs undertaken in children and adolescents with DS have failed to produce measureable changes in cardiovascular capacity despite improvements in performance capabilities (Gonzalez-Aguero et al. 2000). While it is unlikely that individuals with DS have the ability to develop physiological capabilities similar to elite able-bodied athletes, they can certainly improve strength and physical performance through regular training. Whether fuel contributions to exercise are different due to their poor cardiovascular capabilities is unknown.

Individuals with Down syndrome are shorter than the general population by up to 20 cm, or more than two standard deviations below the mean (Angelopoulou et al. 1999; Baptista et al. 2005), primarily due to disproportionate growth retardation of the legs (Barden 2003). As a consequence, growth curves in children and adolescents have been developed specifically for Down syndrome (Hayes and Batshaw 1993) and the validity of body mass index (BMI) as an indicator of obesity may be questionable. Using BMI as a measure of obesity, Melville et al. (2005) found a greater incidence of obesity in adult women with Down syndrome (in fact, only 26% of the women were in the normal range) but not in men compared with non-DS intellectually impaired adults, and higher BMI in DS women but not men was reported compared to nonintellectually impaired controls (Angelopoulou et al. 1999; Baptista et al. 2005). Bronks and Parker (1985) also undertook somatotype ratings in a DS population which classed them as predominantly mesomorphic endomorphs, although this is not entirely surprising considering the relative shortness of their legs would result in low ectomorphy ratings. Estimates of body fat using skinfold and girth measures and a non-population specific equation showed higher percentage body fat than comparison groups. Through undertaking DXA scans, others argue that total body fat levels are not necessarily higher, but rather differently distributed (with a higher fat mass in the truncal region), at least in children and adolescents with Down syndrome (Gonzalez-Aguero et al. 2011a). This has been shown to hold true for adult males despite a significantly lower muscle mass compared to controls, but not for females who displayed both higher fat mass and lower muscle mass (Baptista et al. 2005). Similarly, Usera et al. (2005) found there was a poor relationship between estimating body fat from skinfolds or girths in DS and the percent body fat determined by air displacement plethysmography. Whether there is any relationship between body fat levels and a higher incidence of thyroid dysfunction in DS (Hayes and Batshaw 1993) has not yet been determined, however Allison et al. (1995) reported that the lower resting energy expenditure in DS subjects compared to controls was ameliorated when thyroid function was controlled for. The management of body composition (particularly central adiposity) may be one challenge faced when working with athletes with Down syndrome, however it is also important to undertake a range of anthropometrical assessments to more fully describe their body composition than just body mass and height and to avoid estimating percent body fat from equations that are not validated in this population.

Assessments of energy expenditure in athletes with Down syndrome have not been undertaken. There is mixed evidence regarding resting metabolic rates (RMR) in DS, with some reports indicating reduced RMR in young DS (Luke et al. 1994) whereas others have shown no difference in RMR in a healthy adult DS cohort compared to a control group (Allison et al. 1995; Fernhall et al. 2005). This may be influenced by thyroid dysfunction if present and not appropriately managed. Reduced gait stability increases metabolic rate during walking in individuals with Down syndrome, particularly at higher walking speeds (Agiovlasitis et al. 2011a, 2011b, 2012). The use of pedometers or accelerometers to estimate metabolic rate appears to produce greater variability in results for individuals with Down syndrome compared to the general population, so may not be a valid assessment of exercise energy expenditure (Agiovlasitis et al. 2011, 2012).

Individuals with Down syndrome are at higher risk than the general population of developing Type 1 diabetes (van Goor et al. 1997), coeliac disease (Gale et al. 1997), and as already mentioned, thyroid dysfunction (Hayes and Batshaw 1993; Hasanhodzic et al. 2006). The management of diabetes in athletes has been discussed in Chapter 8. Athletes with coeliac disease must follow a strictly gluten-free diet, and should be educated regarding suitable choices of carbohydrate-rich foods. Following a gluten-free diet can be more difficult when travelling, however the availability of gluten-free options is increasing in many countries. It is therefore important for the sports nutrition practitioner to undertake some research and provide the athlete and support staff with a list of items which are suitable to eat in the countries they may be travelling to. Additionally, local coeliac societies will often have information cards translated into a number of different languages to help communicate with caterers regarding the athlete's specific dietary needs. Finally, thyroid function should be investigated in all athletes with DS since this can influence body composition, bone density, and health. Treatment of thyroid dysfunction normally involves medication (such as thyroxine), although some interest has evolved in dietary therapy for treating thyroid dysfunction (Thiel and Fowkes 2007), and there is acknowledgement of increasing levels of iodine deficiency in developed countries. Therefore the sports nutrition practitioner should actively seek ways to include iodine-containing foods such as seafood and seaweed, dairy foods, eggs, some breads, iodised salt and vegetables grown in iodine rich soils, in the diet of athletes with DS.

Down syndrome is also associated with an increased incidence of low bone mineral density and osteoporosis, independent of gender and height, occurring even in childhood (Angelopoulou et al. 1999; Baptista et al. 2005; Gonzalez-Aguero et al. 2011b). Although the etiology has not been established, there is evidence for a decrease in bone formation markers compared to control (McKelvey et al. 2012), providing further support for regular exercise in this population. The incidence of low bone mineral density in a free living DS population has been reported to be as high as 53% (McKelvey et al. 2012). Therefore it is recommended that athletes with DS be screened for bone mineral density and that all factors related to bone density are optimised, especially when the athlete is still at an age where peak bone mass is being accrued (i.e. <25 y). Nutrition-related factors which optimise bone density include:

1. Adequate vitamin D status (see Chapters 4 and 10).
2. Adequate calcium intake. Dietary recommendations for calcium intake vary between different countries and at different ages. Since dairy foods are the best source of calcium, and have the added advantage of supporting sports nutrition goals, athletes with DS should be encouraged to consume at least three or four serves of dairy foods daily (1000–1300 mg calcium/d). Where the athlete is allergic or intolerant to dairy, appropriate calcium-fortified alternatives (such as calcium fortified soy milk) and other non-dairy sources of calcium (such as fish with edible bones and tofu) should be encouraged before considering calcium supplements.
3. Adequate vitamin K intake. The research regarding vitamin K and bone health is somewhat limited to date, but indications are that adequate vitamin K is necessary for optimal bone health (Fang et al. 2012). Athletes should be encouraged to consume two or more serves of vegetables rich in vitamin K daily (e.g. broccoli, cabbage, spinach, iceberg lettuce).

In summary, when working with athletes with Down syndrome it will be important to screen them for bone density, vitamin D status, thyroid function, coeliac disease and impaired glucose tolerance. Body composition should be assessed using a range of measures and appropriate goals set considering the likelihood of higher body fat levels than able-bodied populations. While formulating a diet to support training needs, the focus should be on ensuring appropriate timing of protein intake post exercise to optimise muscle adaptations to training, and adequate calcium, iodine and vitamin K intakes within an energy budget that is appropriate to their training and body composition requirements.

9.3   AUTISM AND ASPERGER SYNDROME

Autism, or more broadly autism spectrum disorders, are a range of disorders characterised by significant and chronic impairment in a number of different developmental areas, in particular, social interaction (especially the perception of social cues), communication skills (verbal and non-verbal) and repetitive or obsessive behaviour patterns. Asperger syndrome, now believed to be a form of autism, is more uniquely characterised by difficulties specifically with nonverbal communication, restricted and repetitive behaviours, and physical clumsiness, while linguistic skills and cognitive development are preserved.

One aspect that can be challenging with autism disorders is that the repetitive behaviour patterns can include behaviours relating to food and feeding. Some individuals may have a restricted range of food choices (for example, only consuming a specific colour of food or foods of a particular texture) and may be very resistant to introducing new foods or fluids, or new eating behaviours (such as consuming a snack after exercise). The practitioner must ask questions relating to food preferences and understand the willingness of the athlete to change in order to provide the most appropriate advice. Carers will be important to include in consultations.

9.4   PHENYLKETONURIA

Phenylketonuria (PKU) is an inborn error of metabolism in which the metabolism of the amino acid phenylalanine is disrupted. High blood phenylalanine concentrations are neurotoxic as it inhibits the transport of free L-amino acids required for protein and neurotransmitter synthesis (Giovannini et al. 2012). As a result, neuropsychological performance and IQ are impacted unless a low phenylalanine diet is maintained at least through infancy and childhood. The diet may be more flexible in teenagers and adults than in children, although maintaining a low phenylalanine diet as a teenager or adult can also be useful in optimising brain and nervous system functioning, such as concentration and decision making. There is the possibility that some athletes with intellectual impairments have PKU which has been poorly treated in their developing years, and if this is the case it is important to understand that they can still respond favourably to the PKU diet.

PKU is treated with a low protein diet supplemented with a low-phenylalanine protein substitute providing essential amino acids, vitamins and minerals. Therefore, from a sports nutrition perspective, provision of adequate protein overall, and particularly post exercise to support training adaptations, may require more planning and a complete understanding of the diet the athlete should be following. Liaison with the PKU support team is encouraged as they will have the expertise to help you adapt the eating plan to best suit the athlete's sporting needs. Although no research has been undertaken in athletes with PKU, theoretically it is possible that poorly managed PKU would also reduce the protein synthetic response post exercise thereby reducing training adaptations. Furthermore, athletes with PKU are likely to require supplementation of omega-6 and omega-3 fatty acids since dietary sources are limited (Giovannini et al. 2012).

9.5   SPORTS NUTRITION ISSUES WITH INTELLECTUAL IMPAIRMENTS

Only one assessment has been undertaken on nutrition needs of intellectually impaired athletes, and it was limited to those aged 2–13 y, primarily with Down syndrome (Gibson et al. 2011). The most common nutrition problems reported were oral motor problems (difficulty chewing, swallowing or choking), dental problems, food allergies/intolerances, and constipation, with 84% of parents reporting problems with their child eating too much/too little and refusing many foods (Gibson et al. 2011). Although the data may have been skewed by the self-report, voluntary nature of the investigation, managing sports nutrition requirements of athletes with intellectual impairments can be complicated and generally requires patience, some problem solving skills and reiteration. It is imperative that a team approach is utilised, involving parents/carers, the coach and other professionals (such as sport psychologist) to ascertain correct self-reporting, aid reinforcement of messages and resolve any underlying feeding limitations.

Undertaking body composition assessments can be more difficult in athletes with intellectual impairments. Some are not comfortable being touched or are more sensitive to touch, which impacts on the ability to undertake surface anthropometry. It can be useful to demonstrate the techniques to the athletes in advance in order to engage them more proactively in the process. Other athletes may be more likely to have difficulty staying still which makes undertaking DXA scans and air displacement plethysmography more prone to error. It is important for the practitioner and coach to explain the benefits of body composition assessment to the athlete, but also to plan the type and frequency of assessment carefully and develop strategies that optimise the reliability and repeatability of the measurements.

The nature of some intellectual impairments means that athletes can be heavily influenced by any individuals and can therefore be prone to acting on advice which may lead to inappropriate dietary plans or use of supplements. It may be necessary for sporting teams to employ a process of checking athletes' personal possessions, especially where they are subject to anti-doping testing, in order to ensure any supplements used are appropriate and are low risk for inadvertent doping issues (as outlined in Chapter 11). Checking bags when travelling (especially international travel) to ensure the athlete is compliant with all customs requirements is prudent. Examples of unusual behaviours include:

- A parent sending a child to an international competition with several heads of broccoli. Neither the parent nor the athlete informed team staff of this, and the broccoli ended up being taken back home by the athlete at the end of competition. This presented a high risk of being fined since the food was not declared to customs officers in either country.
- An athlete attempting to take home an excessive number of bottles of ready-to-drink sports drink from an international competition (so much so that baggage weight limits were well exceeded).
- An athlete consuming several sports nutrition products, not understanding what they contain or the potential side effects, but not telling anyone because the person who has sold them to the athlete has suggested it's best to "keep it a secret." This behaviour could result in an inadvertent failure of anti-doping tests.

COMMENTARY BOX 9.2

COACH'S INSIGHT: What do you think is the most important thing a sports nutrition practitioner can do to assist your athletes?

Work to educate not only the athlete, but the coach and parent with simple and consistent messages. I find the biggest challenge I have with many athletes I see is their absorption of the information I provide is poor. Coaches and parents are the key to reinforcing and ensuring the information is implemented.

—Emily Nolan, strength and conditioning coach

Finally, educating athletes with an intellectual impairment can require patience and creativity. Many athletes have short attention spans, so education should be undertaken across a number of short-duration sessions, with very direct verbal instructions followed up by written information. Wherever possible, parents or carers and coaches should be involved in this education in order to ensure reinforcement of messages occurs. Some practical suggestions relating to travel are also included in Chapter 13.

REFERENCES

Allison, D.B., Gomez, J.E., Heshka, S., et al. 1995. Decreased resting metabolic rate among persons with Down syndrome. *International Journal of Obesity* 19:858–861.

Agiovlasitis, S., Motl, R.W., Fahs, C.A., et al. 2011a. Metabolic rate and accelerometer output during walking in people with Down syndrome. *Medicine and Science in Sports and Exercise* 43:1322–1327.

Agiovlasitis, S., Motl, R.W., Foley, J.T., and Fernhall, B. 2012. Prediction of energy expenditure from wrist accelerometry in people with and without Down syndrome. *Adapted Physical Activity Quarterly* 29:179–190.

Agiovlasitis, S., Motl, R.W., Ranadive, S.M., et al. 2011b. Energetic optimization during over-ground walking in people with and without Down syndrome. *Gait and Posture* 33:630–634.

Ainsworth, B.E., Haskell, W.L., Herrmann, S.D., et al. 2011. Compendium of Physical Activities: a second update of codes and MET values. *Medicine and Science in Sports and Exercise* 43:1575–1581.

Angelopoulou, N., Souftas, V., Sakadamis, A., and Mandroukas, K. 1999. Bone mineral density in adults with Down's syndrome. *European Radiology* 9:648–651.

Balic, M.G., Mateos, E.C., and Blasco, C.G. 2000. Physical fitness levels of physically active and sedentary adults with Down syndrome. *Adapted Physical Activity Quarterly* 17:310–321.

Baptista, F., Varela, A., and Sardinha, L. 2005. Bone mineral mass in males and females with and without Down syndrome. *Osteoporosis International* 16:380–388.

Barden, H.S. 2003. Growth and development of selected hard tissues in Down syndrome: a review. *Human Biology* 55:539–576.

Bronks, R., and Parker, A.W. 1985. Anthropometric observation of adults with Down syndrome. *American Journal of Mental Deficiency* 90:110–113.

Fang, Y., Hu, C., Tao, X., Wan, Y., and Tao, F. 2012. Effect of vitamin K on bone mineral density: a meta-analysis of randomized control trials. *Journal of Bone Mineral Metabolism* 30:60–68.

Fernhall, B., Figueroa, A., Collier, S., Goulopoulou, S., Giannoploulou, I., and Baynard, T. 2005. Resting metabolic rate is not reduced in obese adults with Down syndrome. *Mental Retardation* 43:391–400.

Fernhall, B., Mendonca, G.V., and Baynard, T. 2013. Reduced work capacity in individuals with Down Syndrome: a consequence of autonomic dysfunction? *Exercise and Sport Sciences Reviews* 41:138–147.

Fernhall, B., and Pitetti, K.H. 2001. Limitations to physical work capacity in individuals with mental retardation. *Clinical Exercise Physiology* 3:176–185.

Frey, G.C., McCubbin, J.A., Hannigan-Downs, S., Kasser, S.L., and Skaggs, S.O. 1999. Physical fitness of trained runners with and without mild mental retardation. *Adapted Physical Activity Quarterly* 16:126–137.

Gale, L., Wimalaratna, H., Brotodiharjo, A., and Duggan, J.M. 1997. Down's syndrome is strongly associated with coeliac disease. *Gut* 40:492–496.

Gibson, J.C., Temple, V.A., Anholt, J.P., and Gaul, C.A. 2011. Nutrition needs assessment of young Special Olympics participants. *Journal of Intellectual and Developmental Disability* 36:268–272.

Giovannini, M., Verduci, E., Salvatici, E., Paci, S., and Riva, E. 2012. Phenylketonuria: nutritional advances and challenges. *Nutrition and Metabolism* 9:1–7.

Gonzalez-Aguero, A., Ara, I., Moreno, L.A., Vicente-Rodriguez, G., and Casajus, J.A. 2011a. Fat and lean masses in youths with Down syndrome: gender differences. *Research in Developmental Disabilities* 32:1685–1693.

Gonzalez-Aguero, A., Vicente-Rodriguez, G., Moreno, L.A., and Casajus, J.A. 2011b. Bone mass in male and female children and adolescents with Down syndrome. *Osteoporosis International* 22:2151–2157.

Gonzalez-Aguero, A., Vicente-Rodriguez, G., Moreno, L.A., Guerra-Balic, M., Ara, I., and Casajus, J.A. 2010. Health-related physical fitness in children and adolescents with Down syndrome and response to training. *Scandinavian Journal of Medicine and Science in Sports* 20:716–724.

Hasanhodzic, M., Tahirovic, H., and Lukinac, L. 2006. Down syndrome and thyroid gland. *Bosnian Journal of Basic Medical Sciences* 6:38–42.

Hayes, A., and Batshaw, M.L. 1993. Down syndrome. *Pediatric Clinics of North America* 40:523–535.

Lante, K., Reece, J., and Walkley, J. 2010. Energy expended in adults with and without intellectual disabilities during activities of daily living. *Research in Developmental Disabilities* 31:1380–1389.

Luke, A., Rolzen, N.J., Sutton, M., and Schoeller, D.A. 1994. Energy expenditure in children with Down syndrome: correcting metabolic rate for movement. *Journal of Pediatrics* 125:829–838.

McKelvey, K.D., Fowler, T.W., Akel, N.S., et al. 2012. Low bone turnover and low bone density in a cohort of adults with Down syndrome. *Osteoporosis International* DOI 10.1007/s00198-012-2109-4.

Melville, C.A., Cooper, S.A., McGrother, C.W., Thorp, C.F., and Collacott, R. 2005. Obesity in adults with Down syndrome: a case-control study. *Journal of Intellectual Disability Research* 49:125–133.

Ohwada, H., Nakayama, T., Suzuki, Y., Yokoyama, T., and Ishmaru, M. 2005. Energy expenditure in males with mental retardation. *Journal of Nutritional Science and Vitaminology* 51:68–74.

Pitetti, K.H., and Tan, D.M. 1991. Effects of a minimally supervised exercise program for mentally retarded adults. *Medicine and Science in Sports and Exercise* 23:594–601.

Thiel, R., and Fowkes, S.W. 2007. Down syndrome and thyroid dysfunction: should nutritional support be the first-line treatment? *Medical Hypotheses* 69:809–815.

Tsimaras, V., Angelopoulou-Sakadami, N., Efstratopoulou, M., and Mandroukas, K. 2001. The influence of a training program on cardiorespiratory capacity of adults with mental retardation. *Exercise and Society* 27:24–31.

Usera, P.C., Foley, J.T., and Yun, J. 2005. Cross-validation of field-based assessments of body composition for individuals with Down syndrome. *Adapted Physical Activity Quarterly* 22:198–206.

Van Goor, J.C., Massa, G.G., and Hirasing, R. 1997. Increased incidence and prevalence of diabetes mellitus in Down's syndrome (Letter to the editor). *Archives of Disease in Childhood* 77:186.

10 Medical Issues, Pharmacology and Nutrient Interactions

Matthias Strupler and Claudio Perret

CONTENTS

10.1 INTRODUCTION

In general, athletes with an impairment are prone to the same medical issues as able-bodied athletes. However, due to the specific nature of their impairments, these athletes may experience some medical conditions and problems that are not found in able-bodied athletes. For example, spinal cord injuries lead to an impairment or a loss of motor, sensory and vegetative function. Depending on the level and completeness of the spinal cord injury, complications such as autonomic dysreflexia, pressure ulcers or urinary tract infections often occur.

This chapter describes some of these impairment-specific medical conditions, presents preventive strategies to keep athletes with an impairment in good health, discusses the role of iron and vitamin D deficiencies, and highlights some common food-drug interactions. Further information can be found in Van de Vliet et al. (2011) and Zaech and Koch (2006).

10.2 MEDICAL CONDITIONS

10.2.1 Neurogenic Bladder

The consequences of spinal cord injury on bladder function depend on the level, duration and severity of the lesion (Cruz and Cruz 2011). Interruption of neuronal circuits of the central and peripheral nervous system affects the voluntary control of bladder function. Lesions of the cervical and thoracic spinal cord are followed by a period of areflexia and urinary retention. Thereafter, voiding is inefficient due to detrusor-sphincter-dyssynergia, a condition characterized by simultaneous contraction of the detrusor and urethral sphincter (Hansen et al. 2010). Ineffective bladder emptying causes the accumulation of large residual volumes of urine and may cause bladder hypertrophy. As a consequence, individuals with neurogenic bladder often have to use intermittent catheterization every 4 to 6 hours or continuous bladder catheterization for emptying their bladder. Implantation of a stimulator for bladder emptying is another method. All individuals with neurogenic bladder are at increased risk for lower urinary tract infections and their complications, so correct management of neurogenic bladder is important to reduce urinary tract infections. Urinary tract infections usually are bacterial infections that must be treated with antibiotics, and both the infection and the treatment have an impact on training and competition. Serious complications such as renal pelvis infection or sepsis often require hospitalization. Frequent fluid intake to produce a sufficient amount of urine and regular emptying of the bladder may prevent these infections.

10.2.2 Bone Density

After spinal cord injury (SCI) bone density is reduced in the paretic limbs. In the femur and tibia bone mass and bone mineral density decrease exponentially. The decreasing bone parameters reach new steady states 3–8 years after injury, depending on the parameter (Eser et al. 2004). The loss of bone mass in the epiphysis is approximately 50% in the femur and 60% in the tibia, while the shafts lose only approximately 35% in the femur and 25% in the tibia. Low bone density increases the risk of fractures even with relatively minor traumas. To reduce bone loss and prevent bone fractures a sufficient supply of calcium (1000 mg/d) and vitamin D (800 IE/d) is required. Bisphosphonates can reduce the loss of bone mass during a treatment of 2 years. Furthermore, a high-volume cycle training with functional electrical stimulation (FES) for 12 months could partially reverse bone loss in chronic SCI and thus may reduce fracture risk of the lower limbs (Frotzler et al. 2008, 2009). Chronic SCI athletes with sensory loss may not report pain after sustaining a fracture, but only spasticity or other unspecific symptoms. Therefore investigation with x-rays is recommended even after minor traumas, to avoid undetected fractures. Bone fractures in individuals with SCI normally have to be treated with surgery to stabilize the bone. After an operation mobilization and independence are more quickly attained than without an operation.

10.2.3 Autonomic Dysreflexia

Autonomic dysreflexia (AD) is a potentially life-threatening condition that occurs in individuals with an SCI at level T6 or above. Due to a massive paroxysmal reflex sympathetic discharge below the lesion level, the constriction of the arteries leads to high blood pressure. The elevated blood pressure causes stimulation of the aortic arch and carotid sinus baroreceptors, which causes inhibition of the vasomotor center and vagal stimulation. Inhibition of vasomotor centers would cause peripheral vasodilation if descending pathways were intact, but in subjects with quadriplegia only the vagal system is effective to control hypertension, which results in bradycardia. Consequently, the symptoms of AD are hypertension, bradycardia, headache, nasal congestion, chills without fever, blurred vision, goose bumps and sweating above the level of injury (Van de Vliet et al. 2011). Noxious stimuli below the level of injury lead to unopposed sympathetic outflow. Noxious stimuli include bladder distention, bowel distention from impaction, skin lesions or skin pressure and many other conditions.

The following steps for treatment are recommended (Sipski and Richards 2006):

1. Sit patient up.
2. Check blood pressure.
3. Treat hypertension with nitroglycerine or nifedipine.
4. Look for and remove noxious stimuli.
5. Monitor symptoms and blood pressure.

Athletes with a SCI above T6 may attempt to use AD to enhance performance. Athletes do not empty their bladder before a competition and in quadriplegics elevation of blood pressure and heart rate leads to an enhancement of performance. This so-called 'boosting' is banned in competition.

10.2.4 PRESSURE ULCERS

Pressure ulcers are a serious complication of SCI, as well as in amputees wearing a prosthesis, and they have the potential to interfere with physical, psychological and social well-being and impact quality of life. In athletes, treatment of pressure ulcers often requires an interruption of sports practice and consequently leads to an impairment in sports performance. Treatment of pressure ulcers is always difficult and takes a long time. Therefore prevention of pressure ulcers is fundamental for athletes. Risk factors for pressure ulcers are lack of sensation, limitation of mobility, moisture from bladder/bowel dysfunction, muscle atrophy, smoking, arteriosclerosis, diabetes and poor nutritional status. Therefore, screening for albumin, ferritin, vitamin B12, folic acid and hemoglobin is mandatory (Cruse et al. 2000). Typical prevention recommendations include daily examination of the skin, keeping skin dry and clean, having regular pressure relief, and having an individually adapted wheelchair cushion. In addition, cessation of smoking, limited alcohol consumption and eating well-balanced meals with regular weight monitoring are recommended. In a systematic review further evidence-based recommendations are electrical stimulation with gluteal electrodes and pressure relief in the forward-leaning position (vertical lift is less effective; Regan et al. 2009).

10.3 PREVENTION

It is important for athletes to stay in good health during preparation and during competition. The duty of a sports medicine doctor is to inform and educate athletes concerning prevention measures that may be effective. Some important issues are discussed below.

10.3.1 HYGIENE

Especially during the cold season the chance to acquire a viral infection is high. The following standard health precautions should be followed to avoid spreading infection:

1. Cover mouth and nose when sneezing or coughing.
2. Wash or disinfect hands regularly, especially before eating.
3. Do not touch or scratch skin, nose, eyes or mouth because an infection can be transmitted this way.
4. Avoid close contact with people (touching, kissing) and avoid crowds.

10.3.2 IMMUNIZATION

The recommendations for immunization are different in each country. Vaccination against tetanus, diphtheria and polio is recommended in most countries. During winter months immunization against flu should be taken into account and planned well in advance. It is important that the support personnel are included in these measures to minimize the possibility of spreading illness.

10.3.3 EXERCISE-INDUCED BRONCHOCONSTRICTION

Exercise-induced bronchoconstriction (EIB) is closely related to asthma and is defined as a transient narrowing of the airways, limiting expiration during strenuous exercise (Parsons and Mastronarde 2009). Asthma and EIB are the most common medical conditions encountered in Olympic athletes, with an overall prevalence of about 8% (Hanstad et al. 2011). However, in endurance sports much higher incidences were found, ranging from 17% to 60% for triathlon, cycling, cross-country skiing, and swimming (Bougault et al. 2011). The high prevalence of EIB in these types of sports is thought to be due to the training/competition environment and ventilatory requirements. For the assessment of EIB and airway hyperresponsiveness various methods such as the mannitol challenge test, the methacholine challenge test and eucapnic voluntary hyperventilation (EVH) are used (Dickinson et al. 2011; Zitt 2005). The value of the different challenge tests for clinical practice is controversial, but EVH seems to be the most specific and methacholine challenge the most sensitive test. A study in our center found that challenge tests are feasible, safe and useful in Paralympic athletes, especially in athletes with spinal cord injury (Osthoff et al. 2013). Different authors conclude that screening for EIB should be used for elite athletes routinely, because a high proportion of previously undiagnosed athletes may benefit from the use of appropriate medication against EIB.

10.4 DEFICIENCIES

Deficiencies of iron and vitamin D are performance-limiting factors.

10.4.1 IRON

Iron is the functional component of hemoglobin and myoglobin and therefore essential for the transport and delivery of oxygen in the body. Iron is also important for mitochondrial enzymes in the context of aerobic metabolism. Therefore declined iron stores can lead to an impairment of sporting performance.

Serum ferritin represents the iron store in the body and is used to screen athletes for iron deficiency. Ferritin is the only parameter that is needed for the detection of an iron deficiency, but C-reactive protein must always be analysed simultaneously, because ferritin may be elevated due to an inflammation in the body. In the literature, iron deficiency is often defined as ferritin levels below 12 µg/L, and iron supplementation is recommended for athletes when ferritin levels fall below 35 µg/L. Iron deficiency is very common, especially in female endurance athletes, with an incidence up to 30% (Verdon et al. 2003; Woolf et al. 2009; Weight et al. 1992). Different factors may cause iron deficiency, such as vegetarianism, insufficient nutrition intake, growth, menstruation, malabsorption, possible loss during exercise (gastrointestinal bleeding, hematuria, sweating and hemolysis) and increased hepcidin levels in athletes, which diminishes iron absorption (Peeling et al. 2008, 2009). All these factors should be investigated before various forms of iron supplementation (oral or repeated injections of iron) are applied. Screening is also necessary to prevent iron overload (Mettler and Zimmermann 2010).

A balanced diet rich in iron and factors that promote iron absorption is paramount for maintaining iron status. Dietary supplements and/or fortified food may also help to prevent iron deficiency, although oral iron supplements must be of sufficient dose and in the form of ferrous sulphate, combined with vitamin C (Deakin 2010). If these precautionary measures are not sufficient, intravenous iron supplementation may be necessary. Iron can be injected intravenously without dilution and not be in conflict with the World Antidoping Agency's (WADA) prohibited list, where infusions of more than 50 ml are not allowed.

Regular screening and sufficient supplementation of iron seem to be important prerequisites for optimal health and performance of athletes.

10.4.2 Vitamin D

Increasing evidence is emerging that vitamin D plays an important role for bone health, immune function, inflammatory regulation and skeletal muscle function (Larson-Meyer and Willis 2010). Recent studies in non-athletes found a correlation between serum 25(OH)D and aerobic fitness, jump height and power (Bischoff-Ferrari 2012). The presence of a vitamin D receptor in the muscle cells supports the proposition that vitamin D is important for muscle function (Hamilton 2011). Recent studies are available concerning the vitamin D status of athletes indicating a high incidence of deficiency, in up to 83% of Australian female gymnasts (Lovell 2008) and 62% of athletes in the United Kingdom during winter (Close et al. 2013).

Vitamin D can be produced sufficiently in the body through endogenous synthesis when the skin is exposed to ultraviolet-B (UVB) radiation. However, cutaneous production depends on different factors, including time of day, cloud cover, smog, latitude, application of sunscreen and skin pigmentation. At latitudes greater than 35° to 37°, UVB is not sufficient in winter months to induce vitamin D production. During summer, exposure of the face and the hands for up to 10 minutes daily is enough to produce 800 to 1000 IU of vitamin D, which is the recommended daily intake for people over 60 yr. Natural sources of vitamin D are salmon, cod liver oil, tuna, cheese and butter. Definitive thresholds for vitamin D status have not been scientifically established. Table 10.1 shows the reference values that are used in literature and for daily practice.

Screening for vitamin D is recommended for athletes as supplementation for vitamin D-deficient athletes can improve performance in various physical parameters, including sprint time and vertical jump (Close et al. 2013). Supplementation with vitamin D is simple, and different products are available over the counter. Usually a daily supply of 800–1000 IU is recommended. An intermittent supply of 5600–7000

TABLE 10.1
Reference Values for Serum 25(OH)D

Deficient	<50 nmol/L	<20 ng/ml
Insufficient	50–75 nmol/L	20–30 ng/ml
Normal	75–220 nmol/L	30–80 ng/ml

IU per week or 24,000–30,000 IU per month seems to have a similar effect. Longer intervals and larger doses are not recommended (Larson-Meyer et al. 2013).

Regular screening and sufficient supplementation of vitamin D seem to be important prerequisites for optimal health and performance of athletes.

10.5 PHARMACOLOGY AND NUTRIENT INTERACTIONS

Paralympic athletes often take medications due to the impairment, associated secondary complications related to the impairment, or to intense sport participation (Van de Vliet et al. 2011). Problems such as exercise-induced bronchoconstriction, urinary tract infections, and pressure ulcers, as discussed previously, are common and must be treated with medications. In this context, athletes and coaches have to be aware of not only the current anti-doping regulations but also the fact that drugs may interact with food and supplement intake. Such interactions are based on changes of pharmacokinetic, pharmacodynamic, and pharmaceutical properties and may lead to severe side effects (Boullata and Hudson 2012; Bushra et al. 2011). The bioavailability of drugs is often altered by concomitant food or supplement ingestion, influencing drug absorption, distribution and metabolism (Bushra et al. 2011; Mason 2010; Rohilla et al. 2013). Absorption of drugs can be affected by foods rich in fat, proteins or dietary fibre (Ayo et al. 2005). In addition, cytochrome P450, one of the most important enzymes in drug metabolism, is significantly inhibited by natural food products such as grapefruit juice, sevillian orange, pomelo or star fruit (Hanley et al. 2011; Kirby and Unadkat 2007). Some drugs build complexes when ingested with milk- or mineral- (e.g. calcium) containing foods, which impedes the gastrointestinal absorption of the drug (Rohilla et al. 2013). In addition, medications can induce side effects and symptoms such as nausea, vomiting, decreased gastro-intestinal motility, diarrhoea, dry mouth or dysgeusia (White 2010) and thus negatively influence dietary habits or performance of an athlete as factors such as taste or appetite change. Taken together, food-drug interactions and drug-food interactions are an important but complex field gaining more interest in the past few years. Some examples of commonly used drugs in para-sports and possible nutritional interactions are discussed in more detail below.

10.5.1 Antacids

The purpose of treatment with antacids is to reduce or neutralize gastric acidity. There exist different substance classes (e.g. H2-antihistamines, proton pump inhibitors), acting differently to reach their therapeutic effect. However, independent of the pharmacological pathway and mechanism, vitamin B12 release from dietary proteins is decreased due to lack of gastric acid, which may lead to a vitamin B12 undersupply with chronic use of antacids (Ruscin et al. 2002). The bioavailability of the proton pump inhibitor omeprazole seems to be increased by soybean ingestion (Singh and Asad 2010), whereas esomeprazole (another proton pump inhibitor) showed a significantly decreased bioavailability when taken 15 minutes before eating a high-fat meal, compared to the fasting state (Sostek et al. 2007).

10.5.2 ANTIBIOTICS

Antibiotics are substances prescribed to treat bacterial infections, which often affect the respiratory system or urinary tract of athletes with an impairment. Several antibiotics (e.g. tetracyclines, ciprofloxacin, norfloxacin and ofloxacin) build insoluble complexes with iron and zinc (Furedi et al. 2009; Lehto et al. 1994; Polk et al. 1989), leading to reduced absorption of the drug as well as the mineral supplement. There is also reduced absorption of tetracyclines when ingested together with milk (Papai et al. 2010), even small amounts added to coffee or tea (Jung et al. 1997). Such interactions can be avoided if the intake of antibiotics is at least two hours before or after iron/zinc supplement or food intake (Mason 2010).

10.5.3 ANTICHOLINERGICS

This medication group includes substances (e.g. oxybutynin, solifenacin, fesoterodine) which block the muscarinic receptors and thus reduce the effect of acetylcholine. The consequence is a relaxing action on the smooth muscles of the bladder and renal tract. Anticholinergics are often applied to treat symptoms of a neurogenic bladder (as described in Section 10.2.1) (Madhuvrata et al. 2012). A common side effect caused by anticholinergic drugs is dry mouth, which influences saliva production and can affect perception of food texture and taste (White 2010). However, a recently published study showed no clinically relevant difference between ingestion of fesoterodine in the fasting state or after a high-fat, high-caloric meal (Malhotra et al. 2009). This supports the hypothesis that anticholinergics can be administered regardless of food intake.

10.5.4 ANTICOAGULANTS

Anticoagulants are used to avoid or treat thromboembolic incidents. One widely used drug of this substance class with a small therapeutic window is warfarin, which influences the coagulation process of the blood. Vitamin K also plays an important role in this process. Ingestion of large amounts of vegetables rich in vitamin K (e.g. broccoli) can interfere with the effectiveness and safety of warfarin intake. The same is true for dietary supplements containing vitamin K. Warfarin has also been reported to interact with other foods such as cooked onions, cranberry juice, chargrilled food, or a high-protein diet (for review see Bushra et al. 2011).

10.5.5 BISPHOSPHONATES

Severe bone loss is a big problem in persons with spinal cord injury and is treated with bisphosphonates such as alendronate (Zehnder et al. 2004). Due to very low bioavailability of this substance class, ingestion 30 minutes before breakfast with water only is recommended to optimize absorption (Porras et al. 1999).

10.5.6   BRONCHODILATORS

Theophylline is a xanthine derivative which induces a bronchodilation. The drug is used for asthma treatment and its bioavailability is influenced by high-fat (increased bioavailability) or high-carbohydrate (decreased bioavailability) meals. The concomitant ingestion of alcohol with theophylline may increase side effects such as nausea or vomiting. Additionally, as caffeine belongs to the group of xanthine derivatives, one must take care when food and drinks containing caffeine (coffee, cola, tea, energy drinks) are consumed together with theophylline, as this may increase drug toxicity (Bushra et al. 2011).

10.5.7   HERBAL PRODUCTS

Many people regularly use herbal products or supplements containing active ingredients such as ginseng, garlic, valerian, gingko, echinacea, or St. John's wort (Peng et al. 2004), without taking into account possible food-drug interactions. The natural origin of such substances does not mean that they are harmless or that no interactions exist. In fact, the effect of a drug can significantly change as transporters and enzymes are influenced by the consumption of herbal supplements, and can induce severe side effects (Bilgi et al. 2010; Peng et al. 2004). St. John's wort, a herbal product commonly used to treat mild to moderate depression, shows a wide spectrum of interactions including, for example, reduced effects of anticoagulants, oral contraceptives or theophylline (Mason 2010). It is important for athletes to discuss their use of any herbal products with a pharmacist or sports medicine practitioner and to carefully check labels/instructions for use.

10.5.8   MYOTONOLYTICS

Myotonolytics were often administered as antispastic medication in subjects with a spinal cord injury. This group of central-acting myotonolytics includes substances such as tizanidine and baclofen (Kheder and Nair 2012). Baclofen is often applied intrathecally via a medication pump and is used chronically in some athletes with spinal cord injury (Van de Vliet et al. 2011). Treatment with this substance class can cause side effects such as nausea and sleepiness. As this substance acts centrally, subjects should refrain from alcohol consumption to avoid intensification of side effects. Athletes should also drive with caution when treated with myotonolytics.

10.5.9   NONSTEROIDAL ANTI-INFLAMMATORY DRUGS (NSAIDs)

NSAIDs (e.g. ibuprofen, diclofenac, ketoprofen, naproxen) are widely used to treat mild to moderate pain and fever but may induce stomach irritation. Ingesting these drugs together with food or milk is indicated as well as abstaining from alcohol, which could increase the risk for liver damage or stomach bleeding (Bushra et al. 2011).

10.5.10 Sildenafil

The incidence of erectile dysfunction is up to 75% in male subjects with a spinal cord injury (Stone 1987). For the treatment of this disorder sildenafil, a selective phosphodiesterase inhibitor, is often prescribed. Sildenafil interacts with grapefruit juice (Jetter et al. 2002) as well as with nitrate (Ishikura et al. 2000; Kloner et al. 2003) which can be found in beetroot juice or spinach juice.

10.5.11 Statins (HMG-CoA Reductase Inhibitors)

Statins are widely used to lower blood cholesterol levels. These substances are metabolized by the enzymatic system called cytochrome P450, one of the most important enzymes in drug metabolism. As grapefruit juice also interacts with cytochrome P450, serum concentrations of some statins (e.g. atorvastatin, lovastatin, simvastatin) are increased (Kantola et al. 1998; Lilja et al. 1998, 1999), whereas others (e.g., pravastatin) are not influenced (Lilja et al. 1999) after grapefruit juice consumption.

10.5.12 Conclusions

Medication and supplement intake in athletes with an impairment is common and bioavailabilty as well as side effects can be influenced based on food-drug interactions. It is therefore important to take into account such possible interactions or to consult an expert before drugs are administered in athletes. This is also true for assumed harmless substances such as herbal products or multivitamin and multimineral supplements and taking these factors into account may help to avoid unexpected and undesirable effects.

COMMENTARY BOX 10.1

ATHLETE INSIGHT: How has sports nutrition advice changed over the years you have been an athlete?

I think over the last 41 years (I used to be an able-bodied swimmer in my earlier years) our entire way of thinking about food and nutrition in general has changed. I think that as an older athlete with a disability I have had to change the way I look at food, as I believe my metabolism has changed as I have gotten older.

—Carol Cooke, cyclist, Paralympic medallist;
ex-rower and able-bodied swimmer

REFERENCES

Ayo, J.A., Agu, H., and Madaki, I. 2005. Food and drug interactions: its side effects. *Nutrition and Food Science* 35:243–252.

Bilgi, N., Bell, K., Ananthakrishnan, A.N., and Atallah, E. 2010. Imatinib and Panax ginseng: a potential interaction resulting in liver toxicity. *Annals of Pharmacotherapy* 44:926–928.

Bischoff-Ferrari, H.A. 2012. "Vitamin D—why does it matter?"—defining vitamin D deficiency and its prevalence. *Scandinavian Journal of Clinical and Laboratory Investigation, Supplement* 243:3–6.

Bougault, V., Turmel, J., and Boulet, L.P. 2011. Airway hyperresponsiveness in elite swimmers: is it a transient phenomenon? *Journal of Allergy and Clinica Immunology* 127:892–898.

Boullata, J.I., and Hudson, L.M. 2012. Drug-nutrient interactions: a broad view with implications for practice. *Journal of the Academy of Nutrition and Dietetics* 112:506–517.

Bushra, R., Aslam, N., and Khan, A.Y. 2011. Food-drug interactions. *Oman Medical Journal* 26:77–83.

Close, G.L., Russell, J., Cobley, J.N., et al. 2013. Assessment of vitamin D concentration in non-supplemented professional athletes and healthy adults during the winter months in the UK: implications for skeletal muscle function. *Journal of Sports Sciences* 31:344–353.

Cruse, J.M., Lewis, R.E., Dilioglou, S., Roe, D.L., Wallace, W.F., and Chen, R.S. 2000. Review of immune function, healing of pressure ulcers, and nutritional status in patients with spinal cord injury. *Journal of Spinal Cord Medicine* 23:129–135.

Cruz, C.D., and Cruz, F. 2011. Spinal cord injury and bladder dysfunction: new ideas about an old problem. *Scientific World Journal* 11:214–234.

Deakin, V. 2010. Iron depletion in athletes. In *Clinical sports nutrition*, ed. L. Burke and V. Deakin, 263–312. 4th ed. Sydney: McGraw-Hill.

Dickinson, J., McConnell, A., and Whyte, G. 2011. Diagnosis of exercise-induced broncho-constriction: eucapnic voluntary hyperpnoea challenges identify previously undiag-nosed elite athletes with exercise-induced bronchoconstriction. *British Journal of Sports Medicine* 45:1126–1131.

Eser, P., Frotzler, A., Zehnder, Y., et al. 2004. Relationship between the duration of paralysis and bone structure: a pQCT study of spinal cord injured individuals. *Bone* 34:869–880.

Frotzler, A., Coupaud, S., Perret, C., et al. 2008. High-volume FES-cycling partially reverses bone loss in people with chronic spinal cord injury. *Bone* 43:169–176.

Frotzler, A., Coupaud, S., Perret, C., Kakebeeke, T.H., Hunt, K.J., and Eser, P. 2009. Effect of detraining on bone and muscle tissue in subjects with chronic spinal cord injury after a period of electrically-stimulated cycling: a small cohort study. *Journal of Rehabilitation Medicine* 41:282–285.

Furedi, P., Papai, K., Budai, M., Ludanyi, K., Antal, I., and Klebovich, I. 2009. [In vivo effect of food on absorption of fluoroquinolones.] *Acta Pharmaceutica Hungarica* 79:81–87.

Hamilton, B. 2011. Vitamin D and athletic performance: the potential role of muscle. *Asian Journal of Sports Medicine* 2:211–219.

Hanley, M.J., Cancalon, P., Widmer, W.W., and Greenblatt, D.J. 2011. The effect of grape-fruit juice on drug disposition. *Expert Opinion on Drug Metabolism and Toxicology* 7:267–286.

Hansen, R.B., Biering-Sorensen, F., and Kristensen, J.K. 2010. Urinary incontinence in spinal cord injured individuals 10–45 years after injury. *Spinal Cord* 48:27–33.

Hanstad, D.V., Ronsen, O., Andersen, S.S., Steffen, K., and Engebretsen, L. 2011. Fit for the fight? Illnesses in the Norwegian team in the Vancouver Olympic Games. *British Journal of Sports Medicine* 45:571–575.

Ishikura, F., Beppu, S., Hamada, T., Khandheria, B.K., Seward, J.B., and Nehra, A. 2000. Effects of sildenafil citrate (Viagra) combined with nitrate on the heart. *Circulation* 102:2516–2521.

Jetter, A., Kinzig-Schippers, M., Walchner-Bonjean, M., et al. 2002. Effects of grapefruit juice on the pharmacokinetics of sildenafil. *Clinical Pharmacology and Therapeutics* 71:21–29.

Jung, H., Peregrina, A.A., Rodriguez, J.M., and Moreno-Esparza, R. 1997. The influence of coffee with milk and tea with milk on the bioavailability of tetracycline. *Biopharmaceutics and Drug Disposition* 18:459–463.

Kantola, T., Kivisto, K.T., and Neuvonen, P.J. 1998. Grapefruit juice greatly increases serum concentrations of lovastatin and lovastatin acid. *Clinical Pharmacology and Therapeutics* 63:397–402.

Kheder, A., and Nair, K.P. 2012. Spasticity: pathophysiology, evaluation and management. *Practical Neurology* 12:289–298.

Kirby, B.J., and Unadkat, J.D. 2007. Grapefruit juice, a glass full of drug interactions? *Clinical Pharmacology and Therapeutics* 81:631–633.

Kloner, R.A., Hutter, A.M., Emmick, J.T., Mitchell, M.I., Denne, J., and Jackson, G. 2003. Time course of the interaction between tadalafil and nitrates. *Journal of the American College of Cardiology* 42:1855–1860.

Larson-Meyer, D.E., Burke, L.M., Stear, S.J., and Castell, L.M. 2013. A-Z of nutritional supplements: dietary supplements, sports nutrition foods and ergogenic aids for health and performance: part 40. *British Journal of Sports Medicine* 47:118–120.

Larson-Meyer, D.E., and Willis, K.S. 2010. Vitamin D and athletes. *Current Sports Medicine Reports* 9:220–226.

Lehto, P., Kivisto, K.T., and Neuvonen, P.J. 1994. The effect of ferrous sulphate on the absorption of norfloxacin, ciprofloxacin and ofloxacin. *British Journal of Clinical Pharmacology* 37:82–85.

Lilja, J.J., Kivisto, K.T., and Neuvonen, P.J. 1998. Grapefruit juice–simvastatin interaction: effect on serum concentrations of simvastatin, simvastatin acid, and HMG-CoA reductase inhibitors. *Clinical Pharmacology and Therapeutics* 64:477–483.

Lilja, J.J., Kivisto, K.T., and Neuvonen, P.J. 1999. Grapefruit juice increases serum concentrations of atorvastatin and has no effect on pravastatin. *Clinical Pharmacology and Therapeutics* 66:118–127.

Lovell, G. 2008. Vitamin D status of females in an elite gymnastics program. *Clinical Journal of Sports Medicine* 18:159–161.

Madhuvrata, P., Cody, J.D., Ellis, G., Herbison, G.P., and Hay-Smith, E.J. 2012. Which anticholinergic drug for overactive bladder symptoms in adults. *Cochrane Database Systematic Review* 1:CD005429.

Malhotra, B., Sachse, R., and Wood, N. 2009. Influence of food on the pharmacokinetic profile of fesoterodine. *International Journal of Clinical Pharmacology and Therapeutics* 47:384–390.

Mason P. 2010. Important drug-nutrient interactions. *Proceedings of the Nutrition Society* 69:551–557.

Mettler, S., and Zimmermann, M.B. 2010. Iron excess in recreational marathon runners. *European Journal of Clinical Nutrition* 64:490–494.

Osthoff, M., Michel, F., Strupler, M., Miedinger, D., Taegtmeyer, A.B., Leuppi, J.D., and Perret, C. 2013. Bronchial hyperresponsiveness testing in athletes of the Swiss Paralympic team. *BMC Sports Science, Medicine and Rehabilitation* 5:7.

Papai, K., Budai, M., Ludanyi, K., Antal, I., and Klebovich, I. 2010. In vitro food-drug interaction study: which milk component has a decreasing effect on the bioavailability of ciprofloxacin? *Journal of Pharmaceutical and Biomedical Analysis* 52:37–42.

Parsons, J.P., and Mastronarde, J.G. 2009. Exercise-induced asthma. *Current Opinion in Pulmonary Medicine* 15:25–28.

Peeling, P., Dawson, B., Goodman, C., Landers, G., and Trinder, D. 2008. Athletic induced iron deficiency: new insights into the role of inflammation, cytokines and hormones. *European Journal of Applied Physiology* 103:381–391.

Peeling, P., Dawson, B., Goodman, C., et al. 2009. Effects of exercise on hepcidin response and iron metabolism during recovery. *International Journal of Sport Nutrition and Exercise Metabolism* 19:583–597.

Peng, C.C., Glassman, P.A., Trilli, L.E., Hayes-Hunter, J., and Good, C.B. 2004. Incidence and severity of potential drug-dietary supplement interactions in primary care patients: an exploratory study of 2 outpatient practices. *Archives of Internal Medicine* 164:630–636.

Polk, R.E., Healy, D.P., Sahai, J., Drwal, L., and Racht, E. 1989. Effect of ferrous sulfate and multivitamins with zinc on absorption of ciprofloxacin in normal volunteers. *Antimicrobial Agents and Chemotherapy* 33:1841–1844.

Porras, A.G., Holland, S.D., and Gertz, B.J. 1999. Pharmacokinetics of alendronate. *Clinical Pharmacokinetics* 36:315–328.

Regan, M.A., Teasell, R.W., Wolfe, D.L., Keast, D., Mortenson, W.B., and Aubut, J.A. 2009. A systematic review of therapeutic interventions for pressure ulcers after spinal cord injury. *Archives of Physical Medicine and Rehabilitation* 90:213–231.

Rohilla, A., Pandey, A., Yadav, S., Chandra Maurya, D., Dahiya, A., and Kushnoor, A. 2013. Drug interactions: a succinct review. *International Journal of Pharmaceutical and Chemical Sciences* 2:297–302.

Ruscin, J.M., Page, R.L., 2nd, and Valuck, R.J. 2002. Vitamin B(12) deficiency associated with histamine(2)-receptor antagonists and a proton-pump inhibitor. *Annals of Pharmacotherapy* 36:812–816.

Singh, D., and Asad, M. 2010. Effect of soybean administration on the pharmacokinetics of carbamazepine and omeprazole in rats. *Fundamental and Clinical Pharmacology* 24:351–355.

Sipski, M.L., and Richards, J.S. 2006. Spinal cord injury rehabilitation: state of the science. *American Journal of Physical Medicine and Rehabilitation* 85:310–342.

Sostek, M.B., Chen, Y., and Andersson, T. 2007. Effect of timing of dosing in relation to food intake on the pharmacokinetics of esomeprazole. *British Journal of Clinical Pharmacology* 64:386–390.

Stone, A.R. 1987. The sexual needs of the injured spinal cord patient. *Problems in Urology* 3:529–536.

Van de Vliet, P., Broad, E., and Strupler, M. 2011. Nutrition, body composition and pharmacology. In *The Paralympic athlete*, ed. Y.C. Vanlandewijck and W.E. Thompson, 172–197. West Sussex, UK: Wiley-Blackwell.

Verdon, F., Burnand, B., Stubi, C.L., et al. 2003. Iron supplementation for unexplained fatigue in non-anaemic women: double blind randomised placebo controlled trial. *British Medical Journal* 326:1124.

White, R. 2010. Drugs and nutrition: how side effects can influence nutritional intake. *Proceedings of the Nutrition Society* 69:558–564.

Woolf, K., St. Thomas, M.M., Hahn, N., Vaughan, L.A., Carlson, A.G., and Hinton, P. 2009. Iron status in highly active and sedentary young women. *International Journal of Sport Nutrition and Exercise Metabolism* 19:519–535.

Zaech, G.A., and Koch, H.G. 2006. *Paraplegie, Ganzheitliche Rehabilitation*. Basel: S. Karger AG.

Zehnder, Y., Risi, S., Michel, D., et al. 2004. Prevention of bone loss in paraplegics over 2 years with alendronate. *Journal of Bone and Mineral Research* 19:1067–1074.

Zitt, M. 2005. Clinical applications of exhaled nitric oxide for the diagnosis and management of asthma: a consensus report. *Clinical Therapeutics* 27:1238–1250.

11 Use of Supplements in Athletes

Claudio Perret and Greg Shaw

CONTENTS

11.1 INTRODUCTION

There is a growing body of nutrients and substances purported to enhance exercise performance, however the practicality of what translates to 'performance enhancement' is now broader than the simple improvement of an isolated competition or training performance. As discussed in Chapter 3, the goal of sports nutrition is to optimise the adaptations to training, and maintaining an athlete's capability to train consistently over a period of time provides a platform for this. A dietary supplement may enhance the ability to train consistently in a number of ways. For example, a probiotic (specific bacteria ingested for the purpose of optimising gut microflora) may be considered ergogenic by reducing the incidence, severity and duration of upper respiratory tract infections (Gleeson et al. 2011; West et al. 2011), thereby allowing the athlete to achieve uninterrupted training. Creatine monohydrate may be considered ergogenic because of its ability to improve training capacity (Maughan et al. 2011) as well as secondary benefits such as enhanced glycogen re-synthesis (van Loon et al. 2004). A formulated sports food such as a carbohydrate gel or formulated protein powder may be considered ergogenic as it can enhance a one-off training performance (Patterson and Gray 2007) and muscle recovery process (Hayes and Cribb 2008), hence optimising the outcome of training in addition to the convenient nutrient source these formulated sports foods provide. It is therefore evident that what traditionally has been held as a definition for performance enhancement needs to be expanded to encompass all areas being identified to contribute to competition performance over acute and chronic time frames. This will also bring clarity to decisions around what constitutes an ergogenic dietary supplement.

It is beyond the scope of this chapter to systematically discuss the full spectrum of dietary supplements for which there is evidence of ergogenic effects. Readers interested in the array of dietary supplements that could be reported as ergogenic, and the current evidence for their use, are directed to a number of excellent review articles, article series and books available in the published literature (Burke et al. 2010, 2012a; Branch 2003; Carr et al. 2011; Doherty and Smith 2004; Hobson et al. 2012). Specifically, readers may be interested in programs like the Sport Supplement Program of the Australian Institute of Sport (AIS) (www.ausport.gov.au/ais/nutrition/supplements) which provides up-to-date information in conjunction with a weight of evidence system (scientific, practical, risk based) to classify supplements. The rest of this chapter will focus on providing a background to the information that needs to be considered by an athlete with an impairment prior to deciding whether to take a new, or continue to take a dietary supplement.

11.2 DEFINITION OF DIETARY SUPPLEMENTS

Dietary supplement is a broad term with numerous definitions both in the literature and in practice. As the definition of what constitutes a dietary supplement is extremely fluid, influenced by reason for use, mode of delivery and the international regulatory framework, a universal definition of dietary supplement can be problematic.

In most countries or regions there is a body (or bodies) that regulates the manufacture and marketing of foods and therapeutic agents. Such organisations provide a working definition of a dietary supplement within their jurisdiction. For example, in the United States a dietary supplement is defined by the Dietary Supplement Health and Education Act of 1994 (DSHEA) as "a product (other than tobacco) intended to supplement the diet that bears or contains one or more of the following dietary ingredients: a vitamin; a mineral; a herb or other botanical; an amino acid; a dietary substance for use by man to supplement the diet by increasing the total dietary intake; or a concentrate, metabolite, constituent, extract, or combination of any ingredient described previously" (US Food and Drug Administration 1994). In Europe a dietary supplement is defined as "foodstuffs the purpose of which is to supplement the normal diet and which are concentrated sources of nutrients (meaning vitamins and minerals) or other substances with a nutritional or physiological effect, alone or in combination, marketed in dose form, namely forms such as capsules, pastilles, tablets, pills and other similar forms, sachets of powder, ampoules of liquids, drop dispensing bottles, and other similar forms of liquids and powders designed to be taken in measured small unit quantities" (European Parliament 2002). These food supplements are unable to claim the ability to cure or treat a disease but may make the claim to affect a physiological function. For example a food supplement cannot claim to cure heart disease but may make the claim that it reduces cholesterol.

In Australia products commonly defined as dietary supplements in the United States or Europe fall into two different categories, regulated by two different bodies. Formulated sports foods are regulated by the Food Standards Australia New Zealand (FSANZ) and are defined as "foods or mixtures of foods specifically formulated to assist sports people in achieving specific nutritional or performance goals" (Food Standards Australia New Zealand 2000). Dietary supplements are regulated by the Therapeutic Goods Administration (TGA) and are not as clearly defined as in other countries (Therapeutic Goods Administration 1989).

Athletes with an impairment need to be aware of what constitutes a dietary supplement in various jurisdictions around the world. Increased international competition and the availability of dietary supplements over the internet mean they are potentially exposed to products and ingredients not approved for sale in their country of residence. In addition, the importation of ingredients/products that are considered supplements in one country may be prohibited by customs laws in another, but breaches of these laws are not always identified.

What constitutes a dietary supplement can often be dictated by the form of the product in question, such as solid foods, drinks, small volume liquids, powders, capsules, and tablets. They may be consumed via two distinct routes: oral or infusion, with the latter route including intramuscular and intravascular administration. While it can be argued that intravascular and intramuscular injection of nutrients should be classified as a medical procedure rather than as a dietary supplement, it is noted that athletes report self-administration of injectable dietary nutrients as a way of supplementing dietary sources (Corrigan and Kazlauskas 2003). The emergence of functional foods (Ozen et al. 2012) and concentrated food sources (Lansley et al. 2011) as ergogenic dietary supplements has blurred the line between foods and traditional dietary supplements even further (Ozen et al. 2012).

A practical definition of sports supplements divides products into nutritional supplements and ergogenic aids based on the intended rationale for their use or mode of action (Burke et al. 2010). This classification includes the sub-category of formulated sports foods. Sports foods are defined as specialised products in a food form with a composition, size or presentation intended to "provide a convenient and practical means of meeting a known nutrient requirement to optimise daily training or competition performance" (Burke et al. 2010). Examples of such products include liquid meal supplements, sports drinks, carbohydrate gels, protein powders and sports bars. It is the purposeful formulation of these foods from specific ingredients that classifies them as dietary supplements, warranting their inclusion in investigations of supplementation practices of athletes. Indeed, they have been shown to provide a substantial contribution to the nutrient intake of athletes (Lun et al. 2009). Micronutrient supplements used to prevent or treat a known nutritional deficiency (for example iron, vitamin D, and multivitamin supplements) are another example of nutritional supplements. By contrast, the classification of ergogenic aid covers all products that claim to provide a direct enhancement of sports performance by mechanisms other than meeting the goals of everyday nutrition. These mechanisms might include effects on the central nervous system (such as caffeine), or supplying metabolites or co-factors that are important in metabolism (such as creatine or sodium bicarbonate). While this classification system may have provided some logical definitions in the days of a smaller supplement industry, the market has now evolved to include large numbers of multi-ingredient sports foods and functional foods which contain ergogenic ingredients in addition to their traditional or regulated nutrient composition. Therefore, there is a blurring of the previously separated categories.

One system that is in everyday use in classifying supplements based on the strength of the evidence for the efficacy of a product when used according to best practice is the Sport Supplement Program of the Australian Institute of Sport (AIS, www.ausport.gov.au/ais/nutrition/supplements). The AIS Sport Supplement Program uses a categorisation system to divide dietary supplements into a series of groups (A, B, C and D). This categorisation is based on the level of scientific evidence available for performance enhancement and the relative risk of a dietary supplement containing (potentially through inadvertent contamination) a banned substance. The most visible component of the program is an education program available to the public via the AIS website. The education program aims to empower athletes and coaches to make informed decisions with background information on the specific dietary supplement, safety guidelines and also evidence-based supplement protocols.

In summary, what defines a dietary supplement is broad, confusing and is changing rapidly. It is therefore the responsibility of athletes, coaches, sports scientists and administrators to ensure programs are in place to help guide and educate athletes on what is effective and safe use of dietary supplements.

11.3   POTENTIAL BENEFITS OF SUPPLEMENT USE

11.3.1   Nutrient Supply in a More Convenient Form (Situation or the Amount)

The simple delivery of nutrients in a convenient form or specific amount, using avenues that have low food safety requirements, a pleasant taste, and long shelf life can be both practical and nutritionally beneficial to athletes (Burke et al. 2010). "Sports foods" may provide convenience, and in certain circumstances may have specific ergogenic benefits over real foods. For example, Burke and colleagues (2012b) showed a potentially smaller anabolic amino acid profile for 20 g of protein from real foods such as steak and eggs compared to other liquid forms of protein (e.g. a dairy-based supplemental liquid meal replacement). Dietary supplements may also provide valuable micronutrients to athletes whose dietary intake is suboptimal due to personal preference, a restricted energy budget (Lun et al. 2009), or as a consequence of altered requirements. While dietary supplementation can provide convenience and a valuable source of specific nutrients, athletes with an impairment should be encouraged to meet their nutritional requirements primarily from whole food sources first and foremost—laziness or poor organization are no justification for using supplements of any type.

11.3.2 EVIDENCE BASE SUPPORTING THE USE OF DIETARY SUPPLEMENTS

The number of dietary supplements that have scientific evidence for effective performance enhancement is small. This is in contrast to the vast number of supplements with proposed 'potential efficacy for use in sporting situations' but for which the scientific evidence is either unavailable or fails to show benefits (Burke et al. 2010). It is important that athletes with an impairment realise that 'potential efficacy' does not always guarantee performance enhancement, nor does it ensure the safety of a supplement. It may also be the case that dietary supplementation negatively impacts athletic training and performance (Ristow et al. 2009).

For a dietary supplement to display potential efficacy, there must be a logical theory demonstrated by which an altered, increased or enhanced outcome of a physiological process would result from the consumption of the dietary supplement. Once the theory is accepted, significant rigor must be employed by researchers worldwide to investigate and elucidate the variety of situations in which the dietary supplement may be effective in changing performance, and provide evidence that this can occur safely (i.e. without substantial side effects). An example of such a process has been demonstrated with the dietary supplement creatine. The efficacy for the consumption of a refined supplemental source of creatine was first published in 1992 by biochemist Roger Harris (Harris et al. 1992). He outlined the theory that the oral consumption of sufficient supplemental creatine monohydrate would increase the cellular (i.e. muscular) phosphocreatine content, a key component of metabolic energy production. In doing so, he hypothesized that creatine supplementation could directly enhance performance in situations where that phosphocreatine was heavily utilised by the contracting muscle. True evidence supporting the effectiveness of creatine supplementation in enhancing athletic performance took longer to demonstrate and well established protocols and situations for use were not available until the mid to late 1990s (Maughan 1995). To this day there is continual addition to the areas in which creatine can be beneficial, expanding now outside of sport into the health and disease arena. Anecdotal reports of British track athletes using dietary creatine supplements surfaced as early as the 1992 Barcelona Olympics, almost simultaneously coinciding with the outlining of the theory but well before the scientific demonstration of effective use occurred. This clearly demonstrates that athletes are reluctant to wait for scientific evidence on the off chance it may improve performance, especially if a sound reasoning is provided for why it might be beneficial. Without effective protocols which are proven to be associated with enhanced performance, athletes may be wasting time and money on ineffective practices, and possibly even endangering their health. One example of this is demonstrated in a study looking at the creatine loading and maintenance practices of Division One collegiate athletes, which reported that athletes utilised supplementation protocols that were outside of scientifically recommended doses (Greenwood et

COMMENTARY BOX 11.1

ATHLETE INSIGHT: How has sports nutrition advice changed over the years you have been an athlete?

> The nutrition advice has become more detailed and specific. Also, the available nutrition supplements/products, testing protocols, and implementation of them has evolved over time. The management and use of accepted supplements such as creatine and caffeine have become more detailed and therefore more effective.

—Hamish Macdonald, track and field, six-time Paralympian

al. 2000). Of the athletes consuming creatine and reporting positive outcomes, 54% used amounts that were below recommended doses (Greenwood et al. 2000). These ineffective supplementation practices may be explained by the timing of this study (late 1990s) when optimal creatine loading and maintenance guidelines were still being developed. It is also recognized that a lack of evidence supporting specific dosing may also lead athletes to consume doses far higher than necessary, and in some cases at potentially toxic and harmful levels (FitzSimmons and Kidner 1998; Prosser et al. 2009). This illustrates the pitfalls athletes with an impairment can face when products are brought to market before substantial evidence is available regarding the ideal supplement dosing protocols, the activities which may benefit the most from the product, and whether the product actually has the effect it is proposed to have.

11.3.3 Enhanced Exercise Capacity vs. Performance Improvement

Recently the distinction between enhanced performance and improved physiological capacity has been presented as an important concept for elite athletes to understand with respect to dietary supplement effectiveness (Hobson et al. 2012). There are some supplements which are most beneficial in improving training capacity and adaptations (such as creatine), whereas the research for others has been confined to specific use in competition (such as sodium bicarbonate). Furthermore, there must be consideration of situations where repeated use may result in a loss of effectiveness or adverse effects (for example, the balance between potential acute benefits of caffeine use and the chronic impact of disrupted sleep over the duration of a swim or athletics meet). It is important for sports nutrition practitioners to consult with coaches and sports medicine and sports science professionals to develop a sound understanding of specific dietary supplement research in order to ensure that if a supplement is used, the protocols for use are effective and its use is timed strategically to take advantage of a specific training focus/period or a particular competitive event.

One current example where there remains confusion as to the primary role and how it is promoted to athletes is the dietary supplement β-alanine. To date, there are several studies which demonstrate β-alanine's ability to enhance the body's capacity to undertake a strenuous exercise bout but there is a distinct lack of evidence regarding its ability to improve performance in an actual sporting event (Hobson et al. 2012). This inability to translate an enhanced physiological capacity into a performance outcome should be a concern to athletes because taking a supplement on the assumption that it will automatically enhance performance may result in missing an opportunity to optimise the potential benefits that the supplement may infer. Athletes with an impairment are encouraged to ensure supplement ingestion protocols are combined with specific training interventions to regularly maximise the impact an enhanced physiological capacity may infer.

11.4   CONCERNS WITH DIETARY SUPPLEMENT USE

11.4.1   EXPENSE

Athletes spend large amounts of money on dietary supplements (Burke and Cox 2010; Slater et al. 2003). Half of Singaporean athletes taking dietary supplements reported spending more than US$30 per month on them, with one athlete spending US$870 a month (Slater et al. 2003). In body builders, where the prevalence of supplement use is high, it was reported in the 1990s that three out of every five athletes spent between US$25 and 100 per month, with a significant proportion spending over US$150 per month on dietary supplements (Brill and Keane 1994). This is not surprising when athletes report cost being of minimal concern when considering the use of dietary supplements (Bayliss et al. 2001), yet it is of concern when athletes are spending more money on dietary supplements than they are on whole foods. In unemployed Sri Lankan athletes, two thirds reported purchasing dietary supplements despite their limited finances (de Silva et al. 2010), with the cost of supplements having increased significantly since the time of the earlier reports. Athletes with an impairment need to ensure that cost is factored into the decision-making process to take a supplement. Athletes should be aware that in many cases real foods may be significantly cheaper and yet have similar outcomes to supplemental sources of nutrients. For example, a serve of skim milk is cheaper than the same amount of protein from a supplemental source and may be just as effective in eliciting a positive protein synthetic response (Burke et al. 2012b).

11.4.2   THE PERCEPTION OF SUPERIOR NUTRITION SOURCES

Dietary supplementation can appear an easy option to athletes, particularly juniors, as a way of enhancing athletic performance. Coaches, sports scientists, sports medicine practitioners and administrators need to ensure that athletes aren't distracted by the allure of dietary supplements. Athletic performance comes from genetic predisposition, long term training, optimal nutritional intake and effective recovery and there is no short cut to success. It is encouraging that in junior athletes from the UK the belief that dietary supplements are necessary to enhance performance was only agreed with by 13% of the 403 athletes surveyed (Nieper 2005).

   It should be noted that, in the general population, dietary supplement intake has been linked to poor health behaviours, including less healthy dietary choices in people taking a placebo which they perceived to be a dietary supplement (Chiou et al.

2011). This perception that a dietary supplement provides a justification for other poor health choices is of concern when translated into an athletic population. If athletes are taking dietary supplements to enhance performance, but as a consequence are neglecting other well established performance enhancing practices (sleep, well planned diet etc.), they are potentially sabotaging overall performance. Athletes with an impairment need to be reminded regularly that dietary supplements are a small component of their athletic development.

11.4.3 NEGATIVE HEALTH CONSEQUENCES

Serbian Paralympic athletes have reported either taking multiple sources of the same vitamins or minerals or consuming dietary supplement and medication combinations that may be detrimental (Suzic Lazic et al. 2011). The literature suggests that polysupplementation is a significant issue across a range of sports and athlete levels, with athletes regularly consuming numerous different supplements without care for potential side effects or detrimental nutrient interactions (Baylis et al. 2001; Corrigan and Kazlauskas 2003; Suzic Lazic et al. 2011; Slater et al. 2003; Tscholl et al. 2010). This should be of concern to athletes with an impairment, particularly those who may be at greater risk of drug-nutrient interactions. For example, an alteration of drug pharmacokinetics can occur after the ingestion of complex mixtures of phytochemicals (e.g. grapefruit juice, fruits, tea) (Bailey and Dresser 2004; Harris 1995; Harris et al. 2003). The concomitant ingestion of caffeine and creatine has been shown to result in a complete elimination of the ergogenic effect of the creatine ingestion (Vandenberghe et al. 1996). And finally, severe, dangerous drops in blood pressure can result from the interaction between phosphodiesterase-5- (PDE5) inhibitors, used to treat erectile dysfunction of neurologic origin in individuals with para- and quadriplegia, and nitrate such as beetroot juice, used to enhance exercise performance (Ishikura et al. 2000; Kloner et al. 2003). Sport nutrition experts need to pay close attention to the dietary supplement practices of athletes with an impairment to ensure polysupplementing is not leading to supplement interactions that could affect the Paralympic athlete's short and long term health.

In addition to the potential risks of polysupplementation or interactions between supplements and medications, the over-consumption of certain dietary supplements may also lead to decrements in performance. Stimulants like caffeine, when consumed in doses higher than recommended, can lead to decrements in performance (Graham and Spriet 1995). Athletes should ascertain that dietary supplement protocols are specifically designed to ensure the minimal amount of individual dietary supplement is consumed for the maximum effect.

11.4.4 CONTAMINATION AND DOPING CONCERNS

The risk of returning a positive doping test due to the inadvertent consumption of a contaminated dietary supplement is a major concern for athletes subjected to doping control. Doping risk regularly rates highly as a concern of athletes in relation to dietary supplementation use (Baylis et al. 2001; Dascombe et al. 2010; de

Silva et al. 2010; Erdman et al. 2007; Slater et al. 2003). The majority of Australian swimmers rated the risk of inadvertent doping as very important (79%) or important (16%) (Baylis et al. 2001). More recently another group of Australian athletes perceived dietary supplements as at risk for a positive doping result (Dascombe et al. 2010). This awareness has emerged from an increase in reported cases of dietary supplement contamination (Geyer et al. 2011; Green et al. 2001; Kamber et al. 2001; Maughan 2004, 2005). The contamination of supplements with banned substances can occur through poor manufacturing quality control or purpose-ful contamination of products by manufacturers (Geyer et al. 2011). The exact source of contamination is difficult to identify when the level of contaminants can vary within single batches, and even within individual containers of a supplement (Maughan 2005). A study of supplements from around the world found that 94 of the 634 (14.8%) supplements sampled contained anabolic or androgenic substances not declared in the ingredient list (Geyer et al. 2004). This demonstrates a real risk athletes should be aware of and concerned about when considering their dietary supplementation practices, as the innocent ingestion of prohibited substances is no excuse for a positive doping outcome and will lead to a penalty according to the anti-doping regulations.

Currently supplement manufacturers have identified contamination as an issue in manufacturing processes (Judkins et al. 2010). Programs have been developed to both internally and externally ensure quality control procedures are in place to remove contamination risk. One such external program is run by HFL Sports Sciences in collaboration with manufacturers (Judkins et al. 2010). This program provides an external testing framework available to manufacturers, testing batches of dietary supplements for banned contaminants before they go to market. A study looking at the effectiveness of this program reported that of 3579 supplements tested in 2008, 14 contained steroids and/or stimulants (Judkins et al. 2010). The following year the program tested 4567 samples. Of the 4196 samples that came from manufacturers involved in the program and who had established quality con-trol practices, only one supplement showed (0.02%) contamination issues (Judkins et al. 2010), demonstrating the potential effectiveness of the program. This sample was identified prior to shipping and hence was removed prior to entering the mar-ketplace. Conversely, of the 371 samples from manufacturers newly enrolled in the program, 10.8% of products showed signs of contamination (Judkins et al. 2010). It should be noted that such programs do have downsides, namely they fail to test for the full spectrum of banned substances named in the WADA code and add a significant cost to companies that engage fully in the testing and auditing process. However, if supplement manufacturers ensure suitable levels of quality control and engage external testing frameworks, they can reduce the risk of contamination to almost zero. The marketing of programs similar to this allows athletes with an impairment to actively seek supplement companies involved in this framework. It is imperative that these programs be continually evaluated in order to help further refine them and enhance their effectiveness.

11.5 SUPPLEMENT USE IN PARALYMPIC ATHLETES

Sports for athletes with an impairment include a large number of different disciplines and impairments. While many athletes may be able to use supplements according to recommendations for able-bodied athletes, greater caution may be warranted in others such as wheelchair athletes suffering from a spinal cord injury (SCI). In this context, one has to be aware that a SCI leads to considerable changes resulting in an impairment or loss of motor, sensory and vegetative functions. Based on the severity of the spinal damage a SCI is classified as complete or incomplete motor or sensory and results in changes in metabolism and body composition, including reduced resting energy expenditure (as outlined in Chapter 4). After the occurrence of a complete SCI, muscles below the lesion are paralysed, sensation for pain and temperature, proprioception and sense of touch are lost, and urologic, sexual and gastrointestinal dysfunctions are common. In addition, gastrointestinal transit time in individuals with a SCI is more prolonged compared to able-bodied controls (Krogh et al. 2000) and these athletes are often treated with medications which might have an impact on the gastrointestinal tract, digestion and resorption of nutrients. For these reasons it seems not advisable to transfer recommendations for nutritional supplements from able-bodied athletes directly into athletes with a SCI. In fact, before using such substances a critical examination, taking into account the special requirements of individuals with SCI, becomes important and necessary, and is discussed in more detail below. Furthermore, possible negative interactions between dietary supplements and medications have to be considered (as discussed previously).

It is surprising that only a limited number of peer-reviewed scientific publications can be found regarding supplement use by athletes with an impairment. To date only a few studies have investigated nutritional behaviors in wheelchair athletes (Goosey-Tolfrey and Crosland 2010; Krempien and Barr 2011, 2012), carbohydrate metabolism (Skrinar et al. 1982) or carbohydrate supplementation (Spendiff and Campbell 2003, 2005). Spendiff and Campbell (2005) reported that a higher concentration of carbohydrate in a sports drink could be advantageous for paraplegic athletes. However, only low (4%) and high (11%) carbohydrate concentrations were tested in this study and it remains unclear whether a drink containing 6–8% carbohydrate might be even more beneficial for performance enhancement in this population, especially when keeping in mind their reduced energy expenditure (Price 2010) and the difficulties they can face in maintaining body mass.

Only one study has been published regarding nutritional ergogenic aid use in athletes with an impairment, which was regarding short term creatine monohydrate supplementation on wheelchair racing performance (Perret et al. 2006). In contrast to several studies in able-bodied subjects (for review please refer to Tarnopolsky 2010), no significant performance enhancement over 800 m was found compared to placebo in these wheelchair athletes. Further investigations of Perret and colleagues leading in to the London 2012 Paralympic Games dealing with caffeine (6 mg.kg^{-1} body mass) and sodium citrate (0.5 g.kg^{-1} body mass) supplementation did not find any improvement in 1500 m wheelchair racing performance compared to placebo (unpublished data), although the data indicated some individual variability in response with some athletes showing improved performance. Five out of nine athletes in this study reported gastrointestinal side effects after the ingestion of sodium citrate. As with creatine, these results stand in contrast to studies in able-bodied athletes, where a clear performance-enhancing effect was found after the ingestion of these supplements (Bird et al. 1995; Oopik et al. 2003; Wiles et al. 1992). This preliminary data highlights the fact that individual responses cannot be ruled out and that data from able-bodied athletes may not be directly transferable into para-sports. Studies critically evaluating potential ergogenic substances (e.g. caffeine, sodium bicarbonate, sodium citrate, β-alanine) in athletes with an impairment are warranted in the future to enable sports nutrition experts to provide evidence-based advice to this specific population of athletes.

11.5.1 PRACTICAL CONSIDERATIONS FOR DIETARY SUPPLEMENTATION IN PARALYMPIC ATHLETES

It is important to adapt recommendations for a supplement to the unique requirements of athletes with an impairment and their specific sport discipline(s). Unfortunately, there remains little data available on fundamental areas like the physiological requirements of various para-sports, which is essential for determining the relevance of or efficacy for any potentially ergogenic nutritional supplement. Further, it is questionable whether the same dosing scheme should be used for athletes in some impaired populations, especially where absolute or lean body mass is substantially different to the able-bodied subjects involved in the original research. Therefore, there may be instances where doses should be applied relative to either total or lean body mass rather than a set absolute dose.

Given that gastrointestinal transit times are prolonged in subjects with a SCI, the timing of supplementation (e.g. time of supplement intake before a competition) and the dosing protocol may need to be modified. However, as the grade and severity of impairment differs from athlete to athlete, no general recommendations can be provided and decisions have to be made individually. The same may also be true for considering the potential side effects of supplements. These effects may differ from the able-bodied population or have a greater impact on athletes with an impairment. Thus it is pragmatic to consider beginning trials of any potential ergogenic supplements with lower doses than would normally be prescribed. For daily practice, it has proven valuable to start with half of the recommended dose (e.g. for sodium bicarbonate) and then to gradually increase the dosage according to an individual's tolerance (see case study). Although this approach is based on trial and error, it is likely to be advantageous in daily sports practice, at least until such time that formal investigations are undertaken in a systematic, scientific manner, together with specifically documenting outcomes (e.g., side effects, tolerance, impact on performance, subjective perception of the athlete). Of course, the individual (grade and severity of impairment, anthropometry, etc.) sport-specific requirements and former experiences from other athletes and coaches should be taken into account.

CASE STUDY—USE OF SODIUM
BICARBONATE IN A HAND CYCLIST

BACKGROUND

The athlete was a male with paraplegia and had been competing in handcycling for 10 years, of which 5 years were at the international level. The athlete had competed in four World Championships, one Paralympic Games, and four World Cups over the 10 year period.

GOAL

The athlete competed in time trials (TTs), road races (RRs) and team relays (TRs) when the right combination of athletes was available to do so. The athlete had been steadily improving his performances at the international level over the previous two years, improving from 11th place to 6th place and then 2nd and 3rd place finishes. He felt that he was doing the maximum that he could training and equipmentwise and was looking for an extra legal edge to help him take the next step, to achieve first place finishes in international competition. He has no desire to use anything illegal in order to improve his performance. His national coach was also a strong anti-doping advocate. In order to achieve this goal he needed to be able to achieve and maintain a higher average speed in TTs and RRs and be able to respond to, or launch, attacks in RRs. Being able to achieve and maintain a higher average speed would also be beneficial to his contribution to any TR events.

PAST HISTORY WITH SODIUM BICARBONATE

The athlete had had one previous experience with using bicarb—a highly inappropriate and very negative one. Without any discussion let alone agreement about it, the athlete's former coach began giving him bottles of water loaded with bicarb during a 24 hour race. As there were no other fluids provided despite his requests, the athlete was forced to drink the fluid provided to him. The consequences were disastrous and distressing. After the race the athlete was "shitting water" (liquid diarrhoea), but had to catch a long flight home. Very distressed, he sought help from the airport doctor who gave him something to stop it so that he could make the flight home without incident. Not surprisingly, after that experience the athlete wasn't keen to try bicarb again.

POTENTIAL REASONS TO CONSIDER
SODIUM BICARBONATE LOADING

The TTs required the athlete to maintain a high steady pace over distances of up to 30 km (although they are generally around 15–20 km); the RRs occur over distances of up to 80 km and may involve a range of different strategies, but frequently involve surging to try and break up a bunch and short, high intensity attacks. The TRs involve teams of three athletes. Each rider completes one or two 2 separate laps of a circuit (the number of laps vary according to the lap distance, which in turn varies according to the courses available to the organiser). TRs generally involve each athlete in a team completing two separate laps of approximately 3 km each. Occasionally the laps are longer and each athlete only completes one lap. The athlete's current national coach felt that the use of bicarb may help him to buffer the build-up and effects of lactic acid and enable him to maintain a higher average speed as well as make him more physically capable of sustaining, or responding to, attacks in RRs. Although sodium bicarbonate has been proven beneficial to sport performance over only 1–7 min in able-bodied individuals, the athlete's description of what limited his performance in these events was considered to be more an issue of buffering high intensity exercise metabolites than a cardiorespiratory limitation.

WHAT INFORMATION WERE YOU GIVEN?

Given the athlete's performance goals, training status and lengthy competition experience, the coach felt that the use of bicarb might be beneficial, under the direction of a sports dietitian/nutritionist. At a meeting early in the training year between the athlete, coach and nutritionist, the athlete's existing race nutrition plan was discussed and strategies for further improving this were considered. The athlete's previous experience with, and concerns about, the use of bicarb were also discussed. The sports dietitian/nutritionist was satisfied that the athlete's existing nutritional approach was appropriate and felt that bicarb may help enhance his performance. Given his past negative experience and reservations, she provided a fact sheet about the use of bicarb and suggested a conservative approach to reintroducing bicarb (i.e. lower than normal dose for weight to start with; trying it at training first—indoor trainer session near a bathroom in case of any gastric upset before trying it at an outdoor training session and then in competition, then gradually increasing the dose if there were no side effects). This information was provided but it was left up to the athlete to consider and decide whether or not he wanted to try bicarb again. There was no pressure put on him to do so.

> Coach: If [athlete] was going to try bicarb again I wanted it to be an informed decision and for him to be comfortable and confident about doing so. I thought the best way for this to happen was to discuss the potential benefits/side effects and strategies with a qualified nutritionist, then leave it up to him to make the decision. I was happy to support him in whatever decision he made.

During an early-season racing block, the athlete decided that he would like to start trialling bicarb. The coach asked the sports nutritionist to recommend a conservative protocol that he could start trialling in the lead-up to the 2012 London Paralympics.

WHAT WAS THE PROCESS?

The sports nutritionist recommended the following very cautious progression/protocol:

Bicarb Trialling Protocol

Theoretical dose at 0.3 mg/kg BM = 23 sodibic capsules.

Initially I would suggest starting with a lower dose to determine tolerance. So, we can start with 15 capsules and see how it goes.

Trial 1

Rest day or morning/afternoon off, where you can be at home (or somewhere close by a bathroom) just in case there are side effects.

Have a small meal/snack based on carbohydrate and consume four capsules with 150 ml water (this is time 0). Always eat with the first dose. What you eat is up to you—you have to bear in mind the training session 2.5 h later. It doesn't need to be big—could be a slice of toast, sandwich, fruit. Make it something you know sits well on your stomach during high intensity exercise.

Every 20 min thereafter, take another four capsules with 150 ml water (the last dose will be three capsules). So, the last dose should be 1 h after the first dose.

Track any symptoms you have and also the food and fluid you consumed. Usually you would do this starting 2.5 h before a race, so track your symptoms for at least 3 h (roughly every 30 min).

Trial 2

Assuming Trial 1 went fine (if it doesn't, report to me and let me know what happened as we can see what might be modified), then do the same before a turbo session at home. The session doesn't have to be a really hard one—this trial is really to see how you then feel during exercise with the bicarb on board, again monitoring for any side effects.

Trial 3

Assuming Trial 2 went fine, then repeat the process before a hard/high intensity turbo session, interval or hills session.

You can do this as many times as you want to under different circumstances. If the first trial goes well, then you can increase the dose up to the 23 capsules (do this in two steps—so take it up to about 19 capsules first, then up to 23).

For 19 capsules, I would do 4 every 15 min rather than every 20 min (4:4:4:4:3), so there's five dosing points over the 1 h period, each with 150 ml water.

For 23 capsules, it would be 5:5:5:4:4 (again, every 15 min with 150–200 ml water). The first time you get to this dose, make it a turbo session at home just in case there are side effects.

Trial 4

In a race situation, same protocol.

Given our race schedule when we returned home (a relatively short period before the races), the sports nutritionist recommended that we complete Trials 1 and 2, as indicated above, during training in Spain and arranged for bicarb to be provided.

Decision

In terms of the progression/protocol, we followed the recommended progression/protocol to the letter in terms of the doses, but the type of training session/environment varied a little. This occurred at the athlete's insistence. The first trial (15-capsule protocol; half the normal recommended dose for the athlete's weight) was completed during a light training session in the lead-up to a World Cup event (the athlete took a towel, water, and change of clothes just in case). When he experienced no side effects except for a few fizzy burps and "gas" afterwards, he decided he wanted to trial the same dose (15 capsules, as indicated in Trial 1) in a race. As the coach I had some reservations about this but given the lack of any real side effects during training, the fact that it was a low dose (half the normal recommended dose for the athlete's weight) and athlete's confidence with the protocol, I allowed him to go ahead.

Outcome

The first race in which the athlete reintroduced bicarb was a World Cup TT one or two days after the training trial. The outcome? The athlete broke through for his first win in international competition. The athlete felt it definitely helped him—he observed: "I didn't get the muscle burn that I previously got and was able to keep riding harder." Again, the only side effects were some fizzy burps and a bit of gas afterwards. He then decided to use the same protocol for the RR. Not far into the race he dropped his chain on a bumpy descent and had to stop to fix it. He then had to "time trial" it to try and catch the bunch again and came close to succeeding. He still managed to finish in a high place in this race despite having to work solo for most of it. He again felt that the bicarb provided him with the extra edge he was looking for and was committed to trialling it further. On returning home, he then trialled the higher doses in the recommended protocol in training before trialling them in competition. He now confidently uses the protocol recommended for his weight in competition.

**Subsequent Question Regarding Use of Bicarb
with Younger, Less Experienced Athletes**

The coach subsequently asked about when it would be appropriate to start
trialling bicarb (or other legal supplements, such as caffeine) with a couple of
younger, less experienced athletes who had competed in one block of international racing. The coach's philosophy is that elements such as bicarb are an
extra that should only be added once everything else has been addressed (i.e.
once bike setup is appropriate, pedalling technique has been mastered, the
athlete is training at the level appropriate for an international athlete and has
competed internationally), but the coach was wondering at what point elements
such as bicarb should be introduced. The sports nutritionist agreed with the
extra philosophy and suggested that it would be best to have the athletes race
for another year so that their pacing strategies without bicarb or caffeine are
mastered before introducing any other elements into the equation.

> Nutritionist: I would probably wait a little while longer to trial this with [these
> athletes]—you need to be sure that they have the ability to pace their race effec-
> tively first before you layer in bicarb or anything else, because it will change
> how they feel in a race and they need to know how to manage this and not "blow
> up." If their current pacing strategies are variable, then this only adds to the
> confusion. So I would probably wait a year of international racing before you
> layered this in [same with caffeine]—let them experience what it's like at inter-
> national level first and get used to how races can be run.
>
> When you feel they're ready to trial it we would start as we did with [older,
> experienced athlete] with a half dose first [according to body mass] and build
> as per tolerance.
>
> This was agreed to as a sensible approach by the coach.

Note: Sodium bicarbonate loading is not necessarily warranted for all hand
cycling events. Care must be taken if using it on consecutive days—repeated
dosing within a day, or on consecutive days, may induce greater side effects.

11.5.2 OTHER CONSIDERATIONS WHEN USING
SUPPLEMENTS IN PARALYMPIC SPORTS

Although the ingestion of supplements never replaces a balanced diet, there might
be special situations in athletes with an impairment (e.g. intense training camps,
high altitude training, quadriplegia with very low energy expenditure) where well-
directed supplementation over a certain time period can make sense to avoid any
potential nutrient insufficiency, such as micronutrients. In this context Krempien
and Barr (2011) reported several nutrient inadequate intakes of calcium, magnesium,
folate and vitamin D in over 25% of elite Canadian athletes with a spinal cord injury.
Targeted provision of individual nutrients can be valuable in correcting documented
deficiencies (such as iron and vitamin D), and as such can indirectly influence exercise performance and health in athletes with an impairment. However, this does not

---

COMMENTARY BOX 11.2

ATHLETE INSIGHT: What sports nutrition practices have had the biggest impact on your training capability or performance?

I have found that keeping a training logbook and nutrition diary has had the biggest impact on me. It has allowed me to see what has worked and what hasn't. Whether I have eaten enough for a certain training block or whether I needed to eat more. By trying different eating practices during training before big races, this has certainly steered me in the right direction.

—Carol Cooke, cyclist, Paralympic medallist;
ex-rower and able-bodied swimmer

I think that the link between body fat levels and my performance is where things have always been focussed for maximising my own performance.

—Michael Milton, five-time Winter Paralympian
and medallist, Summer Paralympic cyclist

In racing, good ol' Gatorade for hydration.

—Richard Nicholson, track and field athlete
and ex-powerlifter, multiple Paralympian

---

mean that the general recommendations for a balanced nutrition can be neglected. Finally, interactions between medication and nutrients have to be specifically taken into account (Perret and Stoffel-Kurt 2011), as many athletes with an impairment require long-term medication as a result of their disability.

KEY READINGS

Branch, J.D. 2003. Effect of creatine supplementation on body composition and performance: a meta-analysis. *International Journal of Sport Nutrition and Exercise Metabolism* 13:198–226.

Burke, L., Broad, E., Cox, G., et al. 2010. Supplements and sports foods. In *Clinical sports nutrition*, ed. L. Burke and V. Deakin, 419–500. 4th ed. Sydney: McGraw-Hill Australia.

Burke, L., Castell, L., and Stear, S. A to Z nutritional supplements (Topic collection). *British Journal of Sports Medicine*. www.bjsm.bmj.com/cgi/collection/bjsm_atoz_nutritional_supplements (accessed December 3, 2012).

Carr, A.J., Hopkins, W.G., and Gore, C.J. 2011. Effects of acute alkalosis and acidosis on performance: a meta-analysis. *Sports Medicine* 41:801–814.

Doherty, M., and Smith, P.M. 2004. Effects of caffeine ingestion on exercise testing: a meta-analysis. *International Journal of Sport Nutrition and Exercise Metabolism* 14:626–646.

Doherty, M., and Smith, P.M. 2005. Effects of caffeine ingestion on rating of perceived exertion during and after exercise: a meta-analysis. *Scandinavian Journal of Medicine and Science in Sports* 15:69–78.

Hobson, R.M., Saunders, B., Ball, G., Harris, R.C., and Sale, C. 2012. Effects of beta-alanine supplementation on exercise performance: a meta-analysis. *Amino Acids* 43:25–37.

Maughan, R.J., Greenhaff, P.L., and Hespel, P. 2011. Dietary supplements for athletes: emerging trends and recurring themes. *Journal of Sports Science* 29(Suppl 1):S57–S66.

Tarnopolsky, M.A. 2010. Caffeine and creatine use in sport. *Annals of Nutrition and Metabolism* 57(Suppl 2):1–8.

REFERENCES

Bailey, D.G. and Dresser, G.K. 2004. Interactions between grapefruit juice and cardiovascular drugs. *American Journal of Cardiovascular Drugs* 4:281–297.

Baylis, A., Cameron-Smith, D., and Burke, L.M. 2001. Inadvertent doping through supplement use by athletes: assessment and management of the risk in Australia. *International Journal of Sport Nutrition and Exercise Metabolism* 11:365–383.

Bird, S.R., Wiles, J., and Robbins, J. 1995. The effect of sodium bicarbonate ingestion on 1500-m racing time. *Journal of Sports Science* 13:399–403.

Branch, J.D. 2003. Effect of creatine supplementation on body composition and performance: a meta-analysis. *International Journal of Sport Nutrition and Exercise Metabolism* 13:198–226.

Brill, J.B., and Keane, M.W. 1994. Supplementation patterns of competitive male and female bodybuilders. *International Journal of Sport Nutrition* 4:398–412.

Burke, L., Broad, E., Cox, G., et al. 2010. Supplements and sports foods. In *Clinical sports nutrition*, ed. L. Burke and V. Deakin, 419–500. 4th ed. Sydney: McGraw-Hill Australia.

Burke, L., Castell, L., and Stear, S. 2012a. A to Z nutritional supplements (Topic collection). *British Journal of Sports Medicine*. www.bjsm.bmj.com/cgi/collection/bjsm_atoz_nutritional_supplements (accessed December 3, 2012).

Burke, L., and Cox, G. 2010. Pills and potions. In *The complete guide to food for sports performance*, 178. Sydney: Allen & Unwin.

Burke, L.M., Winter, J.A., Cameron-Smith, D., et al. 2012b. Effect of intake of different dietary protein sources on plasma amino acid profiles at rest and after exercise. *International Journal of Sport Nutrition and Exercise Metabolism* 22:452–462.

Carr, A.J., Hopkins, W.G., and Gore, C.J. 2011. Effects of acute alkalosis and acidosis on performance: a meta-analysis. *Sports Medicine* 41:801–814.

Chiou, W.B., Yang, C.C., and Wan, C.S. 2011. Ironic effects of dietary supplementation: illusory invulnerability created by taking dietary supplements licenses health-risk behaviors. *Psychological Science* 22:1081–1086.

Corrigan, B., and Kazlauskas, R. 2003. Medication use in athletes selected for doping control at the Sydney Olympics (2000). *Clinical Journal of Sport Medicine* 13:33–40.

Dascombe, B.J., Karunaratna, M., Cartoon, J., Fergie, B., and Goodman, C. 2010. Nutritional supplementation habits and perceptions of elite athletes within a state-based sporting institute. *Journal of Science and Medicine in Sport* 13:274–280.

de Silva, A., Samarasinghe, Y., Senanayake, D., and Lanerolle, P. 2010. Dietary supplement intake in national-level Sri Lankan athletes. *International Journal of Sport Nutrition and Exercise Metabolism* 20:15–20.

Doherty, M., and Smith, P.M. 2004. Effects of caffeine ingestion on exercise testing: a meta-analysis. *International Journal of Sport Nutrition and Exercise Metabolism* 14:626–646.

Erdman, K.A., Fung, T.S., Doyle-Baker, P.K., Verhoef, M.J., and Reimer, R.A. 2007. Dietary supplementation of high-performance Canadian athletes by age and gender. *Clinical Journal of Sport Medicine* 17:458–464.

European Parliament. 2002. Directive 2002/46/EC of the European Parliament and of the Council. Eur-lex.europa.eu/LesUriServe/LexUriServ.do?uri = CONSLEG:2002L0046 :20060421:EN:PDF (accessed November 18, 2012).

FitzSimmons, C.R., and Kidner, N. 1998. Caffeine toxicity in a bodybuilder. *Journal of Accident and Emergency Medicine* 15:196–197.

Food Standards Australia New Zealand. 2000. Standard 2.9.4— Formulated supplementary sports foods. www.comlaw.gov.au/Details/F2011C00549 (accessed November 18, 2012).

Geyer, H., Braun, H., Burke, L.M., Stear, S.J., and Castell, L.M. 2011. A-Z of nutritional supplements: dietary supplements, sports nutrition foods and ergogenic aids for health and performance. Part 22. *British Journal of Sports Medicine* 45:752–754.

Geyer, H., Parr, M.K., Mareck, U., Reinhart, U., Schrader, Y., and Schanzer, W. 2004. Analysis of non-hormonal nutritional supplements for anabolic-androgenic steroids—results of an international study. *International Journal of Sports Medicine* 25:124–129.

Gleeson, M., Bishop, N.C., Oliveira, M., and Tauler, P. 2011. Daily probiotic's (*Lactobacillus casei* Shirota) reduction of infection incidence in athletes. *International Journal of Sport Nutrition and Exercise Metabolism* 21:55–64.

Goosey-Tolfrey, V.L., and Crosland, J. 2010. Nutritional practices of competitive British wheelchair games players. *Adapted Physical Activity Quarterly* 27:47–59.

Graham, T.E., and Spriet, L.L. 1995. Metabolic, catecholamine, and exercise performance responses to various doses of caffeine. *Journal of Applied Physiology* 78:867–874.

Green, G.A., Catlin, D.H., and Starcevic, B. 2001. Analysis of over-the-counter dietary supplements. *Clinical Journal of Sport Medicine* 11:254–259.

Greenwood, M., Farris, J., Kreider, R., Greenwood, L., and Byars, A. 2000. Creatine supplementation patterns and perceived effects in select Division I collegiate athletes. *Clinical Journal of Sport Medicine* 10:191–194.

Harris, J.E. 1995. Interaction of dietary factors with oral anticoagulants: review and applications. *Journal of the American Dietetic Association* 95:580–584.

Harris, R.C., Soderlund, K., and Hultman, E. 1992. Elevation of creatine in resting and exercised muscle of normal subjects by creatine supplementation. *Clinical Science (London)* 83:367–374.

Harris, R.Z., Jang, G.R., and Tsunoda, S. 2003. Dietary effects on drug metabolism and transport. *Clinical Pharmacokinetics* 42:1071–1088.

Hayes, A., and Cribb, P.J. 2008. Effect of whey protein isolate on strength, body composition and muscle hypertrophy during resistance training. *Current Opinion in Clinical Nutrition and Metabolic Care* 11:40–44.

Hobson, R.M., Saunders, B., Ball, G., Harris, R.C., and Sale, C. 2012. Effects of beta-alanine supplementation on exercise performance: a meta-analysis. *Amino Acids* 43:25–37.

Ishikura, F., Beppu, S., Hamada, T., Khandheria, B.K., Seward, J.B., and Nehara, A. 2000. Effects of sildenafil citrate (Viagra) combined with nitrate on the heart. *Circulation* 102:2516–2521.

Judkins, C.M., Teale, P., and Hall, D.J. 2010. The role of banned substance residue analysis in the control of dietary supplement contamination. *Drug Testing and Analysis* 2:417–420.

Kamber, M., Baume, N., Saugy, M., and Rivier, L. 2001. Nutritional supplements as a source for positive doping cases? *International Journal of Sport Nutrition and Exercise Metabolism* 11:258–263.

Kloner, R.A., Hutter, A.M., Emmick, J.T., Mitchell, M.I., Denne, J., and Jackson, G. 2003. Time course of the interaction between tadalafil and nitrates. *Journal of the American College of Cardiology* 42:1855–1860.

Krempien, J.L., and Barr, S.I. 2011. Risk of nutrient inadequacies in elite Canadian athletes with spinal cord injury. *International Journal of Sport Nutrition and Exercise Metabolism* 21:417–425.

Krempien, J.L., and Barr, S.I. 2012. Eating attitudes and behaviours in elite Canadian athletes with a spinal cord injury. *Eating Behaviour* 13:36–41.

Krogh, K., Mosdal, C., and Laurberg, S. 2000. Gastrointestinal and segmental colonic transit times in patients with acute and chronic spinal cord lesion. *Spinal Cord* 38:615–621.

Lansley, K.E., Winyard, P.G., Bailey, S.J., et al. 2011. Acute dietary nitrate supplementation improves cycling time trial performance. *Medicine and Science in Sports and Exercise* 43:1125–1131.

Lun, V., Erdman, K.A., and Reimer, R.A. 2009. Evaluation of nutritional intake in Canadian high-performance athletes. *Clinical Journal of Sport Medicine* 19:405–411.

Maughan, R.J. 1995. Creatine supplementation and exercise performance. *International Journal of Sport Nutrition* 5:94–101.

Maughan, R. 2004. Contamination of supplements: an interview with Professor Ron Maughan by Louise M. Burke. *International Journal of Sport Nutrition and Exercise Metabolism* 14:493.

Maughan, R.J. 2005. Contamination of dietary supplements and positive drug tests in sport. *Journal of Sport Sciences* 23:883–889.

Maughan, R.J., Greenhaff, P.L., and Hespel, P. 2011. Dietary supplements for athletes: emerging trends and recurring themes. *Journal of Sports Sciences* 29(Suppl 1):S57–S66.

Nieper, A. 2005. Nutritional supplement practices in UK junior national track and field athletes. *British Journal of Sports Medicine* 39:645–649.

Oopik, V., Saaremets, I., Medijainen, L., Karelson, K., Janson, T., and Timpmann, S. 2003. Effects of sodium citrate ingestion before exercise on endurance performance in well trained college runners. *British Journal of Sports Medicine* 37:485–489.

Ozen, A.E., Pons, A., and Tur, J.A. 2012. Worldwide consumption of functional foods: a systematic review. *Nutrition Reviews* 70:472–481.

Patterson, S.D., and Gray, S.C. 2007. Carbohydrate-gel supplementation and endurance performance during intermittent high-intensity shuttle running. *International Journal of Sport Nutrition and Exercise Metabolism* 17:445–455.

Perret, C., Mueller, G., and Knecht, H. 2006. Influence of creatine supplementation on 800m wheelchair performance: a pilot study. *Spinal Cord* 44:275–279.

Perret, C., and Stoffel-Kurt, N. 2011. Comparison of nutritional intake between individuals with acute and chronic spinal cord injury. *Journal of Spinal Cord Medicine* 34:569–575.

Price, M. 2010. Energy expenditure and metabolism during exercise in persons with a spinal cord injury. *Sports Medicine* 40:681–696.

Prosser, J.M., Majlesi, N., Chan, G.M., Olsen, D., Hoffman, R.S., and Nelson, L.S. 2009. Adverse effects associated with arginine alpha-ketoglutarate containing supplements. *Human and Experimental Toxicology* 28:259–262.

Ristow, M., Zarse, K., Oberbach, A., et al. 2009. Antioxidants prevent health-promoting effects of physical exercise in humans. *Proceedings of the National Academy of Science USA* 106:8665–8670.

Skrinar, G.S., Evans, W.J., Ornstein, L.J., and Brown, D.A. 1982. Glycogen utilization in wheelchair-dependent athletes. *International Journal of Sports Medicine* 3:215–219.

Slater, G., Tan, B., and The, K.C. 2003. Dietary supplementation practices of Singaporean athletes. *International Journal of Sport Nutrition and Exercise Metabolism* 13:320–332.

Spendiff, O., and Campbell, I.G. 2003. Influence of glucose ingestion prior to prolonged exercise on selected responses of wheelchair athletes. *Adapted Physical Activity Quarterly* 20:80–90.

Spendiff, O., and Campbell, I.G. 2005. Influence of pre-exercise glucose ingestion of two concentrations on paraplegic athletes. *Journal of Sport Science* 23:21–30.

Suzic Lazic, J., Dikic, N., Radivojevic, N., et al. 2011. Dietary supplements and medications in elite sport—polypharmacy or real need? *Scandinavian Journal of Medicine and Science in Sports* 21:260–267.

Tarnopolsky, M.A. 2010. Caffeine and creatine use in sport. *Annals of Nutrition and Metabolism* 57(Suppl 2):1–8.

Therapeutic Goods Administration. 1989. Therapeutic Goods Act 1989. www.tga.gov.au/industry/cm-basics-regulation-overview.htm (accessed November 18, 2012).

Tscholl, P., Alonso, J.M., Dolle, G., Junge, A., and Dvorak, J. 2010. The use of drugs and nutritional supplements in top-level track and field athletes. *American Journal of Sports Medicine* 38:133–140.

U.S. Food and Drug Administration. 1994. Dietary Supplement Health and Education Act 1994. www.fda.gov/RegulatoryInformation/Legislation/FederalFoodDrugandCosmeticActFDCAct/SignificantAmendmentstotheFDCAct/ucm148003.htm (accessed November 18, 2012).

Vandenberghe, K., Gillis, N., Van Lccmputtc, M., Van Hecke, P., Vanstapel, F., and Hespel, P. 1996. Caffeine counteracts the ergogenic action of muscle creatine loading. *Journal of Applied Physiology* 80:452–457.

van Loon, L.J., Murphy, R., Oosterlaar, A.M., et al. 2004. Creatine supplementation increases glycogen storage but not GLUT-4 expression in human skeletal muscle. *Clinical Science (London)* 106:99–106.

West, N.P., Pyne, D.B., Cripps, A.W., et al. 2011. *Lactobacillus fermentum* (PCC(R)) supplementation and gastrointestinal and respiratory-tract illness symptoms: a randomised control trial in athletes. *Nutrition Journal* 10:30.

Wiles, J.D., Bird, S.R., Hopkins, J., and Riley, M. 1992. Effect of caffeinated coffee on running speed, respiratory factors, blood lactate and perceived exertion during 1500-m treadmill running. *British Journal of Sports Medicine* 26:116–120.

12 Assessing Body Composition of Athletes

Gary Slater

CONTENTS

12.1 INTRODUCTION

There may be several reasons for undertaking physique assessment amongst athletes with an impairment, including general health screens, appropriate sizing/fitting or design of prostheses, talent identification initiatives, or routine monitoring of adaptation to training and diet. The rationale for assessment and outcome measures of interest will play a key role in ascertaining which physique assessment technique and normative data to use in assisting to interpret the data collected. Consideration must also be given to the individual athlete and their specific impairment. This may have implications in either the practical administration of the assessment technique and/or the unique physical characteristics which violate underlying assumptions associated with a specific physique assessment technique. For example, the spasm often associated with multiple sclerosis (MS) would corrupt dual energy x-ray absorptiometry (DXA) scan integrity but have little impact on data captured using air displacement plethysmography (BOD POD) (Rosendale and Bartok 2012; Tegenkamp et al. 2011). In contrast, it would be logistically easier to position an athlete with quadriplegia on a DXA scanner than a BOD POD where they would be unable to maintain body position, nor maximally exhale whilst underwater, both requirements for assessment when using hydrodensitometry. Marked changes in total body water (TBW) content and/or the ratio of intracellular to extracellular water, common amongst individuals with a spinal cord injury (Kocina 1997), may preclude body composition assessment using bioelectrical impedance analysis (BIA) (Strauss et al. 2000), but less so for BOD POD (Clascy and Gater 2005). Thus the choice of technique or equipment is a very important aspect to consider when undertaking physique assessment amongst athletes with an impairment.

A relationship between competitive success and physique traits has been identified amongst athletes across a range of sports, including football codes (Olds 2001), aesthetically judged sports (Claessens et al. 1999), swimming (Siders et al. 1993), track and field events (Claessens et al. 1994), skiing (White and Johnson 1991; Stoggl et al. 2010; Larsson and Henriksson-Larsen 2008), and rowing (Shephard 1998). The specific physique traits associated with competitive success vary with the sport. For athletes participating in sports where frontal surface area, power-to-weight ratio, and/or thermoregulation are important, maintenance of low body fat levels is associated with positive outcomes (Norton et al. 1996). However, in sports demanding high force production, muscle mass may be more closely associated with performance outcomes (Olds 2001; Siders et al. 1993; Brechue and Abe 2002; Kyriazis et al. 2010; Stoggl et al. 2010), with specific distribution of muscle mass also important (Stoggl et al. 2010; Larsson and Henriksson-Larsen 2008). Likewise, in sports such as rowing, other physique traits like a shorter sitting height (relative to stature) and longer limb lengths are related to competitive success (DeRose et al. 1989). Because of these relationships, it has become common practice to monitor physique traits of athletes.

Similar relationships likely exist between physique traits and competitive success amongst athletes with an impairment, especially those in which physique traits are not impacted by the condition, such as athletes with intellectual or vision impairment. Less is known about the unique population of athletes with an impairment in which the condition impacts on physique traits, such as those with spinal cord injuries, cerebral palsy, short stature and amputees, but there is at least some evidence confirming physique traits do impact performance in this population (Ide et al. 1994). The impact of the later conditions on presenting physique traits and response to interventions such as diet and exercise are addressed in earlier chapters specific to these conditions. What is more pertinent in the current chapter is the impact a presenting condition may have on the techniques (or their associated assumptions) available for physique assessment, classification of physique traits and disease risk cut-offs or the broader application of physique assessment to specific populations such as the fitting of prostheses for amputees.

12.2 PHYSIQUE ASSESSMENT TECHNIQUES

A wide array of techniques is available for the measurement of body composition, including anthropometric, radiographic (computed tomography (CT), DXA) and other medical imaging techniques (magnetic resonance imaging (MRI), ultrasound),

---

COMMENTARY BOX 12.1

COACH'S INSIGHT: What are the biggest nutrition challenges your athletes face?

This depends on the classification, which relates to the duration of their specific events and the amount of training required. Probably one of the biggest challenges is the athlete's knowledge of how to achieve the best relationship between energy and protein/carbohydrate requirements and the need to control/reduce body fat.

—Peter Day, Paralympic cycling head coach

---

metabolic (creatinine, 3-methylhistidine), nuclear (total body potassium, total body nitrogen) and BIA techniques. When selecting the most appropriate technique, a range of factors should be considered, including:

- Technical issues such as the safety, validity, precision and accuracy of measurement
- Practical issues such as availability, financial implications, portability, invasiveness, time-effectiveness, and technical expertise necessary to conduct the procedures
- The ability of body composition assessment methodologies to accommodate the unique physique traits characteristic of some athletes with an impairment, including particularly tall, broad, and muscular individuals or those with extremely low body fat or skeletal muscle mass
- The athlete's impairment and the impact this may have on the assessment itself or subsequent estimation of body composition, and assumptions associated with this

Table 12.1 provides an overview of assessment techniques potentially available for the assessment of body composition (i.e. fat and fat-free mass) and broader physique traits (i.e. body fat, muscle mass, bone mass, limb lengths, breadths, proportionality etc.) among athletes with an impairment. Consideration is also given to the unique characteristics of these athletes and the impact these can have on viable techniques for assessment.

This chapter reviews the most common techniques used to assess the physique traits of athletes with an impairment with a focus on the technical or procedural aspects associated with their use. Brief consideration is also given to emerging technologies that may have wider application to athletes with an impairment into the future, such as three-dimensional photonic scanning. The rationale for assessment and outcome measures of interest will play a key role in ascertaining which physique assessment technique to use.

TABLE 12.1

Physique Assessment Techniques Potentially Available for Assessment of Body Composition and Physique Traits of Athletes with an Impairment

Technique	Information Provided	Unsuitable for ...
BOD POD	FM, FFM	SCI, amputee
DXA	FM, FFM, BMD	MS, CP with spasm
BIA	FM, FFM, TBW	Oedema, lower body or unilateral amputee, SCI
Anthropometry	Skinfolds, girths, bone breadths and lengths	If absolute FM and FFM measures are required Modifications to protocol may be required

Note: Consideration is given to the unique characteristics of these athletes and the impact this has on techniques available for assessment.

BOD POD = air displacement plethysmography, DXA = dual energy x-ray absorptiometry, BIA = bioelectrical impedance, FM = fat mass, FFM = fat free mass, BMD = bone mineral density, TBW = total body water, SCI = spinal cord injury (complete), MS = multiple sclerosis with spasm, CP = cerebral palsy.

12.2.1 BODY COMPOSITION MODELS: TWO-, THREE-, AND FOUR-COMPARTMENT MODELS

A number of well accepted two-compartment body composition assessment models are available to monitor body composition, including hydrodensitometry, BOD POD and deuterium dilution. These methods are based on the premise that the body can be separated into two chemically distinct compartments, that is, fat mass (FM) and fat free mass (FFM) (Withers et al. 1999). However, each of these methods carries with it some degree of error, most of which lies not in the technical accuracy of the measurements but in the biological variability of the assumptions associated with each technique in the generation of body composition data from raw measures like body density and total body water (TBW). This is especially the case for FFM estimates, and may be exacerbated amongst some athletes with an impairment, such as those with a spinal cord injury where there are substantial changes in bone mineral, muscle mass, and thus water content of the FFM below the spinal cord lesion (Kocina 1997). The combination of data from several of these two-compartment models into a multi-compartment model reduces the number of assumptions made and is now recognized as the current reference method in body composition assessment (Withers et al. 1999).

A three-compartment model approach adjusts the body density obtained from hydrodensitometry or BOD POD (Millard-Stafford et al. 2001) for FFM hydration or TBW using isotope dilution, rather than assume a FFM TBW content of 73.72% (Brozek et al. 1963). Variation in FFM hydration from the assumed constant, as occurs in states of hypohydration and hyperhydration respectively, increases and decreases FFM density with associated under and over estimation of percentage body fat via hydrodensitometry by as much as 10% (Hewitt et al. 1993). Furthermore, measurement of FFM hydration is particularly relevant given that it has by far the lowest density of any FFM component, yet occupies the largest percentage of the FFM.

The introduction of DXA has afforded the creation of a four-compartment model, controlling for biological variability in both TBW and bone mineral content. While this model is theoretically more valid than the three-compartment model because it controls for biological variability in both bone mineral content and TBW, work by Withers and associates (Withers et al. 1998) indicates the additional control for inter-individual variation in bone mineral mass achieves little extra accuracy among able-bodied individuals. This may not be the case for athletes with accelerated bone density loss, such as those with spinal cord lesions (Kocina 1997). Thus multi-compartment models likely offer the most valid index of body composition amongst some classifications of athletes with an impairment. However, their application may be limited to scientific investigations where absolute measures of FM and FFM are key outcome variables. Other techniques with wider availability, less cost implications and time requirement for assessment may be deemed suitable for the routine monitoring of athletes where relative, rather than absolute, changes in body composition are desired (Figure 12.1).

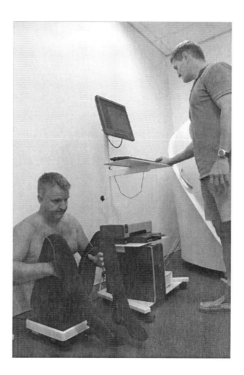

FIGURE 12.1 Weighing athletes with a spinal cord injury without a set of seated scales.

12.2.2 AIR DISPLACEMENT PLETHYSMOGRAPHY

Air displacement plethysmography utilizes basic gas laws to describe the inverse relationship between pressure and volume in two enclosed chambers, consequently allowing for the calculation of body density and body composition. Measurement involves sitting briefly in an enclosed chamber, which accommodates a range of subject types (Dempster and Aitkens 1995), while the volume of air displaced by the body is measured. Thereafter, lung functional residual capacity is measured using pulmonary plethysmography or, if this is not possible, predicted based on age, gender and height. Body density is then calculated by dividing the measured body mass by corrected body volume, with subsequent calculation of percent body fat using either the Siri (Siri 1993) or Brozek (Brozek et al. 1963) equations. As such, the BOD POD is constrained by the same issues as hydrodensitometry when converting a measure of body density into body composition. However the procedures are much less labour intensive for both subjects and technicians and lower the risk of complications in populations such as those with a spinal cord injury, where aspiration and autonomic dysreflexia are possible (Clasey and Gater 2005). The measurement of functional residual capacity using pulmonary plethysmography is both reliable and valid in able-bodied populations (Davis et al. 2007), but this may not be the case for individuals with a spinal cord lesion (Clasey and Gater 2005), impacting on estimates of body composition. As such, residual capacity should be measured wherever possible and never used interchangeably with predicted thoracic gas volumes (Minderico et al. 2008).

The BOD POD compares favourably as a substitute for hydrodensitometry when a measure of body density is desired (Fields et al. 2000), although it has been observed to underestimate body fat slightly in males ($-1.2 \pm 3.1\%$) and overestimate body fat in females ($1.0 \pm 2.5\%$), independent of age, weight or height (Biaggi et al. 1999). This effect is evident amongst athletic populations as well, with BOD POD-derived estimates of body fat consistently lower than those obtained via hydrodensitometry, DXA and a three-compartment model for male collegiate football athletes (Collins et al. 1999). Among female athletes, the BOD POD overestimates body fat when compared against hydrodensitometry but either compares favourably (Ballard et al. 2004) or underestimates body fat when contrasted against DXA (Bentzur et al. 2008). These differences may also be influenced by presenting body composition, with the BOD POD overestimating body fat as fat mass increases yet underestimating body fat in leaner athletes when compared against a multi-compartment reference method (Moon et al. 2009). Amongst a spinal cord injury population with widely varying physical characteristics, the BOD POD produced higher estimates of fat mass compared to hydrodensitometry, although individual differences were small (Dempster and Aitkens 1995) and the validity of hydrodensitometry in this population is uncertain.

While the ability to measure absolute characteristics is an important attribute of a physique assessment technique, equally important is the ability to identify small but potentially important changes in body composition in response to diet, training or other interventions. Research using the artificial manipulation of body composition by the addition of one to two litres of oil, water or a combination of both substances to the BOD POD chamber among normal weight individuals suggests the technology has the ability to pick up changes in either component within the range of 2 kg (Le Carvennec et al. 2007; Secchiutti et al. 2007). When the BOD POD has been used in conjunction with DXA to monitor body composition changes in response to lifestyle interventions, BOD POD estimates of fat mass are typically lower, with concomitant higher estimates of FFM (Minderico et al. 2006; Weyers et al. 2002). However, agreement between techniques was high for identifying the changes in body composition in response to lifestyle interventions (Frisard et al. 2005; Minderico et al. 2006; Weyers et al. 2002).

As with other physique assessment tools, subject presentation can influence results, and thus suitable protocols must be implemented to avoid the impact of these on the reliability of data. Specifically, uncompressed facial and scalp hair underestimate body fat due to trapped isothermal air in body hair (Higgins et al. 2001). Similarly, loose fitting clothing worn during assessment influences body density measurements, underestimating body fat percentage by upwards of 9% (Vescovi et al. 2002; Fields et al. 2000). Consequently, subjects are advised to wear standardized tight fitting swimsuits (Fields et al. 2000; King et al. 2006; Vescovi et al. 2002) in conjunction with a silicone swim cap (Peeters and Claessens 2011) and to remove excess facial hair (Higgins et al. 2001). Changes in body temperature and moisture content may also influence BOD POD data (Fields et al. 2004), suggesting that assessments should be undertaken independent of exercise. This is further supported by the fact that acute dehydration (within the range often experienced by athletes) also influences BOD POD results, underestimating both body fat percentage and FFM, although the effect is within the range of 1% body fat (Utter et al. 2003). Slight body movements during testing, not dissimilar to those likely from tremor, do not appear to influence BOD POD estimates of body composition (Tegenkamp et al. 2011) (Figures 12.2 and 12.3).

Minimizing the influence of these variables enhances the ability of the BOD POD to track small, but potentially important, changes in body composition. While the test-retest reliability of the BOD POD is excellent (Noreen and Lemon 2006), this does not provide insight into the biological variability evident between test measures. The between-day coefficient of variation for body fat using the BOD POD is within the range of 2.0–5.3% (Anderson 2007), although large discrepancies (up to 12%) between trials have been reported in a small percentage of individuals (Noreen and Lemon 2006), for reasons still yet to be determined. In practice, technicians are encouraged to undertake repeat measurements and if these two tests show a difference in percent body fat greater than 0.5%, then a third test may be appropriate (Collins and McCarthy 2003). While reliability between individual BOD POD systems is very good (Ball 2005), athletes should be assessed using the same machine each time when evaluating change.

12.2.3 Dual Energy X-Ray Absorptiometry

DXA was originally developed for the diagnosis of osteoporosis and remains the reference method for this assessment (Lewiecki 2005). It may also have application as a screening tool in identifying athletes at risk of stress fractures (Prouteau et al.

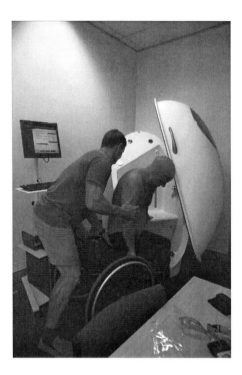

FIGURE 12.2   Assisting a subject into a BOD POD. Note the silicone cap used on the head.

2004; Kelsey et al. 2007). Furthermore, DXA technology is also able to measure soft tissue body composition and has rapidly gained popularity in recent years as one of the most widely used and accepted laboratory-based methods for body composition analysis. DXA not only provides a measure of FM and FFM but also provides information on regional body composition (e.g. arms, legs, trunk) and differences between left and right sides, making it unique among physique assessment tools and particularly appealing for athletes with an impairment such as those with spinal cord injuries where regional changes in fat, bone and muscle mass can be marked but somewhat masked at a whole-body level. Furthermore, whole-body scans are rapid, non-invasive and associated with very low radiation doses, making the technology safe for longitudinal monitoring of body composition, and considered valid amongst those with a spinal cord injury (Jones et al. 1998). Because of its application in the assessment of bone mineral density, DXA technology is also becoming increasingly available through commercial imaging centres. However, longitudinal monitoring should be undertaken on the same machine (Hull et al. 2009; Soriano et al. 2004; Tothill et al. 2001), and using the same technician (Burkhart et al. 2009), especially if regional body composition changes are of interest.

   DXA technology is based on the differential attenuation of transmitted photons at two energy levels by bone, fat and lean tissue (Mazess et al. 1990). The differential attenuations are then expressed as a ratio, the outcome of which is specific to different molecular components, including fatty acids, protein and bone. In theory, assessment of all three components would require measurement at three different photon

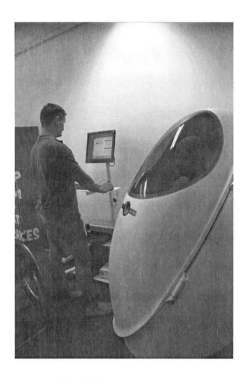

FIGURE 12.3 Undertaking a BOD POD assessment.

energies. The dual energy system can thus only be used to estimate the fractional masses of two components in any one pixel. That is, in bone-containing pixels, bone mineral and soft tissue can be measured, while in non-bone-containing pixels, fat and bone-mineral-free lean can be measured (Pietrobelli et al. 1996). The proportion of fat and bone-mineral-free lean in bone-containing pixels is assumed to be the same as the adjacent non-bone-containing pixels (Pietrobelli et al. 1996), with the software subsequently converting individual pixel data into whole-body output. This assumed ratio of fat to bone-mineral-free lean in soft tissue pixels is applied to upwards of one-third of pixels in a whole-body scan and particularly evident in regions of low bone-free pixels such as the thorax, arm or head, resulting in less reliable identification of composition changes in these regions (Lands et al. 1996; Roubenoff et al. 1993). This will likely be an issue for accurately measuring absolute body composition in several para-sport athletes, including those with a spinal cord lesion or cerebral palsy, because of the greater number of regions of low bone-free pixels. How this impacts on the ability of DXA to accurately track changes in body composition longitudinally remains to be established.

DXA technology has been compared to the modern-day reference body composition assessment tool, the four-compartment model, which accounts for variation in the water and mineral fractions and the associated density of the FFM. While there are some data suggesting good agreement between DXA-derived measures of body composition and the four-compartment model in healthy, young males and females (Prior et al. 1997), others have reported that DXA underestimates body fat

(Deurenberg-Yap et al. 2001), especially among leaner individuals (Van Der Ploeg et al. 2003; Withers et al. 1998). This underestimation has been attributed to variation in FFM hydration (Deurenberg-Yap et al. 2001) or differences in anterior-posterior tissue thickness (Van Der Ploeg et al. 2003). Conversely, DXA has been shown to overestimate fat mass in females, with this bias increasing as body fat levels increase (Moon et al. 2009; Silva et al. 2006). Despite this, amongst athletes where the primary focus is on monitoring change in body composition, DXA appears to offer sufficient sensitivity to identify small changes in body composition.

The precision of measurement for DXA in sedentary populations has been shown to be superior to hydrodensitometry and surface anthropometry (Pritchard et al. 1993), with a coefficient of variation of less than 1.0 kg for FM, FFM, and total mass (Mazess et al. 1990; Tothill et al. 1994). Variability of results achieved by DXA can be divided into two categories: technical and biological error. In an effort to enhance precision of measurement, special consideration should be given to subject positioning (Lambrinoudaki et al. 1998; Lohman et al. 2009), which may be particularly challenging for those with lordosis or congenital conditions affecting the spine, spasticity or other conditions associated with uncontrolled movement. Clothing should be kept to a minimum (Koo et al. 2004), with all metal objects removed. While small amounts of food and fluid do not appear to influence results (Vilaca et al. 2009), larger volumes influence measurement of lean body mass (Horber et al. 1992), and thus measurements should be undertaken in a fasted state wherever possible, preferably soon after waking in a euhydrated state (Going et al. 1993). The altered water distribution and associated oedema of the lower limbs common amongst spinal cord injury athletes (Buchholz et al. 2003) can result in a significant overestimation of FFM. The reliability of regional measurements is inferior to total body results (Calbet et al. 1998; Lohman et al. 2009) (Figures 12.4 and 12.5).

Of particular relevance to athletic populations is the defined scanning area available for assessment, typically within the range of 60–65 cm × 193–198 cm depending on the manufacturer (Genton et al. 2002). It is therefore difficult to perform whole-body DXA scans on particularly tall or broad and very muscular athletes, physique traits perhaps less common within sport for athletes with an impairment but nonetheless still present in sports such as rowing, basketball, and powerlifting. Taller individuals should have two partial scans (one scan of the upper body, with the other scan measuring the remainder of the body) with the body divided at the neck or femoral necks, depending on the specific scanner, resulting in the most accurate estimates of bone and soft tissue composition (Evans et al. 2005; Nana et al. 2012b). Until recently, very broad individuals were 'mummy wrapped' in a sheet, bringing the arms forward, so as to fit within the scanning area. While this afforded a whole-body scan to be undertaken, the number of bone-containing pixels was significantly increased whilst limiting the ability to assess body composition at particular regions of interest, such as the arms and torso. Newer DXA instruments like the iDXA from GE Lunar (Madison, Wisconsin) not only have larger scanning areas (66 cm wide) but also come with software that allows an estimate of whole-body composition from a half-body scan (Rothney et al. 2009), a concept validated previously in obese individuals (Tataranni and Ravussin 1995). The use of foam pads and straps that are not identified by the DXA scanner are recommended to enhance the reliability of DXA

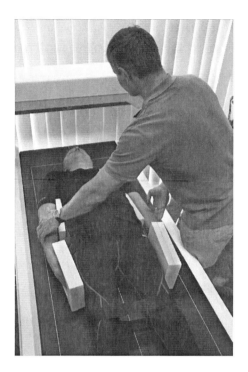

FIGURE 12.4   Standardizing the positioning of an athlete for a DXA scan. Note the use of foam pads to enable consistent positioning and separation of limbs. The foam is not detectable by the DXA scanner.

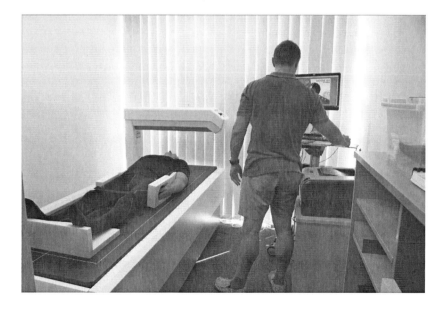

FIGURE 12.5   Undertaking a DXA scan.

measurements (Nana et al. 2012a), and may be particularly valuable for athletes with an impairment who experience tremor, spasticity or other movement during measurement, which, if left uncontrolled, would corrupt results. Given these limitations, DXA technology can and has been used to assess the body composition of individuals across a range of para-sport classifications, including spinal cord lesions (Sutton et al. 2009; Mojtahedi et al. 2009).

12.2.4 BIO-ELECTRICAL IMPEDANCE ANALYSIS

BIA has become increasingly popular as a tool for assessing the body composition of athletes given its relative ease of use, portability and cost effectiveness. It is a safe and non-invasive method to assess body composition that is based on the differing electrical conductivity of FM and FFM (NIH 1996; Kyle et al. 2004a). FFM contains water and electrolytes and is a good electrical conductor, while anhydrous FM is not. The method involves measuring the resistance (R) to flow of a low level current/s (Kyle et al. 2004a). Resistance is proportional to the length (L) of the conductor (in this case the human body) and inversely proportional to its cross sectional area (A). A relationship then exists between the impedance quotient (i.e. L^2/R) and the volume of water (total body water) which contains electrolytes that conduct the electrical current. In practice, height in centimetres is substituted for length. Therefore, a relationship exists between FFM (approximately 73% water) and height $(cm)^2/R$. FM is obtained from FFM by subtracting the value for FFM from total body mass (Kyle et al. 2004a).

Although the relationship between FFM and impedance is readily accepted, there are several assumptions associated with the use of BIA to measure body composition. First, the human body is assumed to be a cylinder with a uniform length and cross sectional area. Rather, the human body more closely resembles several cylinders. The body parts with the smallest FFM (the limbs) have the greatest influence on whole-body resistance, and this may be accentuated in some classifications. The trunk, which is a shorter, thicker segment, contains ~50% of body weight, but contributes a minor amount to the overall resistance. Second, it is assumed the conducting material within the cylinder is homogeneous, which it isn't. Finally, the resistance to current flow per unit length of a specific conductor is assumed to be constant. However, this will vary depending on tissue structure, hydration status and electrolyte concentration of the tissue (Kushner 1992).

Due to the relevance of body water to conductivity of electrical current, there is substantial evidence that BIA is not valid for assessment of individuals with abnormal hydration such as visible oedema, ascites, kidney, liver and cardiac disease and pregnancy (Kyle et al. 2004b). Oedema in particular may be common amongst some athletes with an impairment, including those with a spinal cord lesion (Kocina 1997), with this effect exacerbated by changes in hydration status as a consequence of exercise-induced hypohydration and acute food/fluid intake. Exercise-induced hypohydration to a level of 3% body mass has been shown to decrease the estimate of FM via BIA by 1.7%. Conversely, acute rehydration increased estimates of FM by 3.2%, with a further increase in the estimate of FM as a state of hyperhydration was achieved (Saunders et al. 1998). Even the ingestion of relatively small volumes of fluid (591 ml) has been shown to increase estimates of FM (Dixon et al. 2009). Consequently, athletes should remain fasted for at least 8 h prior to assessment (Kyle et al. 2004b). Given this, it would be prudent to undertake assessments in the morning prior to breakfast wherever possible, with athletes encouraged to present in a well-hydrated state, assessment of which could be done via the collection of a first morning urine sample.

Given the impact of acute changes in hydration status to resistance and thus estimates of TBW and body composition, it has been suggested that BIA could be used to assess acute changes in hydration status. However results to date suggest BIA is only able to predict half of the body water loss resulting from exercise (Koulmann et al. 2000). Other factors reported to influence BIA results include posture and positioning of the limbs, prior exercise, skin temperature (Kushner et al. 1996) and electrode placement (Dunbar et al. 1994). A detailed description of factors to consider when undertaking assessments using BIA are described elsewhere (Kyle et al. 2004a, 2004b). Consideration of these issues will assist in reducing measurement error but errors may still be moderate with this technique, prompting some to suggest BIA may be most appropriate for estimating body composition of groups rather than individuals (Houtkooper et al. 1996). Kyle and associates (2004b) suggest prediction of errors of less than 3.0 kg for males and 2.3 kg for females would be considered good.

Within an athletic population, BIA has been shown to overestimate FFM in smaller males, and underestimate FFM in heavier athletes competing in a weight category sport (Utter and Lambeth 2010). Similarly, BIA has been shown to underestimate fat mass in team sport athletes (Svantesson et al. 2008). If BIA were used to calculate a minimum weight prediction for these athletes, errors of as much as 6–7 kg are possible—greater than those identified with other physique assessment techniques such as DXA, hydrodensitometry and surface anthropometry (Clark et al. 2004). The selection of appropriate prediction equations for the conversion of raw impedance results into FFM is an important consideration, with equations derived from untrained individuals likely to be inappropriate for an athletic population (Pichard et al. 1997). Kyle and associates (2004b) provide an excellent summary of prediction equations derived from healthy subjects, and published since 1990, for adults for FFM, body fat and TBW. To date, no equations have been established from populations with character traits similar to those likely amongst athletes with an impairment, making the conversion of raw impedance data into estimates of body composition lacking validation.

12.2.4.1 Single versus Multi-Frequency Systems

The measurement of difference in electrical properties of various body tissues is not a new concept. The original studies were conducted by Thomasset in the 1960s using two subcutaneous inserted needles (Thomasset 1963). The technique was subsequently refined in the 1970s to four surface electrodes, and resulted in commercially available single-frequency analysers (Kyle et al. 2004a). Since this time, there have been significant advances in BIA with options of single-frequency, multi-frequency and segmental BIA.

Foot-to-foot BIA analysers are the most readily available for public purchase (Jaffrin 2009). These inexpensive body fat 'scales' are popular amongst the general public, being promoted as a simple, portable method of measuring body fatness. However, there are a number of limitations with foot-to-foot devices as current is only circulated through the legs and lower part of the trunk with results extrapolated to the whole body (Jaffrin 2009). This equipment is also limited to those individuals who can freely stand on both legs, limiting its application amongst several classifications of athletes with an impairment. Furthermore, raw impedance data is rarely reported, making selection of population-specific equations impossible. While many systems come with an 'athletic' mode option, this does not enhance the predictive accuracy of BIA when compared to a reference method (Dixon et al. 2006).

Single-frequency BIA (50 kHz) is most commonly used as a field technique to measure body composition. It usually consists of four electrodes placed on the wrist, hand, ankle and foot, though foot-to-foot and hand-to-hand analysers are also available. The two source electrodes are placed on the dorsal surface of the right hand and foot proximal to the metacarpophalangeal and metatarsophalangeal joints respectively. The two voltage electrodes are placed on the midpoint between the distal prominences of the radius and ulna of the right wrist and between the medial and lateral malleoli of the right ankle (Wagner and Heyward 1999).

Multi-frequency BIA consists of measurement of impedance at various frequencies (0, 1, 5, 50, 100, 200 and 500 kHz). At a low single frequency, an electrical current will not fully penetrate the cell membrane, passing only through extracellular water, whereas at high frequencies the current will penetrate the cell membrane (Cornish et al. 1996). By measuring various components across a number of frequencies, a mathematical model can be derived that can be used to predict TBW and subsequently FFM instead of using standard regression equations. This may be more appropriate for individuals where there is variation in standard hydration status or body composition (Martinoli et al. 2003), as may be common amongst some athletes with an impairment. The results of various studies comparing multifrequency BIA to single-frequency BIA and other methods such as DXA have reported mixed results (Pateyjohns et al. 2006; Sun et al. 2005).

12.2.5 SURFACE ANTHROPOMETRY

For reasons of timeliness, practicality and cost-effectiveness, the routine monitoring of body composition among athletic populations is most often undertaken using anthropometric characteristics such as body mass plus subcutaneous skinfold thicknesses and girths at specific anatomical landmarks. Unlike other techniques requiring expensive laboratory-based equipment, surface anthropometry only requires relatively inexpensive equipment that is easily portable. However, highly skilled technicians are required if reliable data are to be collected. Technicians need to be meticulous in terms of both accurate site location and measurement technique. Measurements just 1–2 cm away from a defined site can produce significant differences in results (Ruiz et al. 1971; Hume and Marfell-Jones 2008). Furthermore, if repeat measurements are to be taken over time, it is important that the same technician collect the data (Hume and Marfell-Jones 2008).

The measurement of 'skinfolds' or a double layer of skin and subcutaneous tissue as an index of whole-body fat would appear to be reasonable. However, what is really being measured is the thickness of a double fold of skin and compressed subcutaneous adipose tissue (Martin et al. 1985). To infer from this the mass or percentage of total body fat requires a number of assumptions to be made, including:

- Constant compressibility of skinfolds across sites on the body
- The skin thickness at any one site is negligible or a constant fraction of a skinfold
- Fixed adipose tissue patterning across the body
- A constant fat fraction in adipose tissue
- Fixed proportion of internal to external fat

When assessed via cadaver analysis, few of these assumptions hold true (Clarys et al. 2005). For example, skinfold compressibility is not constant between sites and as a consequence, similar thicknesses of adipose tissue may yield different caliper values due to different degrees of tissue compressibility (Marfell-Jones et al. 2003). Furthermore, the patterning of adipose tissue varies markedly between individuals (Mueller and Stallones 1981), and as such, multiple skinfold sites should be used, including both upper and lower body landmarks (Eston et al. 2005). The impact of spinal cord lesions on body fat distribution above and below the lesion remains to be fully elucidated, making it difficult to ascertain if assessments should include sites both above and below the lesion. Furthermore, while it is estimated that subcutaneous fat comprises one-third of total body fat, this can range from 20–70% depending on gender, degree of fatness and age (Lohman 1981). Despite an obvious violation of these assumptions, a strong relationship does exist between subcutaneous adiposity and whole-body adiposity, and between direct skinfold thickness measures and whole-body adiposity (Clarys et al. 2005).

Estimates of body density, FM and/or FFM can be derived from raw skinfold data using one of many available regression equations. Altogether, more than 100 equations to predict body fat from skinfolds have been produced (Clarys et al. 1987, 1999; Lohman 1981; Martin et al. 1985). However, these equations are typically based on a single measurement, between-subject, cross-sectional comparison of anthropometric parameters and laboratory-based techniques such as hydrodensitometry (Cisar et al. 1989), increasing the assumptions made. Furthermore, these predictive equations have been proven to lack validity in both male (Bulbulian et al. 1987) and female (Sutton et al. 2009) athletes with a spinal cord injury, with the exception of the modified equation by Withers and colleagues, which incorporated waist girth measurement into estimates of body composition (Withers et al. 1987). However, the ability of these equations to track changes in body composition in response to training and/ or dietary interventions has not been widely assessed (Cisar et al. 1989; Wilmore et al. 1970). Preliminary data suggests popular skinfold-based models, including those derived from athletes, lack the sensitivity to track small but potentially important changes in body composition (van Marken Lichtenbelt et al. 2004; Silva et al. 2009). As such, it seems unreasonable to introduce further error by transforming raw skinfold data into estimates of fat mass or percentage body fat. Thus, despite the advancement in physique assessment techniques, and the notable desire of many athletes wishing to know their 'body fat percentage', the conclusions of Johnston (1982) remain true to this date; that is, practitioners are better off to continue using raw anthropometric data rather than attempt to make estimates of whole-body composition from available equations.

While sums of skinfolds are highly correlated with body fat percentage, FFM correlates poorly with skinfolds (Roche 1996). It has been proposed that combining skinfolds with certain body circumferences leads to a better estimate of FFM (Forbes 1999). In theory, skinfold-corrected circumferences offer a more direct assessment of muscle mass, assuming that the skinfold thickness accurately partitions fat and lean components at a specific site (Reid et al. 1992). However, the skinfold-corrected girth estimates have been shown to be less accurate in monitoring changes in muscle mass than predictions using skinfolds alone (Stewart and Hannan 2000; Cisar et al. 1989). This imprecision may be explained, at least in part, by the fact that muscle hypertrophy does not occur uniformly throughout each body region (Abe et al. 2003), yet the anthropometric fractionation estimate of muscle mass places equal weighting on each of five girth measurements (Drinkwater and Ross 1980). Consequently, anthropometric fractionation may not be appropriate when attempting to quantify skeletal muscle mass in athletes with significant muscle hypertrophy (Keogh et al. 2007).

Aside from the convenience of surface anthropometry for assessing physique traits of athletes, parameters such as skinfolds are robust, not readily influenced by factors such as hydration status of the athlete. However, measurement of body composition using surface anthropometry is typically undertaken in conjunction with the measurement of body mass (Table 12.2) and it is body mass that can be acutely influenced by an array of factors, independent of changes in FM or skeletal muscle mass. Consequently, body mass measurements should preferably be made at the same time of day (preferably before breakfast or training but after voiding the bladder and bowel), and wearing minimal clothing (Maughan and Shirreffs 2004), so as to minimize the influence of extraneous factors that can impact on body mass.

TABLE 12.2
Interpretation of Changes in Body Composition Based on Skinfold and Body Mass Data

Anthropometric Trait		Interpretation—Body Composition	
Body Mass	**Skinfolds**	**Muscle Mass**	**Body Fat**
Increase	Stable	Gain	No change
Decrease	Stable	Loss	No change
Stable	Increase	Loss	Gain
Stable	Decrease	Gain	Loss
Increase	Increase	Potential gain	Gain
Increase	Decrease	Gain	Loss
Decrease	Increase	Loss	Gain
Decrease	Decrease	Potential loss	Loss

Other issues to consider include consistency in the scales used (Stein et al. 2005), the phase of the menstrual cycle in females (Bunt et al. 1989), and hydration status. Amongst amputees, the body mass proportions of different limb segments afford an ability to estimate a corrected body mass (as outlined in Chapter 6), which may be of relevance when contrasting results against normative data for performance and/ or health assessments. This proportionality of body segments can also be used to estimate height of individuals (Hickson and Frost 2003).

While surface anthropometry does not offer a direct measure of total fat mass or FFM, its robustness in the field, convenience and low cost ensure it remains a popular method of body composition monitoring amongst athletes. Newer technologies like DXA or the combination of technologies in a three- or four-compartment model offer an opportunity to better interpret surface anthropometry data. Preferably, this should be developed around interpretation of changes in body composition over time rather than a one-off assessment. Such longitudinal investigations also create opportunities to help better understand the association between physique traits and competitive success.

Precise assessment of anthropometric traits, in particular skinfold thickness, can be difficult, and therefore extreme care in site location and measurement is required if meaningful results are to be obtained. Prior to assessment, the tester should develop the appropriate technique, reducing the level of error in repeated measurements, and thus enhancing the ability to detect small but potentially important changes. The standard assessment protocol of the International Society for the Advancement of Kinanthropometry (ISAK) (Stewart et al. 2011) is recommended. Professionals wishing to monitor the physique traits of athletes using surface anthropometry are strongly encouraged to undertake professional training through accredited courses (Figure 12.6).

12.2.6 ALTERNATE TECHNOLOGIES

A range of alternate technologies are also available with potential application in the assessment and monitoring of physique traits of athletes, including ultrasound and three-dimensional photonic scanning. Use of ultrasound for measurement of subcutaneous fat is proposed to overcome some of the drawbacks of subcutaneous skinfold assessment using calipers, particularly error associated with the compressibility and elasticity of skinfolds (Ramirez 1992). The recent availability of higher-resolution, portable and more affordable ultrasound equipment has created renewed interest in this technology for body composition assessment in field settings. A recent investigation in a mixed-athlete population reported strong correlations for both males and females when body fat estimates measured by ultrasound were compared with DXA (Pineau et al. 2009). Similar estimates of FFM have been observed in wrestlers when assessed by ultrasound and hydrodensitometry (Utter and Hager 2008). Consequently, ultrasound may also have application in tracking changes in skeletal muscle mass as a result of injury or training adaptations (Uremovic et al. 2004). More research is required to assess the reliability and validity of the method before it can be considered in routine athlete monitoring.

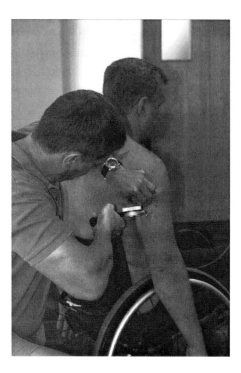

FIGURE 12.6 Undertaking skinfold measurements. Note the landmarking of sites as per ISAK requirements.

Three-dimensional photonic scanning (3DPS) was initially developed for use in the clothing industry to capture information about body surface topography but soon after it was recognized that the technology has potential application within the medical (Wells et al. 2000) and sports environments. It has several potential advantages over traditional anthropometric measurement techniques, capturing a much wider range of anthropometric dimensions in a more time-efficient and noninvasive manner (Schranz et al. 2010).

The method provides information on regional as well as whole-body volume and surface area plus various body dimensions and potentially body composition. Validation work on this approach for measurement of body composition is limited (Wells et al. 2000; Wang et al. 2006) but the technology has already been applied to contrast differences in physique traits between elite athletes and the general population (Schranz et al. 2010). The expense and poor portability of 3DPS systems ensure the technology is not currently practical for field use and thus only used within the research environment.

12.3 FACTORS INFLUENCING RELIABILITY OF METHODS

A wide range of tools are available to assess the physique traits of athletes. Aside from talent identification initiatives and the identification of a preferred physique for a given sport and player position, the primary focus is given to the longitudinal monitoring of physique traits. As such, techniques that are cost- and time-effective, portable, reliable, safe and provide insight into all physique traits, including both fat and muscle mass, are a priority.

Irrespective of the test chosen, all physique assessment tools carry with them some degree of assumption and measurement error. Having an appreciation of this measurement error helps to distinguish between measurement error and real changes in body composition (i.e. documented changes being greater than reported measurement error). While issues associated with equipment contributing to measurement error are often beyond the control of technicians, athlete presentation can also contribute to the error of repeat assessments. As such, factors such as time of day, hydration status and gastrointestinal tract contents should be standardized wherever possible; fasted early morning assessments may be the most reliable where practical. Minimizing the error or noise associated with a test enhances its reliability, making it easier to identify small but potentially important changes. Reliability of measurement also influences the frequency of assessment. In general, physique assessments should not be undertaken any more regularly than every 4–8 weeks, depending on the individual athlete and their body composition goals.

When collecting data, the physical and emotional well-being of the athlete should remain a priority. Sensitivity should be shown to cultural beliefs and tradition. Procedures should be explained to those unfamiliar, with information provided in advance on what testing is to be undertaken, the reason for profiling, what measurements are to be taken and any specific requirements such as clothing to be worn. Where appropriate, consideration should be given to gender comparability between the technician and athlete, with privacy in data collection and reporting always ensured. With this in mind, consideration should be given to the establishment of not only electronic databases which provide a secure means of data collection but also automating reports that provide invaluable historical data as well as interpretation of existing results against previous assessments. Finally, where resources permit, the collection of data in duplicate should be considered, enhancing the reliability of measurement.

Aligned with this, developing a better understanding of factors influencing the noise or error associated with body composition assessment tools will enable the development of protocols which afford a much greater resolution of measurement. Ultimately, this will help to create techniques and protocols that are able to detect small but potentially meaningful changes in body composition. Once established, this will also create an opportunity to have better resolution for assessing interventions (i.e. dietary, training) or unforeseen situations (i.e. injury, illness, detraining) proposed to influence body composition which ultimately will have application within not only the sports environment but also the wider community.

12.4   SUMMARY AND CONCLUSION

Body composition is just one of an array of fitness traits that may contribute to the overall success of an athlete with an impairment. As such, the association between physique traits and competitive success should not be over emphasized. However, the regular monitoring of body composition amongst athletic populations can offer insight into adaptations to training and/or dietary interventions, as well as optimization of body composition for specific sports and playing positions. An array of tools is available for the measurement of body composition, the test of choice being influenced by technical issues like safety, validity, precision and accuracy of measurement as well as practical issues such as availability, cost, portability, invasiveness, time-effectiveness and technical expertise necessary to conduct the assessment. Among athletes with an impairment, consideration must also be given to the unique physique traits these individuals may possess, including particularly tall, broad and/or muscular individuals as well as those with very low body fat levels. These factors considered together, the routine monitoring of body composition amongst athletes with an impairment, continues to be undertaken with the use of surface anthropometry, although BIA, DXA and the BOD POD are becoming more popular as their accessibility increases. However the unique physical characteristics of some athletes may violate the assumptions associated with some of these techniques or introduce substantial measurement error, making it difficult to identify small to moderate changes in physique traits.

Refinement of protocols such as the standardization of how subjects present for assessment and an improved awareness of the limitations of each technique will allow more informed protocols to be developed. This will offer greater insight into acute and longitudinal monitoring of body composition changes, their importance to competitive success, as well as tailoring interventions that can assist in the appropriate manipulation of body composition. The continued monitoring of physique traits amongst athletes with an impairment will help facilitate the establishment of normative data across sports, positions and classifications, allowing greater insight into the importance of physique traits to competitive success in this athletic population.

Despite the array of tools available to assess body composition, surface anthropometry also remains the most practical tool at present to monitor the body

---

COMMENTARY BOX 12.2

ATHLETE INSIGHT: What are the biggest nutrition challenges you face?

My biggest challenge was how to eat enough to train hard but also lose weight while doing it. There is a fine line between trying to drop kilos but having enough for the right fuel/food to train at the top level.

—Carol Cooke, cyclist, Paralympic medallist;
ex-rower and able-bodied swimmer

I have been very lucky as an athlete and have had access to nutrition information specific to my sport for most of my athletic career. The biggest change for me was changing sports (from powerlifting to track and field) as I was using different body systems. Even now, as a track and field athlete, my races vary from 3 s to a wheelchair marathon, which requires completely different fuels!

—Richard Nicholson, track and field athlete
and ex-powerlifter, multiple Paralympian

composition of athletes longitudinally. However, given the ever increasing interest in the relationship between body composition and competitive sporting success, new, more refined assessment tools with greater reliability and resolution of measurement are likely to emerge in the future.

REFERENCES

Abe, T., Kojima, K., Kearns, C.F., Yohena, H., and Fukuda, J. 2003. Whole body muscle hypertrophy from resistance training: distribution and total mass. *British Journal of Sports Medicine* 37:543–545.

Anderson, D.E. 2007. Reliability of air displacement plethysmography. *Journal of Strength and Conditioning Research* 21:169–172.

Ball, S.D. 2005. Interdevice variability in percent fat estimates using the BOD POD. *European Journal of Clinical Nutrition* 59:996–1001.

Ballard, T.P., Fafara, L., and Vukovich, M.D. 2004. Comparison of Bod Pod and DXA in female collegiate athletes. *Medicine and Science in Sports and Exercise* 36:731–735.

Bentzur, K.M., Kravitz, L., and Lockner, D.W. 2008. Evaluation of the BOD POD for estimating percent body fat in collegiate track and field female athletes: a comparison of four methods. *Journal of Strength and Conditioning Research* 22:1985–1991.

Biaggi, R.R., Vollman, M.W., Nies, M.A., et al. 1999. Comparison of air-displacement plethysmography with hydrostatic weighing and bioelectrical impedance analysis for the assessment of body composition in healthy adults. *American Journal of Clinical Nutrition* 69:898–903.

Brechue, W.F., and Abe, T. 2002. The role of FFM accumulation and skeletal muscle architecture in powerlifting performance. *European Journal of Applied Physiology* 86:327–336.

Brozek, J., Grande, F., Anderson, J.T., and Keys, A. 1963. Densitometric analysis of body composition: revision of some quantitative assumptions. *Annals of the New York Academy of Sciences* 110:113–140.

Buchholz, A.C., McGillivray, C.F., and Pencharz, P.B. 2003. The use of bioelectric impedance analysis to measure fluid compartments in subjects with chronic paraplegia. *Archives of Physical Medicine and Rehabilitation* 84:854–861.

Bulbulian, R., Johnson, R.E., Gruber, J.J., and Darabos, B. 1987. Body composition in paraplegic male athletes. *Medicine and Science in Sports and Exercise* 19:195–201.

Bunt, J.C., Lohman, T.G., and Boileau, R.A. 1989. Impact of total body water fluctuations on estimation of body fat from body density. *Medicine and Science in Sports and Exercise* 21:96–100.

Burkhart, T.A., Arthurs, K.L., and Andrews, D.M. 2009. Manual segmentation of DXA scan images results in reliable upper and lower extremity soft and rigid tissue mass estimates. *Journal of Biomechanics* 42:1138–1142.

Calbet, J.A., Moysi, J.S., Dorado, C., and Rodriguez, L.P. 1998. Bone mineral content and density in professional tennis players. *Calcified Tissue International* 62:491–496.

Cisar, C.J., Housh, T.J., Johnson, G.O., Thorland, W.G., and Hughes, R.A. 1989. Validity of anthropometric equations for determination of changes in body composition in adult males during training. *Journal of Sports Medicine and Physical Fitness* 29:141–148.

Claessens, A.L., Hlatky, S., Lefevre, J., and Holdhaus, H. 1994. The role of anthropometric characteristics in modern pentathlon performance in female athletes. *Journal of Sports Sciences* 12:391–401.

Claessens, A.L., Lefevre, J., Beunen, G., and Malina, R.M. 1999. The contribution of anthropometric characteristics to performance scores in elite female gymnasts. *Journal of Sports Medicine and Physical Fitness* 39:355–360.

Clark, R.R., Bartok, C., Sullivan, J.C., and Schoeller, D.A. 2004. Minimum weight prediction methods cross-validated by the four-component model. *Medicine and Science in Sports and Exercise* 36:639–647.

Clarys, J.P., Martin, A.D., Drinkwater, D.T., and Marfell-Jones, M.J. 1987. The skinfold: myth and reality. *Journal of Sports Sciences* 5:3–33.

Clarys, J.P., Martin, A.D., Marfell-Jones, M.J., Janssens, V., Caboor, D., and Drinkwater, D.T. 1999. Human body composition: a review of adult dissection data. *American Journal of Human Biology* 11:167–174.

Clarys, J.P., Provyn, S., and Marfell-Jones, M.J. 2005. Cadaver studies and their impact on the understanding of human adiposity. *Ergonomics* 48:1445–1461.

Clasey, J.L., and Gater, D.R., Jr. 2005. A comparison of hydrostatic weighing and air displacement plethysmography in adults with spinal cord injury. *Archives of Physical Medicine and Rehabilitation* 86:2106–2113.

Collins, A.L., and McCarthy, H.D. 2003. Evaluation of factors determining the precision of body composition measurements by air displacement plethysmography. *European Journal of Clinical Nutrition* 57:770–776.

Collins, M.A., Millard-Stafford, M.L., Sparling, P.B., et al. 1999. Evaluation of the BOD POD for assessing body fat in collegiate football players. *Medicine and Science in Sports and Exercise* 31:1350–1356.

Cornish, B.H., Ward, L.C., Thomas, B.J., Jebb, S.A., and Elia, M. 1996. Evaluation of multiple frequency bioelectrical impedance and Cole-Cole analysis for the assessment of body water volumes in healthy humans. *European Journal of Clinical Nutrition* 50:159–164.

Davis, J.A., Dorado, S., Keays, K.A., Reigel, K.A., Valencia, K.S., and Pham, P.H. 2007. Reliability and validity of the lung volume measurement made by the BOD POD body composition system. *Clinical Physiology and Functional Imaging* 27:42–46.

Dempster, P., and Aitkens, S. 1995. A new air displacement method for the determination of human body composition. *Medicine and Science in Sports and Exercise* 27:1692–1697.

DeRose, E.H., Crawford, S.M., Kerr, D.A., Ward, R., and Ross, W.D. 1989. Physique characteristics of Pan American Games lightweight rowers. *International Journal of Sports Medicine* 10:292–297.

Deurenberg-Yap, M., Schmidt, G., van Staveren, W.A., Hautvast, J., and Deurenberg, P. 2001. Body fat measurement among Singaporean Chinese, Malays and Indians: a comparative study using a four-compartment model and different two-compartment models. *British Journal of Nutrition* 85:491–498.

Dixon, C.B., Deitrick, R.W., Cutrufello, P.T., Drapeau, L.L., and Lovallo, S.J. 2006. Effect of mode selection when using leg-to-leg BIA to estimate body fat in collegiate wrestlers. *Journal of Sports Medicine and Physical Fitness* 46:265–270.

Dixon, C.B., Ramos, L., Fitzgerald, E., Reppert, D., and Andreacci, J.L. 2009. The effect of acute fluid consumption on measures of impedance and percent body fat estimated using segmental bioelectrical impedance analysis. *European Journal of Clinical Nutrition* 63:1115–1122.

Drinkwater, D.T., and Ross, W.D. 1980. Anthropometric fractionation of body mass. In *Kinanthropometry II*, ed. M. Ostyn, G. Beunen, and J. Simons, 178–189. Baltimore: University Park Press.

Dunbar, C.C., Melahrinides, E., Michielli, D.W., and Kalinski, M.I. 1994. Effects of small errors in electrode placement on body composition assessment by bioelectrical impedance. *Research Quarterly for Exercise and Sport* 65:291–294.

Eston, R.G., Rowlands, A.V., Charlesworth, S., Davies, A., and Hoppitt, T. 2005. Prediction of DXA-determined whole body fat from skinfolds: importance of including skinfolds from the thigh and calf in young, healthy men and women. *European Journal of Clinical Nutrition* 59:695–702.

Evans, E.M., Prior, B.M., and Modlesky, C.M. 2005. A mathematical method to estimate body composition in tall individuals using DXA. *Medicine and Science in Sports and Exercise* 37:1211–1215.

Fields, D.A., Higgins, P.B., and Hunter, G.R. 2004. Assessment of body composition by air-displacement plethysmography: influence of body temperature and moisture. *Dynamic Medicine* 3:3.

Fields, D.A., Hunter, G.R., and Goran, M.I. 2000. Validation of the BOD POD with hydrostatic weighing: influence of body clothing. *International Journal of Obesity and Related Metabolic Disorders* 24:200–205.

Forbes, G.B. 1999. Body composition: overview. *Journal of Nutrition* 129:270S–272S.

Frisard, M.I., Greenway, F.L., and Delany, J.P. 2005. Comparison of methods to assess body composition changes during a period of weight loss. *Obesity Research* 13:845–854.

Genton, L., Hans, D., Kyle, U.G., and Pichard, C. 2002. Dual-energy X-ray absorptiometry and body composition: differences between devices and comparison with reference methods. *Nutrition* 18:66–70.

Going, S.B., Massett, M.P., Hall, M.C., et al. 1993. Detection of small changes in body composition by dual-energy X-ray absorptiometry. *American Journal of Clinical Nutrition* 57:845–850.

Hewitt, M.J., Going, S.B., Williams, D.P., and Lohman, T.G. 1993. Hydration of the fat-free body mass in children and adults: implications for body composition assessment. *American Journal of Physiology* 265:E88–E95.

Hickson, M., and Frost, G. 2003. A comparison of three methods for estimating height in the acutely ill elderly population. *Journal of Human Nutrition and Dietetics* 16:13–20.

Higgins, P.B., Fields, D.A., Hunter, G.R., and Gower, B.A. 2001. Effect of scalp and facial hair on air displacement plethysmography estimates of percentage of body fat. *Obesity Research* 9:326–330.

Horber, F.F., Thomi, F., Casez, J.P., Fonteille, J., and Jaeger, P. 1992. Impact of hydration status on body composition as measured by dual energy X-ray absorptiometry in normal volunteers and patients on haemodialysis. *British Journal of Radiology* 65:895–900.

Houtkooper, L.B., Lohman, T.G., Going, S.B., and Howell, W.H. 1996. Why bioelectrical impedance analysis should be used for estimating adiposity. *American Journal of Clinical Nutrition* 64:436S–448S.

Hull, H., He, Q., Thornton, J., et al. 2009. iDXA, Prodigy, and DPXL dual-energy X-ray absorptiometry whole-body scans: a cross-calibration study. *Journal of Clinical Densitometry* 12:95–102.

Hume, P., and Marfell-Jones, M. 2008. The importance of accurate site location for skinfold measurement. *Journal of Sports Sciences* 26:1333–1340.

Ide, M., Ogata, H., Kobayashi, M., Tajima, F., and Hatada, K. 1994. Anthropometric features of wheelchair marathon race competitors with spinal cord injuries. *Paraplegia* 32:174–179.

Jaffrin, M.Y. 2009. Body composition determination by bioimpedance: an update. *Current Opinion in Clinical Nutrition and Metabolic Care* 12:482–486.

Johnston, F.E. 1982. Relationships between body composition and anthropometry. *Human Biology* 54:221–245.

Jones, L.M., Goulding, A., and Gerrard, D.F. 1998. DEXA: a practical and accurate tool to demonstrate total and regional bone loss, lean tissue loss and fat mass gain in paraplegia. *Spinal Cord* 36:637–640.

Kelsey, J.L., Bachrach, L.K., Procter-Gray, E., et al. 2007. Risk factors for stress fracture among young female cross-country runners. *Medicine and Science in Sports and Exercise* 39:1457–1463.

Keogh, J.W., Hume, P.A., Pearson, S.N., and Mellow, P. 2007. Anthropometric dimensions of male powerlifters of varying body mass. *Journal of Sports Sciences* 25:1365–1376.

King, G.A., Fulkerson, B., Evans, M.J., Moreau, K.L., McLaughlin, J.E., and Thompson, D.L. 2006. Effect of clothing type on validity of air-displacement plethysmography. *Journal of Strength and Conditioning Research* 20:95–102.

Kocina, P. 1997. Body composition of spinal cord injured adults. *Sports Medicine* 23:48–60.

Koo, W.W.K., Hockman, E.M., and Hammami, M. 2004. Dual energy X-ray absorptiometry measurements in small subjects: conditions affecting clinical measurements. *Journal of the American College of Nutrition* 23:212–219.

Koulmann, N., Jimenez, C., Regal, D., Bolliet, P., Launay, J.C., Savourey, G., and Melin, B. 2000. Use of bioelectrical impedance analysis to estimate body fluid compartments after acute variations of the body hydration level. *Medicine and Science in Sports and Exercise* 32:857–864.

Kushner, R.F. 1992. Bioelectrical impedance analysis: a review of principles and applications. *Journal of the American College of Nutrition* 11:199–209.

Kushner, R.F., Gudivaka, R., and Schoeller, D.A. 1996. Clinical characteristics influencing bioelectrical impedance analysis measurements. *American Journal of Clinical Nutrition* 64:423S–427S.

Kyle, U.G., Bosaeus, I., De Lorenzo, A.D., et al. 2004a. Bioelectrical impedance analysis. Part I. Review of principles and methods. *Clinical Nutrition* 23:1226–1243.

Kyle, U.G., Bosaeus, I., De Lorenzo, A.D., et al. 2004b. Bioelectrical impedance analysis. Part II. Utilization in clinical practice. *Clinical Nutrition* 23:1430–1453.

Kyriazis, T., Terzis, G., Karampatsos, G., Kavouras, S., and Georgiadis, G. 2010. Body composition and performance in shot put athletes at preseason and at competition. *International Journal of Sports Physiology and Performance* 5:417–421.

Lambrinoudaki, I., Georgiou, E., Douskas, G., Tsekes, G., Kyriakidis, M., and Proukakis, C. 1998. Body composition assessment by dual-energy X-ray absorptiometry: comparison of prone and supine measurements. *Metabolism—Clinical and Experimental* 47:1379–1382.

Lands, L.C., Hornby, L., Hohenkerk, J.M., and Glorieux, F.H. 1996. Accuracy of measurements of small changes in soft-tissue mass by dual-energy X-ray absorptiometry. *Clinical and Investigative Medicine* 19:279–285.

Larsson, P., and Henriksson-Larsen, K. 2008. Body composition and performance in cross-country skiing. *International Journal of Sports Medicine* 29:971–975.

Le Carvennec, M., Fagour, C., Adenis-Lamarre, E., Perlemoine, C., Gin, H., and Rigalleau, V. 2007. Body composition of obese subjects by air displacement plethysmography: the influence of hydration. *Obesity (Silver Spring)* 15:78–84.

Lewiecki, E.M. 2005. Clinical applications of bone density testing for osteoporosis. *Minerva Medica* 96:317–330.

Lohman, M., Tallroth, K., Kettunen, J.A., and Marttinen, M.T. 2009. Reproducibility of dual-energy X-ray absorptiometry total and regional body composition measurements using different scanning positions and definitions of regions. *Metabolism—Clinical and Experimental* 58:1663–1668.

Lohman, T.G. 1981. Skinfolds and body density and their relation to body fatness: a review. *Human Biology* 53:181–225.

Marfell-Jones, M., Clarys, J.P., Alewaeters, K., Martin, A.D., and Drinkwater, D.T. 2003. The hazards of whole body fat prediction in men and women. *Journal de Biometrie Humanaine et Anthropologie* 21:103–118.

Martin, A.D., Ross, W.D., Drinkwater, D.T., and Clarys, J.P. 1985. Prediction of body fat by skinfold caliper: assumptions and cadaver evidence. *International Journal of Obesity* 9(Suppl 1):31–39.

Martinoli, R., Mohamed, E.I., Maiolo, C., et al. 2003. Total body water estimation using bioelectrical impedance: a meta-analysis of the data available in the literature. *Acta Diabetologica* 40(Suppl 1):S203–S206.

Maughan, R., and Shirreffs, S. 2004. Exercise in the heat: challenges and opportunities. *Journal of Sports Sciences* 22:917–927.

Mazess, R.B., Barden, H.S., Bisek, J.P., and Hanson, J. 1990. Dual-energy X-ray absorptiometry for total-body and regional bone-mineral and soft-tissue composition. *American Journal of Clinical Nutrition* 51:1106–1112.

Millard-Stafford, M.L., Collins, M.A., Evans, E.M., Snow, T.K., Cureton, K.J., and Rosskopf, L.B. 2001. Use of air displacement plethysmography for estimating body fat in a four-component model. *Medicine and Science in Sports and Exercise* 33:1311–1317.

Minderico, C.S., Silva, A.M., Fields, D.A., et al. 2008. Changes in thoracic gas volume with air-displacement plethysmography after a weight loss program in overweight and obese women. *European Journal of Clinical Nutrition* 62:444–450.

Minderico, C.S., Silva, A.M., Teixeira, P.J., Sardinha, L.B., Hull, H.R., and Fields, D.A. 2006. Validity of air-displacement plethysmography in the assessment of body composition changes in a 16-month weight loss program. *Nutrition and Metabolism* 3:32.

Mojtahedi, M.C., Valentine, R.J., and Evans, E.M. 2009. Body composition assessment in athletes with spinal cord injury: comparison of field methods with dual-energy X-ray absorptiometry. *Spinal Cord* 47:698–704.

Moon, J.R., Eckerson, J.M., Tobkin, S.E., et al. 2009. Estimating body fat in NCAA Division I female athletes: a five-compartment model validation of laboratory methods. *European Journal of Applied Physiology* 105:119–130.

Mueller, W.H., and Stallones, L. 1981. Anatomical distribution of subcutaneous fat: skinfold site choice and construction of indices. *Human Biology* 53:321–335.

Nana, A., Slater, G.J., Hopkins, W.G., and Burke, L.M. 2012a. Effects of daily activities on dual-energy X-ray absorptiometry measurements of body composition in active people. *Medicine and Science in Sports and Exercise* 44:180–189.

Nana, A., Slater, G.J., Hopkins, W.G., and Burke, L.M. 2012b. Techniques for undertaking dual-energy X-ray absorptiometry whole-body scans to estimate body composition in tall and/or broad subjects. *International Journal of Sport Nutrition and Exercise Metabolism* 22:313–322.

NIH. 1996. NIH consensus statement. Bioelectrical impedance analysis in body composition measurement. National Institutes of Health Technology Assessment Conference statement. December 12–14, 1994. *Nutrition* 12:749–762.

Noreen, E.E., and Lemon, P.W. 2006. Reliability of air displacement plethysmography in a large, heterogeneous sample. *Medicine and Science in Sports and Exercise* 38:1505–1509.

Norton, K., Olds, T., Olive, S., and Craig, N. 1996. Anthropometry and sports performance. In *Anthropometrica*, ed. K. Norton and T. Olds, 287–364. Sydney: University of New South Wales Press.

Olds, T. 2001. The evolution of physique in male rugby union players in the twentieth century. *Journal of Sports Sciences* 19:253–262.

Pateyjohns, I.R., Brinkworth, G.D., Buckley, J.D., Noakes, M., and Clifton, P.M. 2006. Comparison of three bioelectrical impedance methods with DXA in overweight and obese men. *Obesity* 14:2064–2070.

Peeters, M.W., and Claessens, A.L. 2011. Effect of different swim caps on the assessment of body volume and percentage body fat by air displacement plethysmography. *Journal of Sports Sciences* 29:191–196.

Pichard, C., Kyle, U.G., Gremion, G., Gerbase, M., and Slosman, D.O. 1997. Body composition by X-ray absorptiometry and bioelectrical impedance in female runners. *Medicine and Science in Sports and Exercise* 29:1527–1534.

Pietrobelli, A., Formica, C., Wang, Z., and Heymsfield, S.B. 1996. Dual-energy X-ray absorptiometry body composition model: review of physical concepts. *American Journal of Physiology* 271:E941–E951.

Pineau, J.C., Filliard, J.R., and Bocquet, M. 2009. Ultrasound techniques applied to body fat measurement in male and female athletes. *Journal of Athletic Training* 44:142–147.

Prior, B.M., Cureton, K.J., Modlesky, C.M., et al. 1997. In vivo validation of whole body composition estimates from dual-energy X-ray absorptiometry. *Journal of Applied Physiology* 83:623–630.

Pritchard, J.E., Nowson, C.A., Strauss, B.J., Carlson, J.S., Kaymakci, B., and Wark, J.D. 1993. Evaluation of dual energy X-ray absorpiometry as a method of measurement of body-fat. *European Journal of Clinical Nutrition* 47:216–228.

Prouteau, S., Ducher, G., Nanyan, P., Lemineur, G., Benhamou, L., and Courteix, D. 2004. Fractal analysis of bone texture: a screening tool for stress fracture risk? *European Journal of Clinical Investigation* 34:137–142.

Ramirez, M. 1992. Measurement of subcutaneous adipose tissue using ultrasound images. *American Journal of Clinical Nutrition* 89:347–357.

Reid, I.R., Evans, M.C., and Ames, R. 1992. Relationships between upper-arm anthropometry and soft-tissue composition in postmenopausal women. *American Journal of Clinical Nutrition* 56:463–466.

Roche, A.F. 1996. Anthropometry and ultrasound. In *Human body composition*, ed. A.F. Roche, S.B. Heymsfield, and T.G. Lohman, 167–190. Champaign, IL: Human Kinetics.

Rosendale, R.P., and Bartok, C.J. 2012. Air-displacement plethysmography for the measurement of body composition in children aged 6–48 months. *Pediatric Research* 71:299–304.

Rothney, M.P., Brychta, R.J., Schaefer, E.V., Chen, K.Y., and Skarulis, M.C. 2009. Body composition measured by dual-energy X-ray absorptiometry half-body scans in obese adults. *Obesity* 17:1281–1286.

Roubenoff, R., Kehayias, J.J., Dawson-Hughes, B., and Heymsfield, S.B. 1993. Use of dual-energy X-ray absorptiometry in body-composition studies: not yet a "gold standard." *American Journal of Clinical Nutrition* 58:589–591.

Ruiz, L., Colley, J.R., and Hamilton, P.J. 1971. Measurement of triceps skinfold thickness. An investigation of sources of variation. *British Journal of Preventive and Social Medicine* 25:165–167.

Saunders, M.J., Blevins, J.E., and Broeder, C.E. 1998. Effects of hydration changes on bioelectrical impedance in endurance trained individuals. *Medicine and Science in Sports and Exercise* 30:885–892.

Schranz, N., Tomkinson, G., Olds, T., and Daniell, N. 2010. Three-dimensional anthropometric analysis: differences between elite Australian rowers and the general population. *Journal of Sports Sciences* 28:459–469.

Secchiutti, A., Fagour, C., Perlemoine, C., Gin, H., Durrieu, J., and Rigalleau, V. 2007. Air displacement plethysmography can detect moderate changes in body composition. *European Journal of Clinical Nutrition* 61:25–29.

Shephard, R.J. 1998. Science and medicine of rowing: a review. *Journal of Sports Sciences* 16:603–620.

Siders, W.A., Lukaski, H.C., and Bolonchuk, W.W. 1993. Relationships among swimming performance, body composition and somatotype in competitive collegiate swimmers. *Journal of Sports Medicine and Physical Fitness* 33:166–171.

Silva, A.M., Fields, D.A., Quiterio, A.L., and Sardinha, L.B. 2009. Are skinfold-based models accurate and suitable for assessing changes in body composition in highly trained athletes? *Journal of Strength and Conditioning Research* 23:1688–1696.

Silva, A.M., Minderico, C.S., Teixeira, P.J., Pietrobelli, A., and Sardinha, L.B. 2006. Body fat measurement in adolescent athletes: multicompartment molecular model comparison. *European Journal of Clinical Nutrition* 60:955–964.

Siri, W.E. 1993. Body composition from fluid spaces and density: analysis of methods. 1961. *Nutrition* 9:480–491.

Soriano, J.M., Ioannidou, E., Wang, J., et al. 2004. Pencil-beam vs fan-beam dual-energy X-ray absorptiometry comparisons across four systems: body composition and bone mineral. *Journal of Clinical Densitometry* 7:281–289.

Stein, R.J., Haddock, C.K., Poston, W.S., Catanese, D., and Spertus, J.A. 2005. Precision in weighing: a comparison of scales found in physician offices, fitness centers, and weight loss centers. *Public Health Report* 120:266–270.

Stewart, A.D., and Hannan, W.J. 2000. Prediction of fat and fat-free mass in male athletes using dual X-ray absorptiometry as the reference method. *Journal of Sports Sciences* 18:263–274.

Stewart, A.D., Marfell-Jones, M.J., Olds, T., and de Ridder, J.H. 2011. *International standards for anthropometric assessment.* Wellington, New Zealand: International Society for the Advancement of Kinanthropometry.

Stoggl, T., Enqvist, J., Muller, E., and Holmberg, H.C. 2010. Relationships between body composition, body dimensions, and peak speed in cross-country sprint skiing. *Journal of Sports Sciences* 28:161–169.

Strauss, B.J., Gibson, P.R., Stroud, D.B., Borovnicar, D.J., Xiong, D.W., and Keogh, J. 2000. Total body dual X-ray absorptiometry is a good measure of both fat mass and fat-free mass in liver cirrhosis compared to "gold-standard" techniques. Melbourne Liver Group. *Annals of the New York Academy of Sciences* 904:55–62.

Sun, G., French, C.R., Martin, G.R., et al. 2005. Comparison of multifrequency bioelectrical impedance analysis with dual-energy X-ray absorptiometry for assessment of percentage body fat in a large, healthy population. *American Journal of Clinical Nutrition* 81:74–78.

Sutton, L., Wallace, J., Goosey-Tolfrey, V., Scott, M., and Reilly, T. 2009. Body composition of female wheelchair athletes. *International Journal of Sports Medicine* 30:259–265.

Svantesson, U., Zander, M., Klingberg, S., and Slinde, F. 2008. Body composition in male elite athletes, comparison of bioelectrical impedance spectroscopy with dual energy X-ray absorptiometry. *Journal of Negative Results in Biomedicine* 7:1.

Tataranni, P.A., and Ravussin, E. 1995. Use of dual-energy X-ray absorptiometry in obese individuals. *American Journal of Clinical Nutrition* 62:730–734.

Tegenkamp, M.H., Clark, R.R., Schoeller, D.A., and Landry, G.L. 2011. Effects of covert subject actions on percent body fat by air-displacement plethysmography. *Journal of Strength and Conditioning Research* 25:2010–2017.

Thomasset, A. 1963. [Bio-electric properties of tissues. Estimation by measurement of impedance of extracellular ionic strength and intracellular ionic strength in the clinic.] *Lyon Medicine* 209:1325–1350.

Tothill, P., Avenell, A., Love, J., and Reid, D.M. 1994. Comparisons between Hologic, Lunar and Norland dual-energy X-ray absorptiometers and other techniques used for whole-body soft-tissue measurements. *European Journal of Clinical Nutrition* 48:781–794.

Tothill, P., Hannan, W.J., and Wilkinson, S. 2001. Comparisons between a pencil beam and two fan beam dual energy X-ray absorptiometers used for measuring total body bone and soft tissue. *British Journal of Radiology* 74:166–176.

Uremovic, M., Bosnjak Pasic, M., Seric, V., et al. 2004. Ultrasound measurement of the volume of musculus quadriceps after knee joint injury. *Collegium Antropologicum* 28(Suppl 2):227–283.

Utter, A., and Hager, M. 2008. Evaluation of ultrasound in assessing body composition of high school wrestlers. *Medicine and Science in Sports and Exercise* 40:943–949.

Utter, A.C., Goss, F.L., Swan, P.D., Harris, G.S., Robertson, R.J., and Trone, G.A. 2003. Evaluation of air displacement for assessing body composition of collegiate wrestlers. *Medicine and Science in Sports and Exercise* 35:500–505.

Utter, A.C., and Lambeth, P.G. 2010. Evaluation of multifrequency bioelectrical impedance analysis in assessing body composition of wrestlers. *Medicine and Science in Sports and Exercise* 42:361–367.

Van Der Ploeg, G.E., Withers, R.T., and Laforgia, J. 2003. Percent body fat via DEXA: comparison with a four-compartment model. *Journal of Applied Physiology* 94:499–506.

van Marken Lichtenbelt, W.D., Hartgens, F., Vollaard, N.B., Ebbing, S., and Kuipers, H. 2004. Body composition changes in bodybuilders: a method comparison. *Medicine and Science in Sports and Exercise* 36:490–497.

Vescovi, J.D., Zimmerman, S.L., Miller, W.C., and Fernhall, B. 2002. Effects of clothing on accuracy and reliability of air displacement plethysmography. *Medicine and Science in Sports and Exercise* 34:282–285.

Vilaca, K.H., Ferriolli, E., Lima, N.K., Paula, F.J., and Moriguti, J.C. 2009. Effect of fluid and food intake on the body composition evaluation of elderly persons. *Journal of Nutrition Health and Aging* 13:183–186.

Wagner, D.R., and Heyward, V.H. 1999. Techniques of body composition assessment: a review of laboratory and field methods. *Research Quarterly in Exercise and Sport* 70:135–149.

Wang, J., Gallagher, D., Thornton, J., Yu, W., Horlick, M., and Pi-Sunyer, F. 2006. Validation of a 3-dimensional photonic scanner for the measurement of body volumes, dimensions, and percentage body fat. *American Journal of Clinical Nutrition* 83:809–816.

Wells, J., Douros, I., Fuller, N., Elia, M., and Dekker, L. 2000. Assessment of body volume using three dimensional photonic scanning. *Annals of the New York Academy of Science* 904:247–254.

Weyers, A.M., Mazzetti, S.A., Love, D.M., Gomez, A.L., Kraemer, W.J., and Volek, J.S. 2002. Comparison of methods for assessing body composition changes during weight loss. *Medicine and Science in Sports and Exercise* 34:497–502.

White, A.T., and Johnson, S.C. 1991. Physiological comparison of international, national and regional alpine skiers. *International Journal of Sports Medicine* 12:374–378.

Wilmore, J.H., Girandola, R.N., and Moody, D.L. 1970. Validity of skinfold and girth assessment for predicting alterations in body composition. *Journal of Applied Physiology* 29:313–317.

Withers, R.T., Laforgia, J., and Heymsfield, S.B. 1999. Critical appraisal of the estimation of body composition via two-, three-, and four-compartment models. *American Journal of Human Biology* 11:175–185.

Withers, R.T., LaForgia, J., Pillans, R.K., et al. 1998. Comparisons of two-, three-, and four-compartment models of body composition analysis in men and women. *Journal of Applied Physiology* 85:238–245.

Withers, R.T., Whittingham, N.O., Norton, K.I., La Forgia, J., Ellis, M.W., and Crockett, A. 1987. Relative body fat and anthropometric prediction of body density of female athletes. *European Journal of Applied Physiology and Occupational Physiology* 56:169–180.

13 Practical Sports Nutrition Issues

Siobhan Crawshay and Jeanette Crosland

CONTENTS

13.1 INTRODUCTION

Working with an athlete with an impairment will present new challenges for the sports nutritionist. There is a need to understand and take into consideration practical issues that may arise for the athlete or team, and it is important to be able to think beyond the way one would when dealing with issues in an able-bodied setting.

A good understanding of specific impairment categories is paramount when working with these athletes. This will allow the sports nutritionist to understand the physiological needs and practical factors that should be considered when making suggestions to the athlete. It also provides the knowledge needed to be able to tailor the nutrition consultation better (i.e. certain questions may be triggered by knowing the type of issues athletes may face as a result of their particular impairment). Ultimately, this can lead to a more holistic and satisfactory service for the athlete. It is also important for the health professional to understand and consider the practicalities of the lifestyle of someone with a specific impairment. An effective sports nutritionist will be able to convey important and relevant nutrition messages to the athlete in a practical and meaningful manner.

Most athletes will already have their home environment set up for their needs, and will have ways of completing their daily activities that suit their specific requirements. The athletes are often remarkably adaptable, and are ultimately the most knowledgeable about their own personal needs. For example, it is not uncommon for athletes who use a wheelchair to use escalators, or even to wheel their chairs down a set of stairs, rather than use an elevator when elevators are slow or busy. The athlete therefore provides the best resource and learning opportunity for the service provider and listening to the specific needs and practical issues that may arise in their daily environment is a key skill.

With the home environment being well set up to suit the athlete, the job of the sports nutritionist is to consider the daily training environment or the environment in which the competition is being held, and ensure that the athlete is able to simulate as much as possible their home environment. Specifically, food access, meal times and locations, whether shopping or self-catering for food is required, buffet setup and travel time to training and competition venues need to be considered in addition to regular sports nutrition principles.

Some athlete groups have been coupled together below in order to discuss some common practical issues. However, just as we cannot make generalisations about a team of able-bodied footballers all having similar nutrition requirements, we cannot assume that two athletes who happen to be classed in the same impairment group share the same practical issues or have the same nutritional requirements.

13.2   COMMON PRACTICAL ISSUES WHEN TRAVELLING

- Travel times for athletes with an impairment can often be longer than anticipated. Usually, more equipment needs to be carried (e.g. wheelchairs, specific competition equipment), and wheelchair athletes are often the first to board flights and the last to disembark.
- When planning flight travel, consider whether it is best to travel as a whole group of athletes, or whether it may be better to split the team into two or more groups. Splitting the team can be a practical way to travel, especially with wheelchair athletes, as it reduces the logistics required by flight and team staff to ensure all chairs and equipment have been loaded on and off. Wheelchair athletes may also require assistance during the flight, so fewer athletes in each group will make travel much more manageable.
- The location of meals during a training camp or competition needs to be considered. Ideally, this should be close to where the athletes are sleeping or to the training venue, to limit the distance the athletes need to travel for meals. Amputees, wheelchair athletes and those athletes who expend more energy in ambulation will be at risk of getting tired and suffering overuse injuries if they need to travel some distance to eat their meals.
- If athletes are self-catering, they may need more time to prepare their meals, and may require assistance with purchasing and transporting food to the accommodation. However, self-catering may not be practical for all athletes, as cooking equipment and facilities may not be appropriate, especially in confined spaces.

- Allowances will need to be made for other activities the athletes on the camp may need to do around meal times. For example, it may take athletes a long time to shower and get ready in the mornings (including time needed for a potential bowel management regime); therefore scheduling an early breakfast may not allow the athlete to get enough sleep and recovery. Similarly, a meal time late in the evening may not suit an athlete with a bowel management routine which lasts for a couple of hours after the evening meal.

- Maintaining hydration can be a problem for many athletes when travelling, especially non-ambulant athletes and those who intermittently catheterise. Difficulties in toileting on a flight, train or bus may lead many individuals to consciously reduce their fluid intake to avoid bathroom breaks. Dehydration increases the risk of the athlete acquiring a urinary tract infection (UTI), so education around this topic is advised. This may be as simple as suggesting athletes depart for their trip in a better-hydrated state than usual, consume liquid containing electrolyte powders or tablets or other ready-to-drink electrolyte solutions, and reduce the amount drunk at any one time but increasing the frequency of intakes, thereby increasing fluid retention without the need to urinate frequently or large volumes. For those athletes who usually catheterise intermittently, they may choose to use an indwelling catheter (IDC) for short-term use. In addition to this, it is important to emphasise the importance of good hygiene when self-catheterising during travel, as the risk of infection is greater.

- Regular hydration testing using urinary specific gravity is a practical way of monitoring hydration status. It is a useful tool on arrival into a training camp and when a team is about to travel. Having specific hydration protocols for teams on arrival is also a good idea.

- There are several items that individuals in this population must remember to pack. Having a general list for the team can be helpful, but it is ultimately up to the athlete to remember to bring their specific items such as medications and catheters (which can be difficult to source when abroad).

COMMENTARY BOX 13.1

COACH'S INSIGHT: What sports nutrition practices have had the biggest impact on the training capability or performance of your athletes?

Recovery food, and having good food choices available when travelling and in camp.

—Ben Ettridge, wheelchair basketball coach of 8 years, coach of Paralympic medal-winning teams

13.3 PRACTICAL CONSIDERATIONS FOR SPECIFIC IMPAIRMENT GROUPS

13.3.1 SPINAL CORD INJURIES (SCI)

- Ability will vary considerably from those that are completely independent to those who require assistance with tasks of daily living. Most, but not all, SCI athletes will use a wheelchair for ambulation.
- The athlete's own kitchen will often be set up to suit the individual so that they can prepare their meals independently. Some higher-level SCI athletes will require some help to prepare meals, so when advising these athletes on specific types of food, it is a good idea to communicate specific suggestions that the athlete can then give to their carer.
- On-line shopping can be a practical way for the athlete to buy the bulk of their groceries for the week. Assisting the athlete with menu planning over a training week may be a useful process in helping them develop their shopping list.
- In team settings, it is not usually practical to have the athletes self-cater for all meals. One option is to organise for breakfast and snack foods to be available in their rooms, and then eat as a group for lunch and/or dinner at the hotel or a restaurant. This saves time and effort, and also eliminates any potential risk of an accident when preparing food in an environment not set up for the specific needs of the group.
- In terms of hydration, as detailed above, athletes who use wheelchairs often find it inconvenient to go to the bathroom, and therefore voluntarily under-drink to avoid having to go when they are outside of their home environment. This poses issues with dehydration and sports performance, as well as UTIs. Using electrolyte drinks, drinking small amounts across the day and drinking well prior to training and competition all ward against the risk of dehydration. Additionally, when away, ensure the team is aware of accessible toilets at venues, accommodation and at places your team are likely to be visiting.
- Regular monitoring of hydration status when travelling is useful for the athlete. The most practical way to monitor hydration status is using a refractometer if available, or simply getting the athletes to monitor their urine colour and volume in the morning. Providing individualised plans to athletes based on their hydration status assists athletes with achieving euhydration. Despite sport drinks being an effective hydration fluid, the energy content of fluids should always be considered when working with this athlete population due to their likely lower energy expenditure. Low-energy electrolyte drinks during travel are often a better option.
- On flights, wheelchair athletes often need to board airplanes first, and are usually the last to disembark, meaning that travel time can be considerably longer. Aisle seating should be requested for these athletes, enabling them to move to the toilet more easily. In addition, an aisle seat allows staff to access these athletes easily if they need to be moved or assisted with pressure lifts

on the flight (see below). Alternatively, allowing a staff member to occupy an aisle seat next to an athlete can ensure easy access to the bathroom if the athlete uses a catheter bag or bottle that needs to be emptied. Athletes may also carry a disposable bottle for discretely toileting at their seat.

- Pressure areas and skin injuries in this population are common, particularly after long-haul flights or as a result of the increased number of transfers they are performing to equipment that is not their own or does not have appropriate pressure relief measures in place. Ensure there is a plan made between the athlete and team physical therapist, and ensure the athlete has asked a staff member to assist with any movement or pressure lifts that need to be completed.
- Buffet eating at hotels—ensure the buffet tables are at a height that makes the food accessible for wheelchair athletes (this will be considerably lower than the standard buffet servery). In addition, ensure utensils and serving equipment are suitable for use by athletes with a SCI: they should be lightweight and not require a lot of hand rotation.
- Additional time may need to be factored in to the daily program for showering and dressing, as well as for toileting, depending on the individual's bowel management plan.
- It is a good idea to bring snack foods and fluids for use by the team at training and competition venues. This has a double advantage of providing ready access to recovery food immediately after training, and reduces the time spent having to shop for food on the way back to the accommodation, where the main meal will be served.
- Due to reduced sweat rates in this population, it is uncommon to see athletes lose significant fluid while training. In addition to this, obtaining seated scales while on the road can also be challenging. Therefore conducting fluid balance testing in their home training environment may be the most practical solution to educating athletes about their specific losses during training. Ideally, this would be done in a few different environmental conditions so that the athletes can gain an appreciation for their range of fluid losses.
- When undertaking anthropometrical assessments, seated or 'roll on' scales are encouraged for safer and easier transfer. Large base platform scales may also be an option if athletes are willing to transfer down to them, however it is important to check first whether this is possible. Towels may be required to soften the transfer surface, and all surfaces should be carefully checked for sharp edges.

13.3.2 Cerebral Palsy/Acquired Brain Injury

- Cerebral palsy (CP) refers to a range of impairments, and affects people in different ways (as outlined in Chapter 5). Some athletes with CP are non-ambulant or require significant assistance to walk, and so face some similar challenges to SCI athletes, whereas others have minor physical effects and live completely independently.

- Communication boards and various forms of technology provide a way of communicating with those who may find it otherwise difficult. Some CP athletes have speech difficulties, so carrying clear written instructions can be useful when out at meals or when travelling.
- The practicalities of CP athletes eating while travelling need to be considered. Athletes who usually cope adequately with self-feeding at home may need some assistance in the confined space of an airplane seat, especially athletes with a high degree of muscle spasticity who require assistance with transfers and pressure relief. It is important that snacks provided to these athletes are manageable by those who have difficulty chewing.
- Some athletes may have a limited chewing reflex, resulting in them requiring soft foods and/or thickened fluids, and some athletes may even feed using a percutaneous gastroscopic endoscopy (PEG). It is important that these requirements are communicated prior to travelling, including clear instructions for PEG feeding, so that suitable foods and fluids can be organised.
- It may be practical for the group to travel with items such as weighted utensils, plates with lips, and nonslip placemats to assist with feeding CP athletes.
- People with CP often find feeding tiring, so when planning mealtimes, it is important to allow for small, frequent snacks to be consumed. Furthermore, ensuring the snacks are nutrient-dense will help the athlete to achieve their nutritional requirements out of these snacks across the day.
- As is the case with all individuals travelling, dehydration is always an important consideration.

13.3.3 AMPUTEES

- Amputees refer to those who have a partial or total amputation of at least one limb; therefore the range of athletes and their abilities varies dramatically (as outlined in Chapter 6).
- Those athletes who are non-ambulant (e.g. bilateral leg amputees who do not use prostheses) will face similar practical challenges to those of SCI athletes described earlier. However, if the amputee has a fully functional upper body, their ability to prepare and manage food is usually better than that of a quadriplegic. Working from a chair in the kitchen may require a specific kitchen set-up, including lower bench-tops, easy-to-access equipment and appliances that can be easily reached.
- Amputees, particularly bilateral leg amputees who walk with prostheses, can tire more quickly when made to stand and walk for prolonged periods. Cooking and shopping should therefore be organised to be as short in duration as possible. Online shopping with home delivery may be a useful option.
- Arm amputees can find chopping and preparing food more time-consuming, and these athletes will often have specific equipment that makes food preparation easier. Heavy pots and saucepans can also pose problems for arm amputees, so they may cook meals that can be prepared across a few smaller dishes, or may ask for assistance with these items.

COMMENTARY BOX 13.2

COACH'S INSIGHT: For your particular athletes, what are the biggest nutrition challenges they face?

On the whole, general nutrition knowledge, and an understanding of nutrition in particular to support training or an athletic lifestyle is poor. Lack of education and support around proper methods for sustainable weight loss. Trusting someone for advice, sticking to a plan (and following it for extended periods), and understanding the link between nutrition and performance seem to be some other challenges I have observed. Understanding the why's and the concepts behind the information they receive is important so they can become self-sufficient and make informed choices opposed to just following a plan verbatim.

—Emily Nolan, strength and conditioning coach

13.3.4 Vision Impairment

- Athletes who are visually impaired (VI) often use various technologies and strategies to allow them to live independently. Travelling can pose some challenges, as it will mean the athlete may require additional support while orientating themselves to their new environment. VI individuals have such established routines that they rely on for their independence and the impact of these changes when travelling should not be underestimated.
- When working with these athletes, it is important to identify the varying degrees of VI in the group, as this will guide you in the type of considerations that need to be made, as their needs can be very different.
- When creating resources for VI athletes, providing them in electronic format is often the most appropriate. This allows VI athletes to enlarge the font or convert it to an audio format as required. All new touch-screen technologies have adaptive software which translates written information into speech. When providing guidance about meal options while travelling, giving specific detailed directions to cafes, restaurants and supermarkets is useful (e.g. 'turn left out of the hotel, walk 200 m up the road, and a main supermarket will be on your left side'), as well as indicating what type of foods they can find at said eateries.
- Visually impaired athletes may require some assistance with food preparation from staff members while travelling. It can be useful for them to pack foods into specific containers they normally use at home so that they can identify things more easily in transit. In addition, having protein containers labelled with large fonts or preparing protein powders into ready-made portions can be of great help to these athletes.
- Buffet meal settings are not easy environments for visually impaired athletes to dine in, however when travelling with a team, it is quite common for this to be the type of meal service used by venues and hotels. Foods can be difficult to distinguish in bains-marie, the lighting is often not ideal,

and the labels (if present at all) are small, meaning that VI athletes cannot read them. When providing assistance to VI athletes in these settings, it is essential that all of the foods available be read out to the athlete in the first instance, rather than simply reading the first few options. This allows the athletes to plan their meal appropriately, rather than just filling their plate with the food in the first bain-marie and missing their preferred option. When no assistance is given, and the buffet is not clearly set out, athletes have been known to put casserole, peas and apple pie together on their plate or cover their vegetables with custard!

- If liaising with hotels and restaurants regarding menu choices, it is best to avoid fish and meat with bones, as well as other dishes that require 'picking'.
- At restaurants, athletes may have to rely on other people to read out the menu options (unless the menu can be accessed online prior to the meal). They may require assistance once the meal is presented in explaining the positioning of food on their plate, often using a clock system (for example, the meat is at 3 o'clock, vegetables at 9 o'clock). It is important not to move items on the table whose location the athlete has become familiar with, such as fluids.
- Using different utensils, knives and stoves/ovens all pose potential risks to the athlete, meaning that self-catering is rarely a viable option for VI athletes.
- In the home environment, the sports nutrition practitioner should provide very specific advice regarding brand names of foods, and the types of packing the food comes in. The bright lights and various colours in a supermarket make it very challenging for the athletes, as does the fine print on food packages, making it difficult to compare brands when looking for specific nutrient compositions. If a VI athlete is shopping with assistance, giving detailed advice allows them to give specific instructions to their carer.

13.3.5 INTELLECTUAL IMPAIRMENT

- Athletes with an intellectual impairment will vary significantly in how they cope with travel. For some athletes, careful planning with carers may be needed to ensure that the appropriate food and drinks are carried for a journey.
- When working with the athletes to plan food intake in the home environment and when travelling, it may be appropriate to create individualised resources for these athletes. Some athletes may prefer written step-like suggestions, whereas others may work better with picture-based resources.
- Some athletes with an intellectual impairment may cope with their daily life by following a strict routine. While trying to maintain this pattern to a degree whilst travelling might be useful, it may not be totally possible and as a result eating habits can be severely disrupted. Replacing meals with snacks may not always work well and having to eat unfamiliar foods can cause problems. These issues will take careful planning. It is important to monitor such individuals to assess how their food and fluid intake has been affected and aim to correct any problems if possible—even if it can only be successfully done after the journey.

- Athletes with an intellectual impairment may need more encouragement compared with other athletes to choose appropriate food and fluids for their sports performance. Encouragement from carers, family and their friends may be taken onboard more than when advice is given by the professional, therefore educating carers, family and friends can be useful. Guiding the athletes in the right direction but having them make some of their own decisions is an effective way to educate.

In conclusion, it is important for the sports nutritionist to become as involved as possible in the planning of travel, training camp and competition logistics in order to allow consideration of all areas that can impact on the appropriate feeding and nutrition provision to athletes with an impairment. Taking any opportunities to travel with a team or spend time with them in their daily training environment is beneficial.

COMMENTARY BOX 13.3

ATHLETE INSIGHT: Challenges to training consistently and optimising performance?

At this stage of my career it is about life balance with family and work commitments as well as wanting to find the time and energy for training. I think it is a common issue for many athletes with an impairment as they need to work to pay the bills and don't earn the same level of income as our able-bodied peers.

—Michael Milton, five-time Winter Paralympian and medallist, Summer Paralympic cyclist and current triathlete

The biggest challenge is time—there is never enough! As I have worked full time for my entire career, achieving it has been difficult to manage my obligations for sport and work. When I have tried to increase my training load too much I don't have the opportunity to recover properly between sessions as I am at work. Now, as a veteran, I think recovery is more important than extra km's!

—Richard Nicholson, track and field athlete and ex-powerlifter, multiple Paralympian

14 Summary and Future Directions

Elizabeth Broad

CONTENTS

14.1 KEY MESSAGES

Athletes with an impairment are often very different even within a class. With limited specific scientific information available, some practitioners and coaches may feel 'out of their depth' when working with these athletes. Rather than seeing that as a negative, embrace the challenge and be willing to explore. A good grounding in the principles of sports nutrition and in exercise physiology will enable a practitioner to use intuition and experience to support an athlete with an impairment, whether it be someone who is just starting out or an experienced athlete looking to reach the pinnacle of their career. Effective sports nutrition advice that is focussed on performance will help each athlete achieve their own personal goals.

14.2 IMPLICATIONS FOR SPORTS DIETITIANS/NUTRITIONISTS

- Interviews with athletes with an impairment will require more detail than those undertaken with able-bodied athletes. Take the time to understand their impairment, their sport, and any clinical issues they may experience.
- Spend time observing the athletes both in training and competition to understand what their sport involves and how it may differ from the sport for able-bodied athletes.
- Talk to the athletes' coach(es) about their observations regarding their athletes, such as their energy levels for training, speed of recovery, functional limitations and general health.
- Involve carers and family where relevant in education and finding practical solutions to issues which require addressing.

- Collate data over time and network with colleagues to develop sufficient pools of information that can be published or used as benchmarks.
- Be prepared to refer or consult with other nutrition experts, particularly where clinical issues require management.
- Become involved in planning for trips/travel for training and/or competition. The practical considerations required may sometimes seem challenging, however finding solutions will help the athletes deliver their best performances.
- Try new or different ways of providing nutrition advice and be flexible with your nutrition education processes.
- Avoid assumptions. Athletes with an impairment can be highly adaptable.

14.3   IMPLICATIONS FOR ATHLETES AND COACHES

- Actively encourage any opportunity for a sports nutrition practitioner to discuss with you your training methods, your observations of your athletes, and most importantly to observe athletes in training and in competition.
- When it does not interrupt training or competition, provide opportunities for individuals such as physiologists and nutritionists to collect data on you/ your athletes as this may help provide a more targeted and specific nutrition support plan.
- Be aware that some things may require some trial and error to get the strategy right. Open communication from all parties will be necessary in order to make this effective for the individual.

14.4   FUTURE RESEARCH DIRECTIONS

Throughout this book, numerous deficits in our knowledge have been highlighted, which provides a range of options for future research. Due to the relatively small numbers of individuals with similar impairments in one location or one country, there is potential value in collaborative research projects within, or between, nations. Some of this research is of a practical nature and could therefore be undertaken by collating relevant data over an extended period of time, while other projects most

---

COMMENTARY BOX 14.1

COACH'S INSIGHT: What are the biggest nutrition challenges your athletes face?

Poor food choices due to poor nutrition education. Also, a dependence on mum/ dad/caregivers to make nutritional choices for them.

—Ben Ettridge, wheelchair basketball coach of 8 years, coach of Paralympic medal-winning teams

likely will require equipment and expertise that can only be found at universities or specific research institutions. Practitioners are encouraged to develop a network of colleagues with whom they could collaborate and communicate regularly.

The following topics are a summary of some of the key areas that could be explored:

- Physiological requirements of a range of different sporting events and activities undertaken by athletes with an impairment
- Fuel utilisation during exercise in athletes with specific types of impairment, such as cerebral palsy, spinal cord injuries, amputees etc.
- Glycogen storage capacity and utilisation during exercise of athletes with a spinal cord injury
- Protein requirements post exercise for athletes with specific types of impairment (particularly spinal cord injury)
- Energy expenditure both at rest and during exercise in athletes with specific types of impairments
- Validation of methods of hydration assessment and fluid requirements of athletes with an impairment
- Validation, or cross-comparison, of methods of assessing body composition and physique in specific impairment types
- Optimal nutrition to speed wound healing
- Incidence of vitamin D deficiency in athletes with an impairment and optimal prevention and management strategies
- Long term monitoring of a variety of anthropometrical measures using various tools to determine the physique traits of elite athletes with an impairment and provide benchmark data and correlations to performance
- The effectiveness of nutritional supplements and ergogenic aids specifically for athletes with an impairment, including the potential need for modifying protocols to suit specific impairment types
- Nutritional interventions to restrict the progression of eye diseases in visually impaired athletes

In summary, simple practical investigations and more complex clinical or laboratory based studies alike will increase the ability of practitioners to more fully understand and correctly advise athletes with an impairment and their coaches to get more out of their sporting experiences.

Index

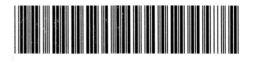